Back Pain in the Young Child and Adolescent

Richard M. Schwend • William L. Hennrikus

Editors

Back Pain in the Young Child and Adolescent

A Case-Based Guide

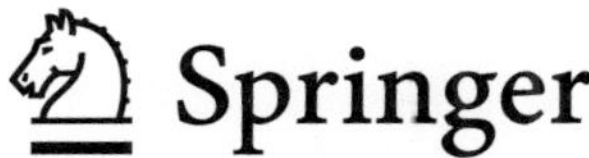 Springer

Editors
Richard M. Schwend
Department of Orthopaedic Surgery
Children's Mercy Hospital
Kansas City, MO
USA

William L. Hennrikus
Department of Orthopaedics
Penn State College of Medicine
Hershey, PA
USA

ISBN 978-3-030-50757-2   ISBN 978-3-030-50758-9   (eBook)
https://doi.org/10.1007/978-3-030-50758-9

This Springer imprint is published by the registered company Springer Nature Switzerland AG
The registered company address is: Gewerbestrasse 11, 6330 Cham, Switzerland

"You can observe a lot by just watching."
Yogi Berra

We dedicate this book to our wives and families, for whose support we are forever grateful.

Preface

Musculoskeletal conditions are a frequent cause of disability and discomfort for children. Back pain is a common complaint presenting to the primary care physician's office, the emergency room, or urgent care and can be a source of great anxiety for the child, parents, and clinician. Many primary care physicians have not received specific education and training on the appropriate workup and referral for pediatric back pain. This book is designed to fill this "gap" in musculoskeletal education.

Multiple physicians who are in the trenches caring for children with back pain have contributed to this text. We designed the book with case-based chapters written in a standardized format to help the reader navigate through the many diagnoses that can present with back pain. The authors have included clinical cases from their practices, common presenting symptoms, physical exam findings, tips on the work up, when to refer, multiple illustrations, and red flags to keep the clinician out of trouble. Each chapter also includes brief practical pearls from the editors.

In addition, we have included introductory chapters on topics such as epidemiology, anatomy, radiology, and medical conditions that contribute to back pain. A common theme throughout the book is that a focused history, physical examination, the use of plain radiographs, and simple laboratory tests are elements of a basic work up for most cases of back pain. Advanced imaging studies and more sophisticated laboratory tests are used on a case-by-case basis as indicated during the collaborative evaluation of the patient by the primary care physician and the spine specialist.

We are indebted to the many outstanding authors for sharing their experience and unique perspective in caring for children. We are also indebted to our editor at Springer, Connie Walsh, who led us through the maze of book publishing with clarity and diplomacy. We also thank our primary care colleagues, for whom this book is written and who typically are the first to see these children with back pain. The eminent pediatric orthopedic surgeon Mercer Rang said that "Preventive orthopaedics is better than reactive orthopaedics. Prevention is wholesale and treatment is retail." Finally, we thank our pediatric patients, who, over the course of our careers in pediatric orthopedics, have taught us the most.

Hopefully this book provides you the reader with new ideas and many clinical pearls to use in your practice. However, if themes in the book confuse or obscure, we welcome your feedback so that we can improve for the second edition of this book. Please email us at: rmschwend@cmh.edu and WLH5k@hotmail.com.

Kansas City, MO, USA
Hershey, PA, USA
Richard M. Schwend
William L. Hennrikus

Contents

Contributor List

John T. Anderson, MD Orthopaedic Surgery, University of Missouri – Kansas City School of Medicine, Kansas City, MO, USA

Orthopaedic Surgery, Children's Mercy – Kansas City, Kansas City, MO, USA

Natasha M. Archer, MD, MPH Department of Pediatrics, Dana Farber/Boston Children's Cancer and Blood Disorders Center, Harvard Medical School, Boston, MA, USA

Nicholas E. Arlas, BA Department of Orthopedic Surgery, University of Colorado – School of Medicine, Colorado Springs, CO, USA

Douglas G. Armstrong, MD Orthopedic Surgery, Orthopedics and Rehabilitation, PennState Health Hershey Medical Center, Hershey, PA, USA

Laurel C. Blakemore, MD Division of Pediatric Orthopedics, University of Florida, Gainesville, FL, USA

Todd J. Blumberg, MD Department of Orthopaedics and Sports Medicine, Seattle Children's Hospital, University of Washington, Seattle, WA, USA

M. Alison Brooks, MD, MPH Department of Orthopedics & Rehabilitation, University of Wisconsin–Madison School of Medicine & Public Health, Madison, WI, USA

Matthew M. Brown, MD, DPT Department of Orthopedics & Rehabilitation, University of Wisconsin–Madison School of Medicine & Public Health, Madison, WI, USA

Greg S. Canty, MD Sports Medicine Center, Pediatric Orthopaedic Surgery, Children's Mercy Kansas City, Kansas City, MO, USA

Department of Orthopaedic Surgery, University of Missouri-Kansas City School of Medicine, Kansas City, MO, USA

Department of Orthopaedic Surgery, University of Kansas School of Medicine, Kansas City, MO, USA

Wojciech L. Czoch, MD Pediatric Orthopaedics, Cohen Children's Medical Center, New Hyde Park, NY, USA

Michael DeFrance, DO Department of Orthopaedic Surgery, Rowan University School of Osteopathic Medicine, Stratford, NJ, USA

Mary E. Dubon, MD Pediatric Sports Medicine, Boston Children's Hospital, Boston, MA, USA

Pediatric Rehabilitation Medicine, Spaulding Rehabilitation Hospital Boston, Charlestown, MA, USA

Physical Medicine and Rehabilitation, Harvard Medical School, Boston, MA, USA

Howard R. Epps, MD Private Practice, Houston, TX, USA

Lorena V. Floccari, MD Department of Orthopedic Surgery, Akron Children's Hospital, Akron, OH, USA

Jesse Galina, BS Pediatric Orthopaedics, Cohen Children's Medical Center, New Hyde Park, NY, USA

David Gendelberg, MD Department of Orthopaedics and Sports Medicine, Harborview Medical Center, University of Washington, Seattle, WA, USA

Nattaly E. Greene, MD Harvard Combined Orthopaedic Residency Program, Boston, MA, USA

Andrew J. M. Gregory, MD Department of Orthopedics, Vanderbilt University Medical Center, Nashville, TN, USA

Arun R. Hariharan, MD, MS Department of Orthopaedics, Nemours/Alfred I. duPont Hospital for Children, Wilmington, DE, USA

Stephanie B. Ihnow, MD, MSEd Division of Pediatric Orthopaedic Surgery, Cincinnati Children's Hospital Medical Center, Cincinnati, OH, USA

Division of Pediatric Orthopaedic Surgery, University of Florida, Gainesville, FL, USA

Jefferson W. Jex, MD Department of Orthopaedic Surgery, Walter Reed National Military Medical Center, Bethesda, MD, USA

Kerwyn C. Jones, MD Department of Orthopedic Surgery, Akron Children's Hospital, Akron, OH, USA

Shannon M. Kelly, MD Division of Orthopaedic Surgery and Sports Medicine, Children's National Health System, Washington, DC, USA

Melanie Kennedy, MD Division of Sports Medicine, Cincinnati Children's Hospital Medical Center, Cincinnati, OH, USA

Department of Pediatrics, University of Cincinnati College of Medicine, Cincinnati, OH, USA

Krishn Khanna, MD Department of Orthopaedic Surgery, University of California – San Francisco, San Francisco, CA, USA

Dana H. Kotler, MD Physical Medicine and Rehabilitation, Harvard Medical School, Boston, MA, USA

Christopher Aaron Kowalski, MD Orthopedic Surgery, PennState Milton S. Hershey Medical Center, Hershey, PA, USA

Cynthia R. LaBella, MD Department of Pediatrics, Northwestern University's Feinberg School of Medicine, Chicago, IL, USA

Institute for Sports Medicine at Ann & Robert H. Lurie Children's Hospital of Chicago, Chicago, IL, USA

Raymond W. Liu, MD Department of Orthopaedic Surgery, University Hospitals Cleveland Medical Center, Rainbow Babies and Children's Hospitals, Case Western Reserve University, Cleveland, OH, USA

Stephen D. Lockey, MD, MBA Department of Orthopaedics, Medstar Georgetown University Hospital, Washington, DC, USA

Kelsey Logan, MD, MPH Division of Sports Medicine, Cincinnati Children's Hospital Medical Center, Cincinnati, OH, USA

Departments of Pediatrics and Internal Medicine, University of Cincinnati College of Medicine, Cincinnati, OH, USA

Teri M. McCambridge, MD Department of Pediatrics and Orthopedics, University of Maryland Medical System, Baltimore, MD, USA

Alicia McCarthy, BSN, MSN Department of Orthopaedics, Nemours/Alfred I. duPont Hospital for Children, Wilmington, DE, USA

Ayesha Maqsood, MD, MBA Department of Surgery, Ann & Robert H. Lurie Children's Hospital of Chicago, Chicago, IL, USA

Kody Moffatt, MD, MS Sports Medicine, Orthopedics, Children's Hospital & Medical Center Omaha, Omaha, NE, USA

James F. Mooney III, MD Shriners Hospital for Children – Springfield, Springfield, MA, USA

Surya N. Mundluru, MD Department of Pediatric Orthopaedic Surgery, University of Texas McGovern School of Medicine, Houston, TX, USA

Robert F. Murphy, MD Department of Orthopaedics and Physical Medicine, Medical University of South Carolina, Charleston, SC, USA

Blaise A. Nemeth, MD Orthopedics and Rehabilitation, American Family Children's Hospital, University of Wisconsin School of Medicine and Public Health, Madison, WI, USA

Matthew E. Oetgen, MD, MBA Division of Orthopaedic Surgery and Sports Medicine, Children's National Health System, Washington, DC, USA

Norman Y. Otsuka, MSc, MD, FRCSC, FAAP, FACS, FAOA Division of Orthopaedic Surgery, Southern Illinois University School of Medicine, Springfield, IL, USA

William A. Phillips, MD Department of Orthopaedic Surgery, Texas Children's Hospital, Baylor College of Medicine, Houston, TX, USA

George J. Richard, MD Department of Orthopaedic Surgery, University of Florida, Gainesville, FL, USA

Natalie Ronshaugen, MD Sports Medicine, Orthopedics, Children's Hospital & Medical Center Omaha, Omaha, NE, USA

Coleen S. Sabatini, MD, MPH Department of Orthopaedic Surgery, University of California San Francisco, UCSF Benioff Children's Hospital Oakland, Oakland, CA, USA

Sanjeev Sabharwal, MD, MPH Department of Orthopaedic Surgery, University of California – San Francisco, Benioff Children's Hospital of Oakland, Oakland, CA, USA

Kristine Santos Martin, APN Department of Surgery, Ann & Robert H. Lurie Children's Hospital of Chicago, Chicago, IL, USA

John F. Sarwark, MD Division of Orthopaedic Surgery & Sports Medicine, Department of Surgery, Ann & Robert H. Lurie Children's Hospital of Chicago, Chicago, IL, USA

Richard M. Schwend, MD Department of Orthopaedic Surgery, Children's Mercy Hospital, Kansas City, MO, USA

Eva Seligman, MD Department of Pediatrics, Johns Hopkins University School of Medicine, Baltimore, MD, USA

Suken A. Shah, MD Division of Spine and Scoliosis, Department of Orthopaedics, Nemours/Alfred I. duPont Hospital for Children, Wilmington, DE, USA

Brian A. Shaw, MD Department of Orthopedic Surgery, University of Colorado – School of Medicine, Colorado Springs, CO, USA

Jessica M. Smith, DO Pediatric Sports Medicine, Children's Mercy Kansas City, Kansas City, MO, USA

Ashley Startzman, DO Department of Orthopaedic Surgery, Texas Children's Hospital, Baylor College of Medicine, Houston, TX, USA

Peter F. Sturm, MD, MBA Spine Surgery, Crawford Spine Center, Division of Pediatric Orthopaedic Surgery, Cincinnati Children's Hospital Medical Center, Cincinnati, OH, USA

Mathew Varghese, MS Department of Orthopaedics, St. Stephen's Hospital, New Delhi, Delhi, India

Morgan B. Weber, MD Department of Orthopaedic Surgery, University Hospitals Cleveland Medical Center, Rainbow Babies and Children's Hospitals, Case Western Reserve University, Cleveland, OH, USA

Part I
Background

Chapter 1
Epidemiology of Pediatric Back Pain

Morgan B. Weber and Raymond W. Liu

Introduction

Back pain in children and adolescents is more common than previously thought. Historically, it has been taught that pediatric back pain is rare, usually associated with underlying pathologic conditions, and necessitates an MRI [1]. Literature over the past 40 years, however, has challenged these notions. Pediatric back pain prevalence has been increasing since the 1980s [2, 3]. Lifetime prevalence of back pain is reported in up to 89% of adolescents [4]. Although the etiology of most pediatric back pain cases is benign and self-limited [5, 6], back pain can have effects on a child's lifestyle including reduction in physical activity and absence from school. Additionally, pediatric back pain is a risk factor for chronic back pain as an adult [7, 8]. In this chapter the prevalence, risk factors, natural history, and potential disability resulting from pediatric back pain are reviewed.

Defining Back Pain

Back pain in the literature is variably reported in terms of generic back pain, spinal pain, neck pain, thoracic pain, upper back pain, or low back pain. The majority of studies, including this chapter, group back pain into neck pain, thoracic or mid-back pain, and low back pain. However, the lack of standardization of terminology about back pain makes it difficult to compare studies. Low back pain (LBP), defined as pain limited to the region between the lower margins of the twelfth rib and gluteal

M. B. Weber · R. W. Liu (✉)
Department of Orthopaedic Surgery, University Hospitals Cleveland Medical Center, Rainbow Babies and Children's Hospitals, Case Western Reserve University, Cleveland, OH, USA
e-mail: Raymond.Liu@UHhospitals.org

© Springer Nature Switzerland AG 2021
R. M. Schwend, W. L. Hennrikus (eds.), *Back Pain in the Young Child and Adolescent*, https://doi.org/10.1007/978-3-030-50758-9_1

folds, is the most common type of back pain [9] and has been most frequently studied. In contrast, there is a relative paucity of literature on pediatric thoracic and neck pain.

Prevalence

Back Pain

Lifetime back pain prevalence estimates range from 5% to 89% of the pediatric population [4, 10, 11]. Severe or permanent back pain is estimated at 3–15% [4, 12, 13].

Neck and Thoracic Pain

Lifetime prevalence of neck pain for children aged 9 and 15 years is 10% and 15%, respectively, and lifetime prevalence for mid-back pain is 20% and 28%, respectively [14]. One-year prevalence of neck pain ranges from 10% to 19% [13, 15, 16], and thoracic pain is estimated at 8% [15].

Low Back Pain

There is variability in LBP prevalence estimates, ranging from 1% to 66% [2]. In a recent meta-analysis, the mean point prevalence was 12%, mean period prevalence for 1 month was 18%, and for 1 year, it was 27%. Mean lifetime prevalence was 40% [2]. LBP point prevalence and recurrent or continuous back pain all increase with age [17]. Back pain is uncommon in children less than 4 years and may signal more alarming conditions in this age group [18]. Both lifetime prevalence and 1-year period prevalence are reported to be around 1% in 7-year-old children [17, 18]. Prevalence increases to 4% (1-month period prevalence) in 8–10-year-old children [19]. One-year period prevalence is reported at 6%, 18%, and 18.4% for 10-, 14-, and 16-year-old patients, respectively [17]. In a systematic review, lifetime prevalence increases from 1% at age 7 to 17% at age 12 years, and there is then a steep increase to 53% at age 15 years [18]. It is estimated that lifetime prevalence rises by about 10% annually from 12% at age 11 to 50% by age 15 years [20]. By age 18 years, lifetime prevalence approaches 70–80%, which is equivalent to that of adults [2].

Incidence

The 2-year incidence of neck pain in a cohort of students aged 13–15 years at follow-up was 60%, mid-back pain was 50%, and LBP was 42% [4]. In a 1-year longitudinal study of 12–13-year-olds, annual incidence of LBP was 18% [21]. In a similar study of children ages 11–14 years known to be free of symptoms at baseline, 19% reported LBP 12 months subsequently [22], and in another study, annual LBP incidence was 17% among adolescents at a mean age of 13.8 years [23]. LBP incidence, similar to prevalence, increases with age [20].

Pain Frequency, Duration, and Intensity

The majority of pediatric back pain is mild, with low frequency, low intensity, and short duration, typically less than a week [4, 17, 24]. The median duration is 3 days [22], and the majority report a duration of 1–2 days [24]. "Frequent" symptoms are present in approximately 25–33% of adolescents [9, 25]. Severe, chronic, or recurrent LBP is present in 5–29% of adolescents [9, 13, 17, 20, 25–27]. Analgesics were utilized by 13–23% of students for LBP [27, 28]. The prevalence of sciatica is estimated at 2–6% of adolescents [26, 27].

Disability

For some patients the effect of back pain can lead to decreased quality of life and interference with daily activities. An estimated 7–29% of adolescents report LBP severe enough to reduce function, disturb sleep, lead to school absence, interfere with leisure activities, or cause sport cessation [9, 13, 24–30]. Neck pain can also interfere with daily activities [13]. The most common reports of disability include difficulty carrying schoolbags, lifting/carrying heavy objects, sitting at school, forward bending, standing for more than 10 minutes, walking over 2 km, getting up from bed, putting socks on, and job/sports activities in leisure time [24, 26, 27]. LBP may influence social, emotional, and mental health. The relationship is likely bidirectional with interactions perpetuating a cycle of pain, negative thoughts, and dissatisfactory mental health [31].

Medical Attention

The prevalence of back pain requiring medical consultation is reported at 6%, 8%, and 34% for schoolchildren aged 9, 13, and 15, respectively [14]. Overall, 6–25% of the pediatric population will see a physician for LBP [27, 28, 30]. Of the adolescents who report LBP, 4–32% will seek medical care [20, 21, 24, 25].

Natural History

The differential diagnosis for back pain is broad and includes trauma, infection, rheumatologic conditions, malignancy, and medical illnesses such as pyelonephritis or sickle cell crisis. Fortunately, the majority of pediatric back pain is benign and self-limiting. In a large prospective study of children with LBP of greater than 3 months, only 21% of children had a definitive underlying diagnosis [32]. Similarly, in a recent study of nearly 22,000 adolescents with back pain, over 80% had no identifiable diagnosis [6]. Adolescent back pain is typically non-specific pain classified as musculoskeletal or mechanical [20, 33]. In both children and adults, large prospective studies have shown that the best predictor of future LBP episodes is a history of prior LBP [34, 35].

Risk Factors

Since the majority of work on the etiology of LBP in childhood is cross-sectional, the temporal nature of exposure and any associated outcome cannot be assessed. Thus, the majority of studies identify factors that are associated with back pain rather than predictors for its development. Current evidence suggests the risk for developing back pain is multifactorial, which are divided here into physical, biological, lifestyle, and psychosocial domains.

Physical Domain

Trunk Muscles

Several cross-sectional studies have found evidence that reduced endurance or strength of trunk extensor [26, 31, 36, 37], trunk flexor [26, 38], and abdominal muscles [9, 26, 34, 38] are associated with pediatric LBP. Reduced back muscle endurance [36], baseline low lumbar extension strength [37], and imbalanced trunk muscle strength [39] have been predictive of future LBP. Trunk muscle function, however, is not consistently associated with LBP [8, 13, 36, 40], nor is it consistently predictive of future LBP [34]. Although evidence suggests trunk muscle function may be independently associated with LBP, deficits in muscle function are also associated with activity level, lifestyle, and psychological factors [40, 41].

Trunk Mobility

Sagittal and coronal plane motions facilitate the spine to absorb force. Back muscles protect the spine from excessive bending, and poor mobility reduces this protection [38]. Multiple prospective studies, however, have not found predictive value in trunk mobility [20, 21, 34, 37].

Posture

Non-neutral postural alignment is theorized to cause LBP through altered mechanical loading and motor control resulting in modified stress distributions, tissue strain, and pain [41, 42]. LBP has been associated with lumbar hyperlordosis [9, 43], loss of lumbar lordosis [43, 44], thoracic kyphosis [42], and both increased and decreased sacral inclination [43, 44]. In contrast, some studies have found no relationship with spinopelvic parameters [21, 45]. More recent studies have classified sitting and standing postures into subgroups [36, 43, 45, 46]. In doing so, non-neutral standing postures have been associated with LBP [36, 46], and there is evidence that extremes of sitting spinal posture (both lordotic and particularly slumped/flexed sitting) may be associated with LBP [28, 31, 47]. Decreased functional trunk stability and postural insufficiency have been associated with adolescent LBP [48], although more recent studies have found no correlation [42, 49].

Trunk Asymmetry

Trunk asymmetry and idiopathic scoliosis have historically been thought to be painless in adolescents [50], but more recently have been recognized as potential risk factors for the development of back pain in adolescents [5, 49, 51]. Adolescents with scoliosis have been found to have a greater than twofold increased odds of back pain versus controls [51], and greater spinal deformity has been recently associated with increased pain intensity [52].

Muscle and Joint Flexibility

Hypermobility has been associated with non-specific chronic pain including LBP [31]. This relationship is inconsistent, however, and generalized joint hypermobility has not been predictive of future back pain [16, 36]. On the other hand, decreased mobility has also been associated with LBP. Decreased hamstring flexibility [8, 34, 53], tight quadriceps [8], and decreased hip mobility [53] have been associated with LBP. Other studies have found no association with back pain and lower extremity flexibility or stiffness [27, 36].

Trunk Stability

Spinal stability refers to the ability to tolerate physiologic loads without structural changes or damage to spinal cord or nerve roots [54]. Stability is conferred by a combination of musculature, flexibility, and posture. The interaction among trunk strength, sagittal and coronal spinal mobility, and posture can contribute to LBP. This may explain conflicting results when these factors are studied independently. For example, high mobility in combination with low strength is predictive of back pain [37]. Posture alters trunk motor control patterns, and non-neutral lumbar postures have been linked with poor back muscle activation and endurance [47, 55]. Posture has also been linked to potential risk factors from biological, lifestyle, and psychosocial domains. For example, slump sitting is associated with higher body mass index (BMI), greater television use, and lower perceived self-image [47].

Biological Domain

Weight and Height

There is some evidence to suggest that children with LBP may be heavier [27, 34, 40, 49, 53, 56], but several studies have reported no significant difference in weight or BMI in children with and without back pain [33, 37, 38, 49, 57–60]. Weight, BMI, or weight gain has not been predictive of future LBP [21, 22, 34, 36].

The relationship between standing height and back pain is controversial [22, 33]. Some evidence suggests increased height may be associated with LBP in boys [21, 34, 61]. Increased sitting height, or trunk length, has been identified as a potential risk factor [13, 21], although the rate of change of sitting height may be more predictive of LBP than the absolute value [9, 38]. Spine growth accelerates relative to lower extremity growth around the time of puberty. The onset of LBP roughly corresponds to puberty, and the increasing height and change in body composition during puberty may impact back pain [56]. Differential growth rates between vertebrae and surrounding muscles and ligaments and the resulting relative lack of lean tissue mass and sudden changes in mechanical loading of the spine may make adolescents more vulnerable to trauma, powerful muscle contractions, and overuse injuries [62]. High school students with a large growth spurt (>5 cm in 6 months) were three times more likely to report LBP [8].

Gender

The prevalence of LBP is higher among female adolescents compared to male adolescents [7, 27, 28, 33, 36, 37, 58, 63, 64]. However, this finding is inconsistent as gender association has been ambiguous in other studies [12, 25, 29].

Family History

Parental LBP has been significantly associated with childhood LBP [9, 12, 25, 40, 49, 58, 65]. Back pain in a parent triples the risk for back pain in girls [49]. A combination of genetics, environmental exposures, and psychosocial factors likely explains this relationship. Evidence suggests parental history may play a more important behavioral role among younger children than among older children [16, 66]. Twin studies demonstrate the shared environment to be a strong component with genetic factors playing a lesser role in children age 11–15 years [16, 66]. In contrast, as individuals grow older (age > 15 years), genetic effects become more evident [66]. With increasing age, psychosocial familial influences decrease, and a more complex and precise individual understanding of pain develops.

Lifestyle Domain

Activity

Physical activity plays a role in back pain in children and adolescents, as either a risk or protective factor [67]. Some authors have described a U- or J-shaped relationship in which both low and high activity levels may be related to increased back pain [29, 61, 64].

Sedentary Activity

There is weak and conflicting evidence for sedentary activities as a risk factor for LBP. Sedentary activities such as computer use, watching television, or playing video games have been associated with LBP [12, 33, 37, 58]. However, other studies have found no relationship between sedentary activities and LBP [27, 29, 49, 59, 60]. Dose-risk relationships are inconsistent, and prospective studies have not found sedentary activities to be predictive of LBP [22, 58, 59, 68].

Physical Activity

Self-reported physical activity has been associated with both increased [36, 37] and decreased [33, 34] risk of back pain. Other studies report inconsistent or absent relationships [17, 58, 59].

Physical activity is traditionally assessed using self-reported survey answers, which may not accurately estimate true physical activity in children. For example, one author found that survey data overestimated time spent in physical activity and underestimated moderate physical activity. Using accelerometers as a measure of activity, the same author found no cross-sectional association, but low physical activity was predictive of back pain 3 years later, and higher physical activity was protective against future LBP [11, 69]. In contrast, a similar study using an activity monitor did not find a cross-sectional or longitudinal association at 2-year follow-up between levels of activity and back pain [70].

Sport

Exercise has been considered a risk factor for LBP and chronic LBP especially if intense, frequent, and competitive [22, 27, 33, 37, 64]. Involvement in sports has been predictive of future LBP [40]. Kamada et al. 2016 found a dose-response relationship between sports activity and musculoskeletal pain, including LBP in adolescents. An increase in sports activity by 1 hour per week led to a 3% higher probability of developing pain 1 year later [71]. The growing spine is vulnerable to overuse injury, and adolescents with high training volume may be particularly at risk for LBP [15, 72]. Activities with greater stresses on the lumbar spine are associated with adolescent LBP and increased frequency of radiological spine abnormalities [73]. Gymnastics, rowing, weight lifting, wrestling, diving, swimming, football, basketball, golf, and racket sports have been associated with LBP [25, 33, 61]. Compression of the spine in the vertical plane (football, weight lifting), rotational or shear force in the horizontal plane (throwing and racket sports, golf, baseball), cyclic tensile stresses from repetitive motions (rowing gymnastics, ballet, cheer), and frequent hyperextension (gymnastics, dance, football, pole-vault, figure skating) are all thought to contribute to LBP [74, 75].

Occupational Activity

Part-time employment has been associated with LBP [27, 60] and has also been predictive of future LBP [8, 22]. The significance of the type of job (physically demanding activity, lifting heavy objects) in relation to adolescent back pain remains unclear [22, 59, 60].

Sleep

The evidence is inconsistent on the effect of sleep quantity and quality and LBP in adolescents [63, 76]. Auvinen et al. found a dose-response relationship in 16-year-olds between level of insufficient sleep and musculoskeletal (low back, neck, and shoulder) pain [64]. Daytime sleepiness and tiredness in the morning have also been associated with LBP [17, 60]. However no association was found between hours of sleep per day and back pain in a separate study [58]. The relationship among pain, psychological factors, and sleep is complex. Insufficient sleep may merely be a risk indicator for psychological distress. Sleep may, however, present an independent physiological risk factor for LBP through activation of the inflammatory process via cortisol and cytokine networks [64].

Smoking and Alcohol

Smoking is associated with LBP [27, 41]. In addition, passive or second-hand smoking has been associated with adolescent back pain [49]. Prospective studies have identified smoking as a risk factor predicting future LBP, and pack-years smoking has been associated with incident and persistent LBP with a dose-response relationship [8, 77]. Smoking can be interpreted as a behavioral marker for psycho-social problems, and it is strongly associated with mental health status [78]. When adjusted for psychosocial variables, smoking as an independent predictor of LBP is less clear [77, 78]. Nicotine is reported to have direct toxic effects on bone metabolism, collagen synthesis, circulation, and wound healing [79]. Animal models suggest smoking works through biological mechanisms affecting intervertebral disk health [80, 81]. Nicotine, through excitatory and pro-inflammatory effects, may also alter the perception and threshold for pain [82]. Similarly, alcohol consumption is associated with psychological factors, and, although alcohol has been independently associated with LBP, results are inconsistent [36, 57, 78].

Backpacks

The relationship of backpacks to back pain is controversial. Despite this controversy, the American Academy of Pediatrics recommends backpack weight less than 10–20% of body weight and symmetric carrying with the use of both shoulder straps. Backpack weight in excess of 10% of body weight may alter posture and gait and increase the risk of LBP [26, 83]. Similarly, asymmetric carrying (carrying a backpack on one shoulder, e.g.) has also been associated with postural changes and increased risk for LBP [58, 84]. In contrast many other studies have found no relationship between schoolbag weight [25, 59, 60] or carrying style [12, 25, 49] and back pain. Relative mechanical loads, type of schoolbag, and carrying method have not been predictive of future back pain [22]. Dianat et al. recently reported that carrying a schoolbag for more than 30 minutes a day was a risk factor for back pain [59]. Interestingly, an increase in LBP is observed in children who perceive their schoolbags to be heavy [68, 84].

Psychosocial Domain

Psychological, Behavioral, and Cognitive Factors

Psychosocial factors play a role in the development of back pain, particularly chronic or severe back pain and back pain leading to disability. Psychological, social, and emotional factors may have a stronger relationship with back pain than physical and mechanical factors [59, 60, 65]. Higher levels of stress, depression, negative behavior, emotional problems, loneliness, poor overall well-being, peer problems, conduct problems, and other somatic complaints have been associated with increased risk for LBP [22, 30, 41, 63]. Adolescents with medium and high values of stress reported more back pain compared to adolescents who reported no stress, and adolescents who reported poorer general well-being also reported more back pain [30]. Poor academic achievement and academic dissatisfaction has also been associated with LBP [9, 25].

Increased risk for LBP has been reported in individuals with higher internalizing (anxiety, depression, nervousness) and externalizing (conduct problems, rule breaking, aggression, disobedience, violence) behaviors [41]. Conduct problems (anger, disobedience, violence) and hyperactivity (restlessness, distraction, lack of concentration) were predictors of future back pain [22]. Answering "yes" to the question "Do you often feel nervous?" in adolescence was predictive of pain in young adulthood [7].

Catastrophizing is a cognitive style characterized by worry, magnification of pain, negative thought patterns, and perceived lack of control. Catastrophizing is one of the most important psychological predictors of pain [85]. The use of catastrophizing as a coping technique is associated with disability in children with chronic back pain [65]. More negative beliefs about LBP are associated with activity modification and care-seeking [86]. Negative thoughts such as dissatisfaction with school chairs and perception of a heavy backpack have been associated with LBP [25, 87]. Poor self-perceived health and fitness may also influence the development of back pain [25, 68].

Parental modeling of pain behavior may influence a child's coping mechanisms, beliefs about pain, and disability secondary to pain. A family history of back pain is associated with higher levels of catastrophizing and increased disability due to pain (missed school, inability to engage in activities) [65]. Behavioral responses to back pain in adolescents (seeking medical attention, use of analgesic pain medications, absence from work, avoidance of physical activity) are aligned with those of their primary caregiver [88].

Low back pain may be a physical manifestation of psychological or emotional distress, known as somatization. Somatic symptoms at baseline including headache, abdominal pain, and sore throat were predictive of future back pain [60]. Somatic complaints increased the odds for LBP with impact [36]. Somatization is a poor prognostic factor and is associated with a higher degree of disability [89].

Social Factors

Multiple social factors have been studied with little evidence to support any factor as an independent risk factor. Family functioning, number of family life stress events (including money problems, residential problems, moving, death of a loved one, job loss, divorce), mother or father education, ethnicity, and household income at age 14 were not predictive of future LBP at age 17 [36]. A higher socioeconomic index for area of residence was associated with decreased odds for both LBP with impact and LBP with minimal impact compared to no LBP [36]. In contrast, social class, as measured by parental occupation, has not been associated with LBP [37]. Social factors have been associated with beliefs about back pain. For example, in one study individuals with higher annual income were more likely to believe one should stay active during an episode of LBP [90]. Geography has not consistently been shown to be associated with LBP [17].

Approaching Back Pain from a Multidimensional Perspective

The majority of back pain in adolescence is non-specific. Epidemiological evidence indicates a combination of risk indicators, rather than a single risk factor, results in back pain (Fig. 1.1). During the workup of an adolescent with back pain, serious spinal and systemic pathology must first be ruled out. Assessment and management may then be tailored to an individual's biopsychosocial profile. O'Sullivan et al. detail a cognitive functional approach in which modifiable risk factors are identified based on interview and exam. Those factors are then targeted under three broad areas including education, functional restoration, and healthy lifestyle behaviors [41].

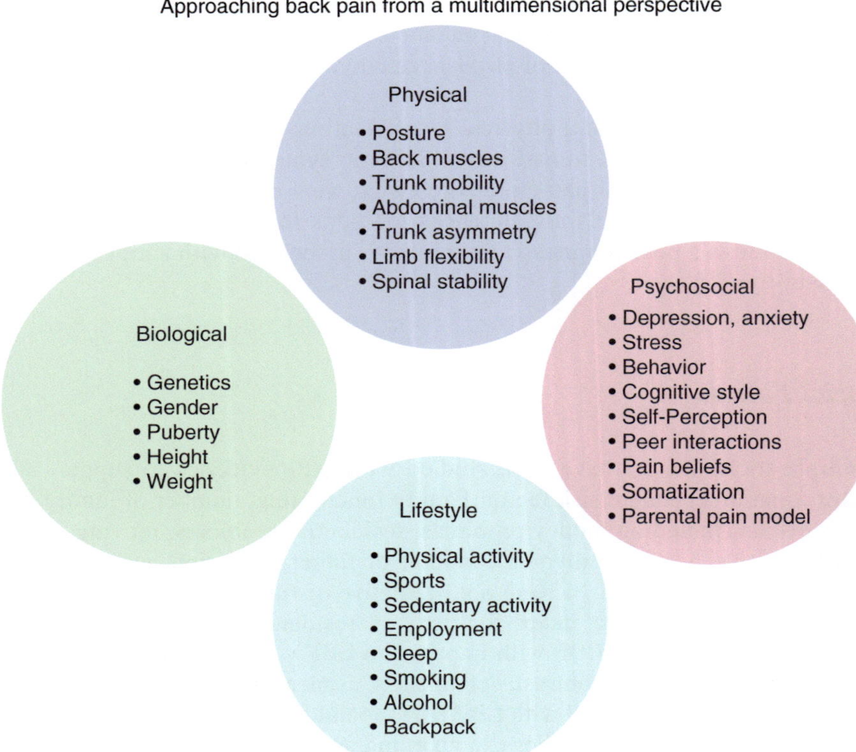

Fig. 1.1 Risk for developing back pain is multifactorial with risk factors in the physical, biological, lifestyle, and psychosocial domains

Prevention

Based on the high prevalence of pediatric back pain and the substantial quality of life reduction in some patients, prevention programs in childhood could reduce the burden of disease in both pediatric and adult populations. The lack of clear risk factors is a challenge to developing prevention programs. Currently there is a lack of strong evidence for successful programs.

Prevention will require multidimensional interventions addressing musculoskeletal, psychological, cognitive, and social systems. A multidimensional approach, including pain education combined with targeted postural and endurance training, was used to successfully reduce the incidence of LBP and disability in adolescent female rowers [91]. Prevention efforts aimed at athletes have included emphasis on preseason conditioning, proper technique, improvements in flexibility, neuromuscular training, and appropriate rest, with gradual increase in frequency and intensity [5, 75]. More research is needed to ascertain the effectiveness of psychosocial prevention efforts and back pain.

Brief Summary

Back pain is common in children. The majority of pediatric back pain is of musculoskeletal etiology with brief and mild episodes. Some children, however, will experience frequent, chronic, or severe back pain resulting in decreased quality of life, reduction in physical activity, decreased sports participation, increased use of medications, and absence from school. The risk for developing back pain is multifactorial including physical, biological, lifestyle, and psychosocial causes. Psychological, behavioral, and cognitive factors can also play a role in the development of back pain. The multifactorial nature of back pain necessitates a detailed and thoughtful assessment, an accurate diagnosis, and appropriate treatment.

Conclusion

- Back pain in children and adolescents is common.
- Back pain in children younger than 4 years old warrants a careful and detailed workup.
- Multiple risk factors exist in the physical, biological, lifestyle, and psychosocial domains.

Editor Discussion

As this comprehensive chapter illustrates, back pain in children and adolescents is common and can stem from physical, biological, lifestyle, and psychosocial causes. Also remember that back pain in children does not have to come from the spine.

W. L. Hennrikus

It has been said that young children are all about activity, teenagers about appearance, and as we age, all about comfort. This chapter outlines the many and varied factors that can present as a painful spine. Back pain when it occurs in its severest and long-standing forms can take over a child's life, leading to decreased activity, weight gain, poor core strength, and depression. This cycle of decreased fitness leading to poor health can continue, with the family unable to free itself from the grasp of despair. The primary care physician is well positioned to recognize this cycle and provide needed intervention.

R. M. Schwend

References

1. Hollingworth P. Back pain in children. Br J Rheumatol. 1996;35(10):1022–8.
2. Calvo-Muñoz I, Gómez-Conesa A, Sánchez-Meca J. Prevalence of low back pain in children and adolescents: a meta-analysis. BMC Pediatr. 2013;13(1):14.
3. Vikat A, Rimpelä M, Salminen JJ, Rimpelä A, Savolainen A, Virtanen SM. Neck or shoulder pain and low back pain in Finnish adolescents. Scand J Public Health. 2000;28(3):164–73.
4. Aartun E, Hartvigsen J, Wedderkopp N, Hestbaek L. Spinal pain in adolescents: prevalence, incidence, and course: a school-based two-year prospective cohort study in 1,300 Danes aged 11–13. BMC Musculoskelet Disord. 2014;15(1):187.
5. MacDonald J, Stuart E, Rodenberg R. Musculoskeletal low back pain in school-aged children. JAMA Pediatr. 2017;171(3):280.
6. Yang S, Werner BC, Singla A, Abel MF. Low back pain in adolescents. J Pediatr Orthop. 2017;37(5):344–7.
7. Brattberg G. Do pain problems in young school children persist into early adulthood? A 13-year follow-up. Eur J Pain. 2004;8(3):187–99.
8. Feldman DE. Risk factors for the development of low back pain in adolescence. Am J Epidemiol. 2001;154(1):30–6.
9. Salminen JJ. The adolescent back. Acta Paediatr. 1984;73(s315):1–122.
10. Jeffries LJ, Milanese SF, Grimmer-Somers KA. Epidemiology of adolescent spinal pain. Spine (Phila Pa 1976). 2007;32(23):2630–7.
11. Wedderkopp N, Kjaer P, Hestbaek L, Korsholm L, Leboeuf-Yde C. High-level physical activity in childhood seems to protect against low back pain in early adolescence. Spine J. 2009;9(2):134–41.
12. Gunzburg R, Balagué F, Nordin M, Szpalski M, Duyck D, Bull D, et al. Low back pain in a population of school children. Eur Spine J. 1999;8(6):439–43.
13. Kujala UM, Salminen JJ, Taimela S, Oksanen A, Jaakkola L. Subject characteristics and low back pain in young athletes and nonathletes. Med Sci Sports Exerc. 1992;24(6):627–32.
14. Kjaer P, Wedderkopp N, Korsholm L, Leboeuf-Yde C. Prevalence and tracking of back pain from childhood to adolescence. BMC Musculoskelet Disord. 2011;12(1):98.
15. Kujala UM, Taimela S, Viljanen T. Leisure physical activity and various pain symptoms among adolescents. Br J Sports Med. 1999;33(5):325–8.
16. El-Metwally A, Mikkelsson M, Ståhl M, Macfarlane GJ, Jones GT, Pulkkinen L, et al. Genetic and environmental influences on non-specific low back pain in children: a twin study. Eur Spine J. 2008;17(4):502–8.
17. Taimela S, Kujala UM, Salminen JJ, Viljanen T. The prevalence of low back pain among children and adolescents. Spine (Phila Pa 1976). 1997;22(10):1132–6.
18. Hill JJ, Keating JL. A systematic review of the incidence and prevalence of low back pain in children. Phys Ther Rev. 2009;14(4):272–84.
19. Wedderkopp N, Leboeuf-Yde C, Andersen LB, Froberg K, Hansen HS. Back pain reporting pattern in a Danish population-based sample of children and adolescents. Spine (Phila Pa 1976). 2001;26(17):1879–83.
20. Burton KA, Clarke RD, McClune TD, Tillotson MK. The natural history of low back pain in adolescents. Spine (Phila Pa 1976). 1996;21(20):2323–8.
21. Nissinen M, Heliövaara M, Seitsamo J, Alaranta H, Poussa M. Anthropometric measurements and the incidence of low back pain in a cohort of pubertal children. Spine (Phila Pa 1976). 1994;19(12):1367–70.
22. Jones GT, Watson KD, Silman AJ, Symmons DP, Macfarlane GJ. Predictors of low back pain in British schoolchildren: a population-based prospective cohort study. Pediatrics. 2003;111(4 Pt 1):822–8.
23. Feldman DE, Rossignol M, Shrier I, Abenhaim L. Smoking. Spine (Phila Pa 1976). 1999;24(23):2492.

24. Watson KD, Papageorgiou AC, Jones GT, Taylor S, Symmons DPM, Silman AJ, et al. Low back pain in schoolchildren: occurrence and characteristics. Pain. 2002;97(1):87–92.
25. Bejia I, Abid N, Salem KB, Letaief M, Younes M, Touzi M, et al. Low back pain in a cohort of 622 Tunisian schoolchildren and adolescents: an epidemiological study. Eur Spine J. 2005;14(4):331–6.
26. Salminen J, Pentti J, Terho P. Low back pain and disability in 14-year-old schoolchildren. Acta Paediatr. 1992;81(12):1035–9.
27. Harreby M, Nygaard B, Jessen T, Larsen E, Storr-Paulsen A, Lindahl A, et al. Risk factors for low back pain in a cohort of 1389 Danish school children: an epidemiologic study. Eur Spine J. 1999;8(6):444–50.
28. Meziat Filho N. Coutinho ES, e Silva GA. Association between home posture habits and low back pain in high school adolescents. Eur Spine J. 2015;24(3):425–33.
29. Skoffer B, Foldspang A. Physical activity and low-back pain in schoolchildren. Eur Spine J. 2008;17(3):373–9.
30. Stallknecht SE, Strandberg-Larsen K, Hestbæk L, Andersen A-MN. Spinal pain and co-occurrence with stress and general well-being among young adolescents: a study within the Danish National Birth Cohort. Eur J Pediatr. 2017;176(6):807–14.
31. O'Sullivan P, Beales D, Jensen L, Murray K, Myers T. Characteristics of chronic non-specific musculoskeletal pain in children and adolescents attending a rheumatology outpatients clinic: a cross-sectional study. Pediatr Rheumatol. 2011;9(1):3.
32. Bhatia NN, Chow G, Timon SJ, Watts HG. Diagnostic modalities for the evaluation of pediatric back pain. J Pediatr Orthop. 2008;28(2):230–3.
33. Masiero S, Carraro E, Celia A, Sarto D, Ermani M. Prevalence of nonspecific low back pain in schoolchildren aged between 13 and 15 years. Acta Paediatr. 2008;97(2):212–6.
34. Salminen JJ, Erkintalo M, Laine M, Pentti J. Low back pain in the young a prospective three-year follow-up study of subjects with and without low back pain. Spine (Phila Pa 1976). 1995;20(19) 2101–7.
35. Hellsing A-L, Bryngelsson I-L. Predictors of musculoskeletal pain in men. Spine (Phila Pa 1976). 2000;25(23):3080–6.
36. Smith A, Beales D, O'Sullivan P, Bear NSL. Low back pain with impact at 17 years of age is predicted by early adolescent risk factors from multiple domains: analysis of the Western Australian Pregnancy Cohort (Raine) study. J Orthop Sport Phys Ther. 2017;47(10):752.
37. Sjölie AN, Ljunggren AE. The significance of high lumbar mobility and low lumbar strength for current and future low back pain in adolescents. Spine (Phila Pa 1976). 2001;26(23):2629–36.
38. Jones MA. Biological risk indicators for recurrent non-specific low back pain in adolescents. Br J Sports Med. 2005;39(3):137–40.
39. Lee J-H, Hoshino Y, Nakamura K, Kariya Y, Saita K, Ito K. Trunk muscle weakness as a risk factor for low back pain. Spine (Phila Pa 1976). 1999;24(1):54–7.
40. Balague F, Bibbo E, Melot C, Szpalski M, et al. The association between isoinertial trunk muscle performance and low back pain in male adolescents. Eur Spine J. 2010;19(4):624–32.
41. O'Sullivan P, Smith A, Beales D, Straker L. Understanding adolescent low back pain from a multidimensional perspective: implications for management. J Orthop Sports Phys Ther. 2017;47(10):741–51.
42. Feng Q, Jiang C, Zhou Y, Huang Y, Zhang M. Relationship between spinal morphology and function and adolescent non-specific back pain: a cross-sectional study. J Back Musculoskelet Rehabil. 2017;30(3):625–33.
43. Dankaerts W, O'Sullivan P, Burnett A, Straker L. Differences in sitting postures are associated with nonspecific chronic low back pain disorders when patients are subclassified. Spine (Phila Pa 1976). 2006;31(6):698–704.
44. Jackson RP, McManus AC. Radiographic analysis of sagittal plane alignment and balance in standing volunteers and patients with low back pain matched for age, sex, and size. Spine (Phila Pa 1976). 1994;19(Supplement):1611–8.

45. Dolphens M, Cagnie B, Coorevits P, Vanderstraeten G, Cardon G, D'Hooge R, et al. Sagittal standing posture and its association with spinal pain: a school-based epidemiological study of 1196 flemish adolescents before age at peak height velocity. Spine (Phila Pa 1976). 2012;37:1657.
46. Dolphens M, Cagnie B, Coorevits P, Vleeming A, Danneels L. Classification system of the normal variation in sagittal standing plane alignment: a study among young adolescent boys. Spine (Phila Pa 1976). 2013;38(16):E1003–12.
47. O'Sullivan PB, Smith AJ, Beales DJ, Straker LM. Association of biopsychosocial factors with degree of slump in sitting posture and self-report of back pain in adolescents: a cross-sectional study. Phys Ther. 2011;91(4):470–83.
48. Cudre-Mauroux N, Kocher N, Bonfils R, Pirlet M, et al. Relationship between impaired functional stability and back pain in children: an exploratory cross-sectional study. Swiss Med Wkly. 2006;136(45–46):721–5.
49. Wirth B, Knecht C, Humphreys K. Spine day 2012: spinal pain in Swiss school children– epidemiology and risk factors. BMC Pediatr. 2013;13(1):159.
50. Ramirez N, Johnston CE, Browne RH. The prevalence of back pain in children who have idiopathic scoliosis. J Bone Joint Surg. 1997;79:364–8.
51. Sato T, Hirano T, Ito T, Morita O, Kikuchi R, Endo N, et al. Back pain in adolescents with idiopathic scoliosis: epidemiological study for 43,630 pupils in Niigata City, Japan. Eur Spine J. 2011;20(2):274–9.
52. Théroux J, Le May S, Hebert JJ, Labelle H. Back pain prevalence is associated with curve-type and severity in adolescents with idiopathic scoliosis. Spine (Phila Pa 1976). 2017;42(15):E914–9.
53. Sjolie AN. Low-back pain in adolescents is associated with poor hip mobility and high body mass index. Scand J Med Sci Sports. 2004;14(3):168–75.
54. Izzo R, Guarnieri G, Guglielmi G, Muto M. Biomechanics of the spine. Part I: spinal stability. Eur J Radiol. 2013;82(1):118–26.
55. Astfalck RG, O'Sullivan PB, Straker LM, Smith AJ, Burnett A, Paulo Caneiro J, et al. Sitting postures and trunk muscle activity in adolescents with and without nonspecific chronic low back pain. Spine (Phila Pa 1976). 2010;35(14):1387–95.
56. Perry M, Straker L, O'Sullivan P, Smith A, Hands B. Fitness, motor competence, and body composition are weakly associated with adolescent back pain. J Orthop Sports Phys Ther. 2009;39(6):439–49.
57. Kovacs FM, Gestoso M, Gil del Real MT, López J, Mufraggi N, Ignacio Méndez J. Risk factors for non-specific low back pain in schoolchildren and their parents: a population based study. Pain. 2003;103(3):259–68.
58. Noll M, Candotti CT, da Rosa BN, Loss JF. Back pain prevalence and associated factors in children and adolescents: an epidemiological population study. Rev Saude Publica. 2016;50:31.
59. Dianat I, Alipour A, Asghari JM. Prevalence and risk factors of low back pain among school age children in Iran. Health Promot Perspect. 2017;7(4):223–9.
60. Watson KD. Low back pain in schoolchildren: the role of mechanical and psychosocial factors. Arch Dis Child. 2003;88(1):12–7.
61. Jones GT. Epidemiology of low back pain in children and adolescents. Arch Dis Child. 2005;90(3):312–6.
62. DiFiori JP, Benjamin HJ, Brenner JS, Gregory A, Jayanthi N, Landry GL, et al. Overuse injuries and burnout in youth sports: a position statement from the American Medical Society for Sports Medicine. Br J Sports Med. 2014;48(4):287–8.
63. Batley S, Aartun E, Boyle E, Hartvigsen J, Stern PJ, Hestbæk L. The association between psychological and social factors and spinal pain in adolescents. Eur J Pediatr. 2019;178(3):275–86.
64. Auvinen J, Tammelin T, Taimela S, Zitting P, Karppinen J. Associations of physical activity and inactivity with low back pain in adolescents. Scand J Med Sci Sports. 2007;18(2):188–94.
65. Lynch AM, Kashikar-Zuck S, Goldschneider KR, Jones BA. Psychosocial risks for disability in children with chronic back pain. J Pain. 2006;7(4):244–51.

66. Hestbaek L, Iachine IA, Leboeuf-Yde C, Kyvik KO, Manniche C. Heredity of low back pain in a young population: a classical twin study. Twin Res. 2004;7(1):16–26.
67. Sitthipornvorakul E, Janwantanakul P, Purepong N, Pensri P, van der Beek AJ. The association between physical activity and neck and low back pain: a systematic review. Eur Spine J. 2011;20(5):677–89.
68. Szpalski M, Gunzburg R, Balague F, Nordin M, Melot C. A 2-year prospective longitudinal study on low back pain in primary school children. Eur Spine J. 2002;11(5):459–64.
69. Wedderkopp N, Leboeuf-Yde C, Bo Andersen L, Froberg K, Steen HH. Back pain in children. Spine (Phila Pa 1976). 2003;28(17):2019–24.
70. Aartun E, Hartvigsen J, Boyle E, Hestbaek L. No associations between objectively measured physical activity and spinal pain in 11-15-year-old Danes. Eur J Pain. 2016;20(3):447–57.
71. Kamada M, Abe T, Kitayuguchi J, Imamura F, Lee I-M, Kadowaki M, et al. Dose–response relationship between sports activity and musculoskeletal pain in adolescents. Pain. 2016;157(6):1339–45.
72. d'Hemecourt PA, Gerbino PG, Micheli LJ. Back injuries in the young athlete. Clin Sports Med. 2000;19(4):663–79.
73. Lundin O, Hellstrom M, Nilsson I, Sward L. Back pain and radiological changes in the thoraco-lumbar spine of athletes. A long-term follow-up. Scand J Med Sci Sports. 2001;11(2):103–9.
74. Patel DR, Kinsella E. Evaluation and management of lower back pain in young athletes. Transl Pediatr. 2017;6(3):225–35.
75. Purcell L, Micheli L. Low back pain in young athletes. Sports Health. 2009;1(3):212–22.
76. Andreucci A, Campbell P, Dunn KM, Are sleep problems a risk factor for the onset of musculoskeletal pain in children and adolescents? A systematic review, Sleep. 2017;40(7), zsx093, https://doi.org/10.1093/sleep/zsx093.
77. Gill DK, Davis MC, Smith AJ, Straker LM. Bidirectional relationships between cigarette use and spinal pain in adolescents accounting for psychosocial functioning. Br J Health Psychol. 2014;19(1):113–31.
78. Heaps N, Davis MC, Smith AJ, Straker LM. Adolescent drug use, psychosocial functioning and spinal pain. J Health Psychol. 2011;16(4):688–98.
79. Abate M. Cigarette smoking and musculoskeletal disorders. Muscles Ligaments Tendons J. 2013;3:63.
80. Uei H, Matsuzaki H, Oda H, Nakajima S, Tokuhashi Y, Esumi M. Gene expression changes in an early stage of intervertebral disc degeneration induced by passive cigarette smoking. Spine (Phila Pa 1976). 2006;31(5):510–4.
81. Holm S, Nachemson A. Nutrition of the intervertebral disc: acute effects of cigarette smoking: an experimental animal study. Ups J Med Sci. 1988;93(1):91–9.
82. Green BN, Johnson CD, Snodgrass J, Smith M, Dunn AS. Association between smoking and back pain in a cross-section of adult Americans. Cureus. 2016;8(9):e806.
83. Sheir-Neiss GI, Kruse RW, Rahman T, Jacobson LP, Pelli JA. The association of backpack use and back pain in adolescents. Spine (Phila Pa 1976). 2003;28(9):922–30.
84. Negrini S, Negrini A. Postural effects of symmetrical and asymmetrical loads on the spines of schoolchildren. Scoliosis. 2007;2(1):8.
85. Sullivan MJL, Thorn B, Haythornthwaite JA, Keefe F, Martin M, Bradley LA, et al. Theoretical perspectives on the relation between catastrophizing and pain. Clin J Pain. 2001;17(1):52–64.
86. Smith AJ, O'Sullivan PB, Beales D, Straker L. Back pain beliefs are related to the impact of low back pain in 17-year-olds. Phys Ther. 2012;92(10):1258–67.
87. Yamato TP, Maher CG, Traeger AC, Wiliams CM, Kamper SJ. Do schoolbags cause back pain in children and adolescents? A systematic review. Br J Sports Med. 2018;52(19):1241–5.
88. O'Sullivan PB, Straker LM, Smith A, Perry M, Kendall G. Carer experience of back pain is associated with adolescent back pain experience even when controlling for other carer and family factors. Clin J Pain. 2008;24(3):226–31.
89. Ailliet L, Rubinstein SM, Knol D, van Tulder MW, de Vet HCW. Somatization is associated with worse outcome in a chiropractic patient population with neck pain and low back pain. Man Ther. 2016;21:170–6.

90. Suman A, Bostick GP, Schaafsma FG, Anema JR, Gross DP. Associations between measures of socio-economic status, beliefs about back pain, and exposure to a mass media campaign to improve back beliefs. BMC Public Health. 2017;17(1):504.
91. Perich D, Burnett A, O'Sullivan P, Perkin C. Low back pain in adolescent female rowers: a multi-dimensional intervention study. Knee Surg Sports Traumatol Arthrosc. 2011;19(1):20–9.

Chapter 2
Anatomy of the Pediatric Spine

Christopher Aaron Kowalski and Douglas G. Armstrong

The spinal column is a series of vertebrae, stacked one on another, forming a central canal to house the spinal cord. The spine serves multiple purposes, including support for the skull, as a scaffold for the appendicular skeleton, and as a conduit which provides protection for the central nervous system. Normally, the spine is straight in the coronal plane and has four curvatures in the sagittal plane – cervical lordosis, thoracic kyphosis, lumbar lordosis, and sacropelvic kyphosis (Fig. 2.1). Thus, the human spine permits bipedal ambulation while maintaining the center of gravity in optimal alignment over the centers of the hip joints. Neuromuscular maturation determines alignment and growth. At birth the spine is aligned in mild kyphosis. Cervical lordosis develops as the infant achieves head control, and lumbar lordosis develops as standing is achieved (Fig. 2.2) [1, 2]. Vertebral and disc growth and development are impaired in children with neuromuscular diseases that prevent ambulation such as cerebral palsy [3].

The vertebral column is divided into five regions based on morphology and location. These are the cervical, thoracic, lumbar regions, the sacrum, and the coccyx (see Fig. 2.1). There are seven cervical vertebrae, with eight associated cervical spinal nerves. The 12 thoracic vertebrae are typically associated with paired ribs that articulate with the thoracic vertebral bodies and disc spaces. Five lumbar vertebrae are below the thoracic spine. The sacrum is composed of five vertebrae, fused at maturity, which articulate with the iliac bones through the sacroiliac joints. The coccygeal segments consist of 3–5 vestigial vertebral bodies caudal to the sacrum and which may be fused to each other.

C. A. Kowalski
Orthopedic Surgery, PennState Milton S. Hershey Medical Center, Hershey, PA, USA

D. G. Armstrong (✉)
Orthopedic Surgery, Orthopedics and Rehabilitation, PennState Health Hershey Medical Center, Hershey, PA, USA
e-mail: darmstrong@pennstatehealth.psu.edu

© Springer Nature Switzerland AG 2021
R. M. Schwend, W. L. Hennrikus (eds.), *Back Pain in the Young Child and Adolescent*, https://doi.org/10.1007/978-3-030-50758-9_2

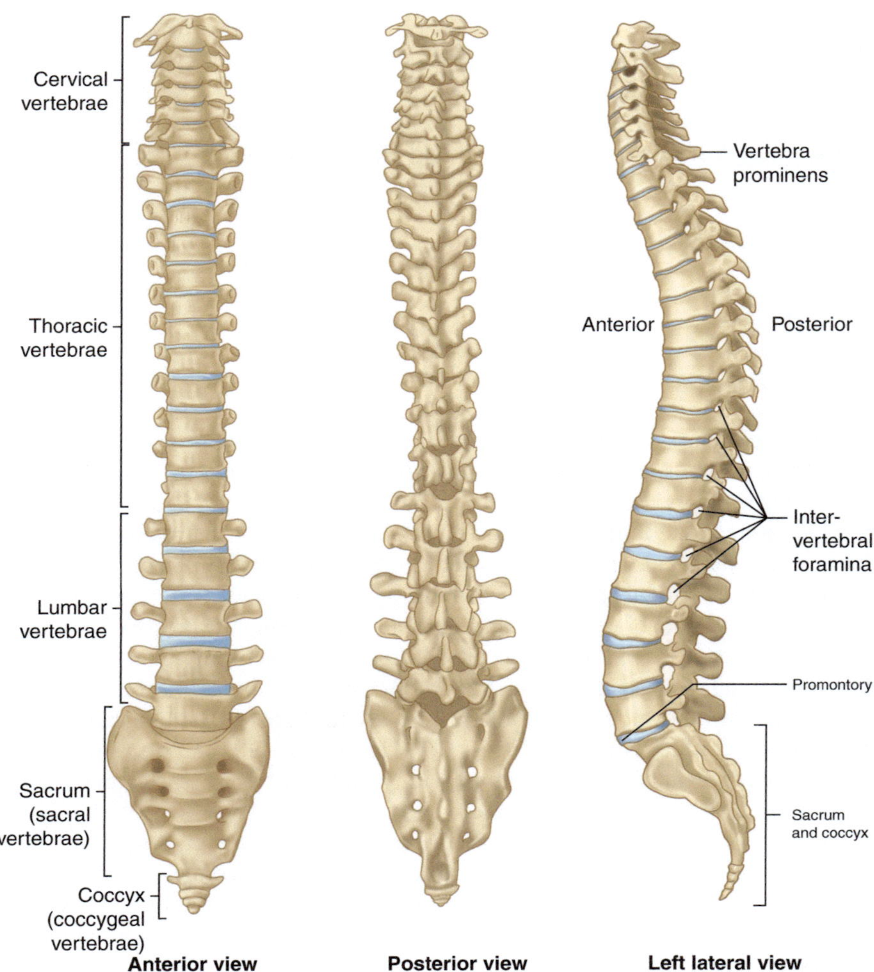

Fig. 2.1 The spinal column

Although there are distinguishing features in each region, much of the bony anatomy is common to each vertebra. An individual vertebra has the following components (Fig. 2.3): the vertebral body, two pedicles projecting posteriorly, two transverse processes project in a lateral direction, and the posterior neural arch which includes the laminae, a spinous process, and superior and inferior articular processes with their associated facet joints [4]. The spinous process is the only structure which can be palpated beneath the skin. The main portion of the vertebra is the cylinder-shaped body, which bears the majority of axial loads applied to the spine. The intervertebral discs are between each of the verte-bral bodies.

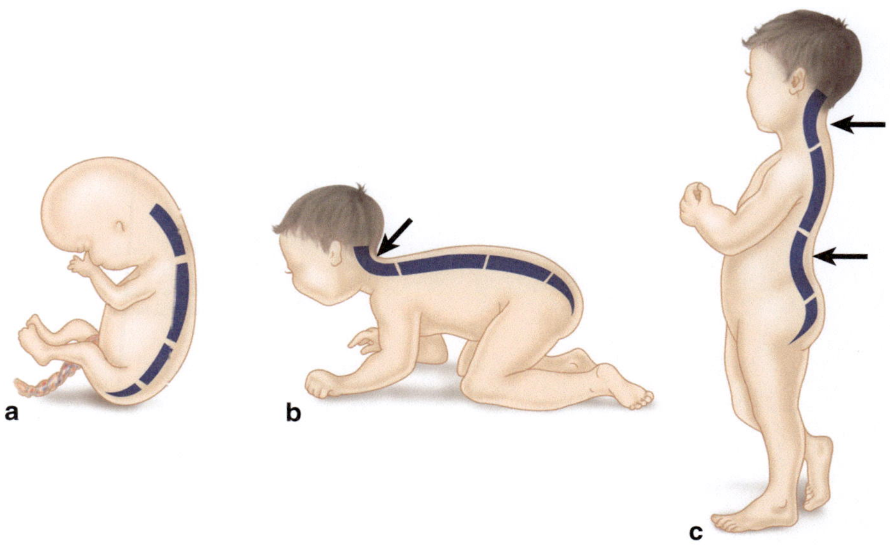

Fig. 2.2 Spine alignment in the fetus (**a**), infant (**b**), and toddler (**c**)

The vertebral segments are stabilized by their bony architecture and by ligaments. Each vertebra typically has six joints: two superior articular facets, two inferior facets, and the disc spaces between vertebral bodies. Further stability is a consequence of ligamentous and muscular attachments (Fig. 2.4). Structurally, the most important ligaments of the spinal column include the anterior and posterior longitudinal ligaments, the annulus fibrosus, the intertransverse ligaments, ligamentum flavum, and interspinous ligaments.

The anterior longitudinal ligament (ALL) is a thick band contiguous with the periosteum along the anterior aspect of the vertebral bodies. It spans from the sacral bodies to the cervical spine where it becomes confluent with the anterior atlanto-occipital membrane at C1. The ALL is an important stabilizer, limiting extension of the spinal column, and serves to reinforce the annulus fibrosus.

Located between each pair of vertebral bodies are the intervertebral discs, each of which is composed of the annulus fibrosus and nucleus pulposus. The annulus fibers are thick and arranged in layers at oblique angles to each other [2]. The annular ligaments are mainly composed of type I collagen, which is optimal for resisting tensile loads [5]. The nucleus pulposus is located within the central portion of the disc and is a gelatinous material made of type II collagen and proteoglycans. The disc anatomy is conducive to the absorption of compression forces, such as axial loading of the spine, while allowing mobility [5].

The posterior longitudinal ligament (PLL) is located on the posterior aspects of the vertebral bodies and annulus within the spinal canal. The PLL prevents excessive flexion and reinforces the intervertebral disc. The intertransverse ligament is located between the transverse processes and limits side bending. The ligamentum

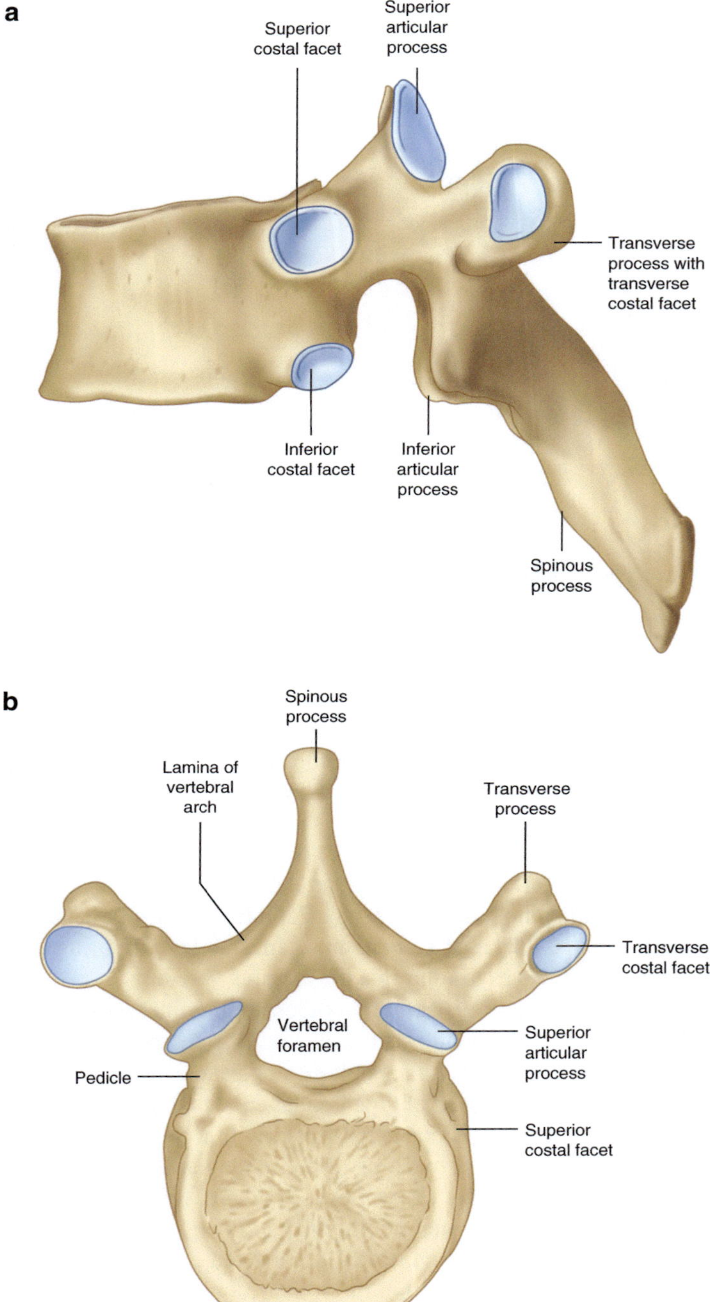

Fig. 2.3 Sixth thoracic vertebra. (**a**) Lateral aspect and (**b**) cranial aspect

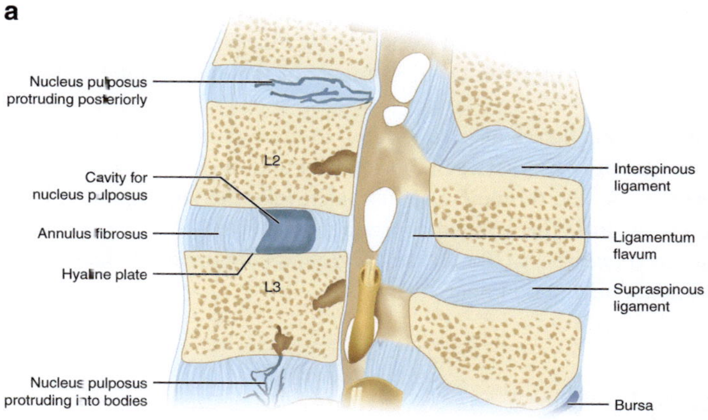

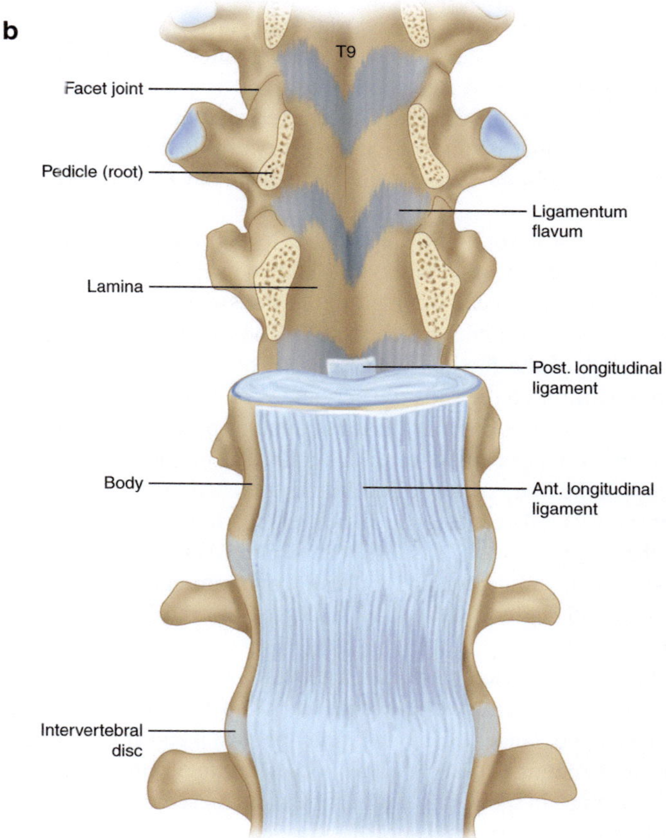

Fig. 2.4 Ligaments of the spine. (**a**) Lateral aspect and (**b**) anterior aspect

flavum, named for its distinctive yellow hue, is oriented in the coronal plane and connects the laminae of adjacent vertebrae. It functions as an important stabilizer and provides some protection to the contents of the spinal canal, especially at the lumbar spine.

The interspinous ligament is superficial to the ligamentum flavum. It is a thick, sagittal oriented ligament between the superior and inferior aspects of adjacent spinous processes. At the thoracic and lumbar levels, the supraspinous ligament is a thin structure, of little mechanical consequence, located between and along the tips of the spinous processes. In the cervical region, the ligament thickens to become the more significant nuchal ligament.

Cervical Spine (Fig. 2.5)

At maturity, the cervical spine is aligned in lordosis of 20–40 degrees [6]. Along with the spinal cord and exiting nerves, the cervical region houses the vertebral arteries, which course from the subclavian arteries into the occipital cortex of the brain. The vertebral arteries travel within the transverse foramina, located at the lateral aspects of the cervical vertebrae. The vertebral arteries can be injured during cervical spine trauma that involves excessive forward flexion or distraction, since the pediatric spinal column can stretch more than the spinal cord or vertebral arteries.

The first two cervical vertebrae are adapted to allow mobility of the skull and upper spine. The first cervical vertebra, also known as the atlas, has two large cup-shaped superior articular facets, oriented in the transverse plane and which articulate with the occipital condyles of the skull. The occipito-atlanto joints permit approximately 50% of the flexion and extension of the head, with the remaining movement coming through the subaxial cervical vertebrae [6, 7]. The second cervical vertebra, also known as the axis, has an odontoid process that projects cranialward from the anterior aspect of its vertebral body. The odontoid articulates with the posterior aspect of the body of atlas. The atlas is attached to the odontoid by several strong ligaments oriented vertically and transversely. In the normal child, the interval between the odontoid and C1 is less than 4 mm (ADI = atlanto-dens interval). Rotation is permitted, and flexion and extension are minimal [2, 7]. Fifty percent of the rotation, about 35 degrees of the total 70 degrees, of the C-spine occurs through the atlanto-axial joints.

During infancy, the cervical vertebrae are ovoid in shape. During childhood the vertebral bodies may appear wedge-shaped on plain lateral radiographs [8]. The naturally wedged appearance occasionally may be mistaken for a compression fracture. As the child matures, the vertebral bodies assume adult configuration and become more squared. In the young child, there is increased mobility of the cervical spine in part because the orientation of the cervical facet joints, particularly at the upper C-spine, is more horizontal. Pseudosubluxation between C2 and C3, caused by the horizontal orientation of the facet joints, occurs between ages 1 and 7 years

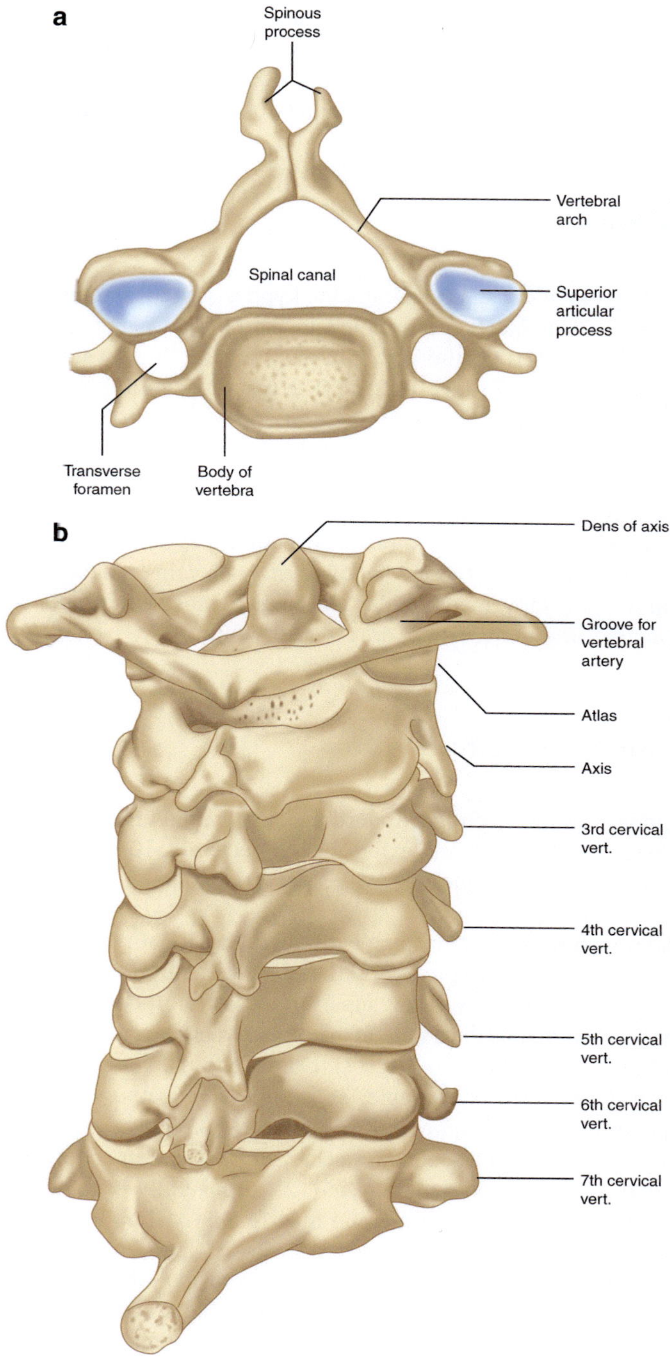

Fig. 2.5 (**a**) The cervical spine. (**b**) Fifth cervical vertebra

[9]. With growth and maturation, the subaxial cervical articular facets become oriented more vertically. Typically, the mature individual has considerable neck mobility including flexion of 80–90 degrees, extension to 70 degrees, 70–90 degrees of axial rotation, and 20–45 degrees of lateral flexion [2, 7].

Thoracic Spine (Fig. 2.3)

The thoracic region of the spine is aligned in kyphosis of 20–50 degrees at maturity. The thoracic articular facets are oriented in the coronal plane at an angle of 60 degrees. This and the fact the thoracic spine supports the chest wall result in limited segmental mobility from T1 to T10 [2, 7]. The upper and mid-thoracic spinous processes each project posteriorly, at an angle of approximately 30 degrees caudally. The thoracic laminae overlap one another, like shingles on a roof, protecting the thoracic spinal cord. Thirty degrees flexion and 20 degrees extension may occur in the thoracic spine of mature individuals [2, 7]. The ribs articulate with the spine at the vertebral bodies and the facet joints, which defines an axis of rotation. The upper ribs rotate upward with respiration; the lower ribs rotate up- and outward. This rotation determines the movement of the chest wall, most noticeable with labored breathing such as in asthma, croup, or respiratory failure.

Lumbar Spine (Fig. 2.6)

The five lumbar vertebrae configure a lordotic curve in the sagittal plane, permitting 30 and 50 degrees of flexion and extension, respectively, 10–20 degrees of lateral bending in each direction, and 10 degrees of axial rotation to the left and right [2, 7, 9].

At birth only about 1/3 of the spine is ossified, the majority being cartilaginous. By age 5 years, 65% of the spine is ossified [1]. Vertical growth of the spine is a consequence of growth plates at the superior and inferior aspects of the vertebral bodies. Each vertebra contributes about 1 mm per year to height, with some variation according to age and region [10, 11]. Damage to the vertebral growth centers may result in deformity. For example, Scheuermann's kyphosis may be result of excessive pressure on the periphery of the vertebral epiphysis [12].

The "ring apophysis" is a secondary center of ossification contained within the periphery of the vertebral body epiphysis [12]. It generally becomes radiographically apparent at 12–15 years of age and may remain visible in the lumbar spine until vertebral growth is complete, up to age 20–22 years in males. Spina bifida occulta is a consequence of failure of bony fusion of the posterior arch. It is most commonly seen at L5 and is considered to be a normal variant [12].

Along with the bony and ligamentous anatomy, muscular attachments provide stability to the spine and allow for motion throughout the spine, as well as the ability

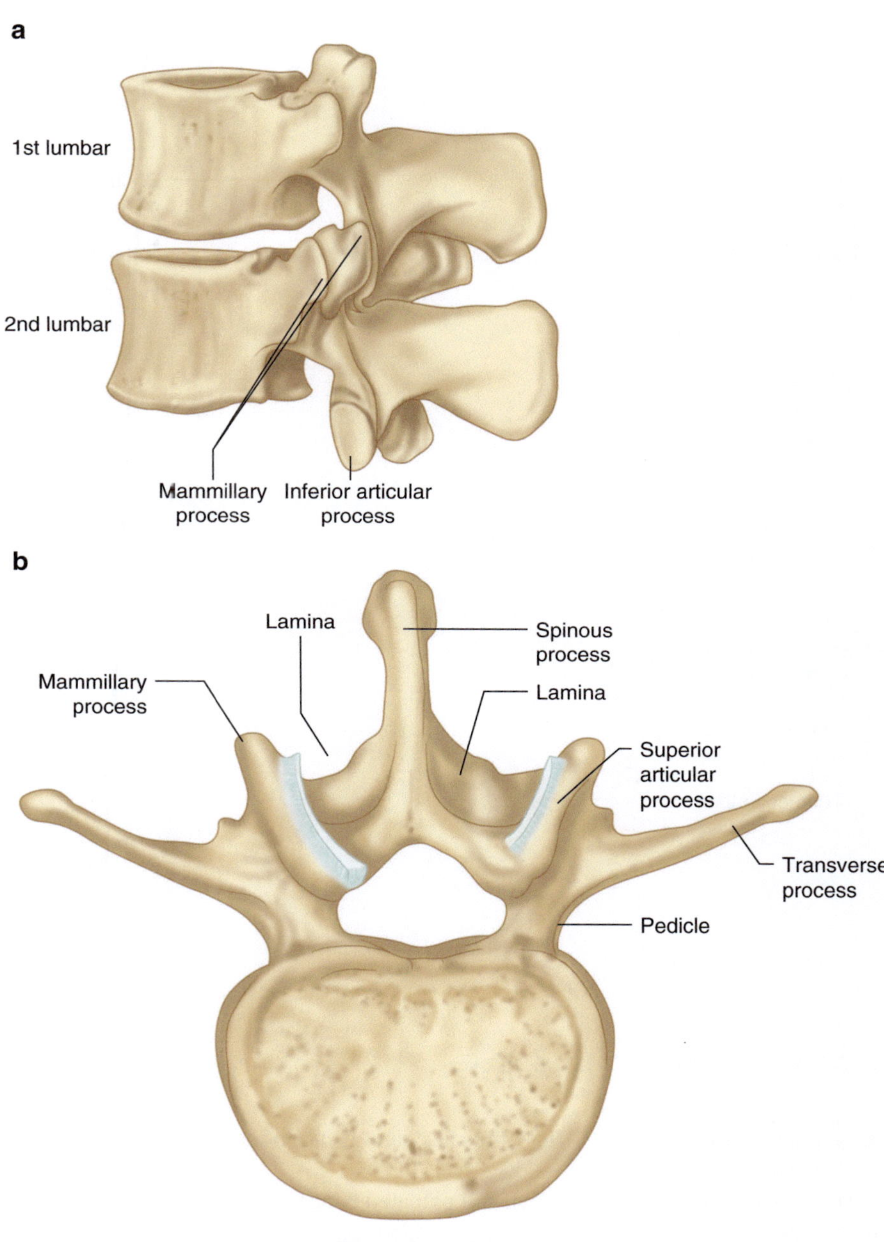

Fig. 2.6 Lumbar vertebrae. (**a**) Lateral aspect and (**b**) cranial aspect

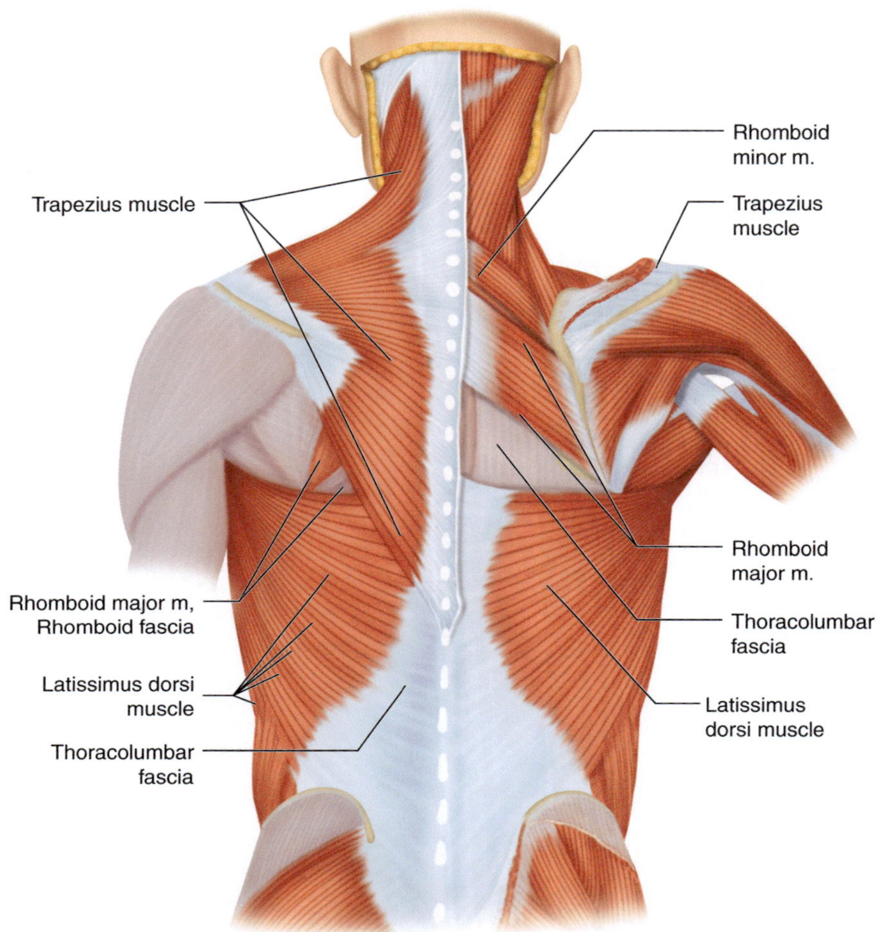

Fig. 2.7 Muscles of the spine – superficial layer

to maintain an erect posture. These muscles can be subdivided into superficial and deep layers.

The superficial layers can be seen and palpated beneath the skin (Fig. 2.7). These are the latissimus dorsi, serratus posterior superior and inferior, levator scapulae, rhomboid major and minor, and the trapezius. Most muscles of this layer attach to the posterior spinal elements and scapula; they are important in stabilizing and providing mobility to the shoulder girdle.

The deep layer of back muscles includes the multifidus, semispinalis, iliocostalis, longissimus, spinalis, and splenius muscles. These muscles are generally categorized as erector spinae muscles and attach from the pelvis, ribs, and skull to the spinal column. Most span the majority of the posterior spinal column and have variations depending on location. These are critical in maintaining an erect posture, as well as contributing to head and neck movement. They are type I fibers and therefore are slow twitch, have high oxidative and low glycolytic capacity, and are relatively resistant to fatigue [13].

The spinal cord is composed of millions of neurons that carry transmissions to and from the brain and which control the diverse functions of the body. It begins at the foramen magnum of the skull and terminates around L1, where it divides into the cauda equina [14]. It has different sections in which specific neurons travel, much like a highway system. Some of these tracts course efferently away from the brain and spinal cord to the body. Other tracts course afferently from the body toward the spinal cord and brain.

The spinal cord is comprised of gray and white matter. Gray matter is central in the cord and is composed of unmyelinated neurons and interneurons and generally is where chemical transmissions occur between neurons. White matter surrounds the gray matter and contains myelinated neurons that are traveling up and down the cord. The specific sections within the white matter include the ventral and lateral corticospinal tracts, dorsal columns, and spinothalamic tracts. The corticospinal tracts contain motor neurons, which transmit efferent signals to muscles throughout the body. The dorsal columns carry afferent sensory fibers from specialized neurons that detect light touch, proprioception, and vibration. Lastly, the spinothalamic tracts carry pain and temperature sensations to the sensory cortex.

Along the length of the spinal cord, spinal nerves exit within the cervical, thoracic, lumbar, and sacral regions. At each of these levels, a ventral and dorsal root are found, which exit the spinal column via the intervertebral or neural foramen. These nerves then combine to form the spinal nerve trunk, after which they again branch off into the ventral and dorsal rami. Housed within the dorsal root is the dorsal root ganglion, which contains the cell bodies of the afferent sensory nerves as they convey signals from the peripheral nerves to the brain. These rami also connect with the sympathetic chain, which houses sympathetic neurons.

Editor Discussion

Although the study of anatomy has been unfortunately de-emphasized by some medical schools, anatomy remains the framework onto which all physicians build their knowledge and learn their craft. Understanding spine anatomy is key to making an accurate diagnosis and planning appropriate treatment for any patient with back pain. The authors of this chapter have written a clear and practical guide to spine anatomy for the primary care physician.

W. L. Hennrikus

Unique to the pediatric spine is developmental anatomy. The spinal column also provides length to the developing thorax. At birth the spine is longer and growing faster than the lower limbs, so there is a bias to early development of the thorax. Thoracic volume in a neonate is only 6% that of an adult. By age 5 years, the growth velocity of the spine decreases, and the lower limbs start to grow faster than the trunk. The spinal canal is 95% the dimensions of the adult, although the chest is only 30% adult volume. By age 10 years, the thorax is still only 50% the volume of an adult. The spine more than doubles in length from birth to adulthood. The pediatric spine also has variations (such as age-dependent different shape of vertebra), anomalies (such as spina bifida occulta of L5 or six instead of five lumbar vertebra), and abnormalities (such as congenital hemivertebra or cervical fusions seen in Klippel Feil syndrome). Parents are often quite nervous about any deviation from normal, so it is important to explain the benign nature of most of these variations and anomalies and to adequately understand and evaluate the significance of abnormalities.

R. M. Schwend

References

1. Dimeglio A. Growth of the spine before age 5 years. J Pediatr Orthop B. 1993;1:102–7.
2. Louis R. Surgery of the spine. New York: Springer Verlag; 1983.
3. Taylor JR. Growth of human intervertebral discs and vertebral bodies. J Anat. 1975;120(1):49–68.
4. McMinn RMH, editor. Last's anatomy. 9th ed. Edinburgh: Churchill Livingstone; 1994.
5. Roberts S, Evans H, Trivedi J, Menage J. Histology and pathology of the human intervertebral disc. J Bone Joint Surg. 2006;88(Suppl 2):10–4.
6. Bogduk N, Mercer S. Biomechanics of the cervical spine. I: normal kinematics. Clin Biomech. 2000;15(9):633–48.
7. Martinez-Lozano AG. Radiographic measurements. In: Weinstein SL, editor. The pediatric spine principles and practice. 2nd ed. Philadelphia: Lippincott Williams & Wilkins; 2001.
8. El-Khoury GY, Sato Y. Imaging modalities. In: Weinstein SL, editor. The pediatric spine. Principles and practice. 2nd ed. Philadelphia: Lippincott Williams & Wilkins; 2001.
9. Bible JE, Biswas D, Miller CP, Whang PG, Grauer JN. Normal functional range of motion of the lumbar spine during 15 activities of daily living. J Spinal Disord Tech. 2010;23(2):106–12.
10. Canavese F, Dimeglio A. Normal and abnormal spine and thoracic cage development. World J Orthop. 2013;4(4):167–74.
11. Sarwark J, Aubin CE. Growth considerations of the immature spine. J Bone Joint Surg. 2007;89(Suppl 1):8–13.
12. Ganey TM, Ogden JA. Development and maturation of the axial skeleton. In: Weinstein SL, editor. The pediatric spine principles and practice. 2nd ed. Philadelphia: Lippincott Williams & Wilkins; 2001.
13. Herbison GJ, Jaweed MM, Ditunno JF. Muscle fiber types. Arch Phys Med Rehabil. 1982;63(5):227–30.
14. Brodal P. The central nervous system: structure and function. 3rd ed. Oxford: Oxford University Press; 2004. p. 369–96.

Chapter 3
Medical and Non-surgical Conditions That Can Cause or Contribute to Back Pain in a Child or Adolescent

Blaise A. Nemeth

While the prevalence of back pain in adolescents has increased, back pain in children <10 years old remains uncommon [1, 2]. As such, attention to defining characteristics of specific pathologic etiologies proves beneficial in developing a differential diagnosis and guiding further work-up to assist in diagnosis and treatment in children of all ages. With causes ranging from skeletal to intra-abdominal disorders, benign tumors to malignancy, and structural issues to systemic disease, understanding important aspects of the history and physical examination for each possible diagnosis helps narrow the differential diagnosis. Plain radiographs identify structural issues from focal or systemic disease and guide the use of advanced imaging and/or laboratory analyses [3, 4]. Chapter 6 discusses additional details regarding the role of radiographs and advanced imaging.

Acute presentations of back pain occur following injury in spondylolysis and disc disease and from muscle strain. Acute onset of back pain without injury raises concern for malignancy or infection. Almost all spine disorders have the potential to present with chronic back pain, so the presence of daily or progressive pain, night pain, systemic symptoms, and/or neurologic findings indicate more concerning pathologic processes [4]. Further aspects of the history and physical exam are discussed in Chap. 5. In the absence of findings, the pain may be referred to as "non-specific" and biomechanical issues or muscular pain attributed as the cause [3]. Outside of disease-specific treatments, physical therapy and modification of exacerbating causes remain mainstays of treatment for non-specific back pain.

B. A. Nemeth (✉)
Orthopedics and Rehabilitation, American Family Children's Hospital,
University of Wisconsin School of Medicine and Public Health, Madison, WI, USA
e-mail: nemeth@ortho.wisc.edu

© Springer Nature Switzerland AG 2021
R. M. Schwend, W. L. Hennrikus (eds.), *Back Pain in the Young Child and Adolescent*. https://doi.org/10.1007/978-3-030-50758-9_3

Mechanical Back Pain (Non-specific or Muscular Back Pain)

In children >10 years old, most commonly, the cause of back pain is without a specific, identifiable, structural etiology or disease process [2]. As a result, the pain may be referred to as "non-specific" and suspected to be due to muscular pain or as a result of biomechanical issues. While mechanical back pain may be suspected, ultimately, it is a determination made after assessing for other etiologies, thus requiring a thorough history and physical exam, as well as radiographs, to exclude other possibilities. Likewise, mechanical back pain is not a definitive diagnosis, and patients should be monitored for lack of improvement or new findings suggestive of an evolving process that warrants further work-up.

Mechanical back pain commonly presents as chronic pain with an insidious onset. Often the pain is episodic, so appears acute in onset if the first complaint occurs around a flare of pain, but the pain improves over time. Other times, pain lasts a month or longer [5]. Frequently, patients continue to experience episodes of back pain over years or into adulthood [6]. Location of pain varies, with mid-back pain more common among children under 10 years and low back pain most common in teenagers [6]. Other than tenderness over the paraspinous muscles, the physical exam should be normal in respect to range of motion of the spine, strength, reflexes, and sensation. Plain radiographs demonstrate no evidence of abnormalities in the vertebral bodies, disc spaces, or pars interarticularis. Alignment of the spine may vary (see "Scoliosis").

Proposed etiologies for mechanical back pain include poor postural alignment due to alterations or imbalances in muscle activation [7–9]. Anything that alters mechanics may contribute to symptoms, such as low levels of physical activity, prolonged sedentary time (especially if sitting posture is poor and/or screen use), obesity, and use of heavy backpacks [10–13]. Incidence of back pain increases as backpack weight exceeds 10–15% of body weight [14, 15].

Physical therapy to address postural mechanics is the mainstay of treatment. Frequency of visits with the therapist may be less important than the specific guidance on how to improve strength and mobility, as well as physical conditioning [16, 17]. Parents of pediatric patients sometimes seek chiropractic care for their child's back pain. However, studies in the medical literature are limited regarding benefit or safety [18]. Analgesics may provide short-term relief in some patients, but opioid use should be minimized to avoid side effects.

Scoliosis

Scoliosis deserves special attention as a cause of back pain. While 20-year follow-up studies demonstrated a slightly higher rate of back pain among patients with scoliosis, both after surgery and bracing, pain was typically mild and did not affect quality of life [19, 20]. Low back pain occurred more commonly in patients following surgery, and patients who received bracing but did not undergo surgery experienced pain in the lower back and/or thoracic region. Commonly pain occurs around the paraspinous prominence, representing the apex of the curve on the convex side [21] (Fig. 3.1). Back pain also occurs in patients wearing an orthosis for scoliosis management and may occur more often in patients with progressive curves [22]. The pain in patients with scoliosis is essentially "non-specific." In the presence of a scoliotic curve, evaluation for other causes of pain and/or scoliosis, including spinal cord dysraphism, benign or malignant tumors, infection, and spondylolysis, should be considered before attributing the pain to a muscular cause related to the scoliosis, especially if the curve is progressive or other signs or symptoms are present (Fig. 3.2). Treatment of mechanical back pain in patients with scoliosis is the same as for those without scoliosis, relying primarily on physical therapy [23].

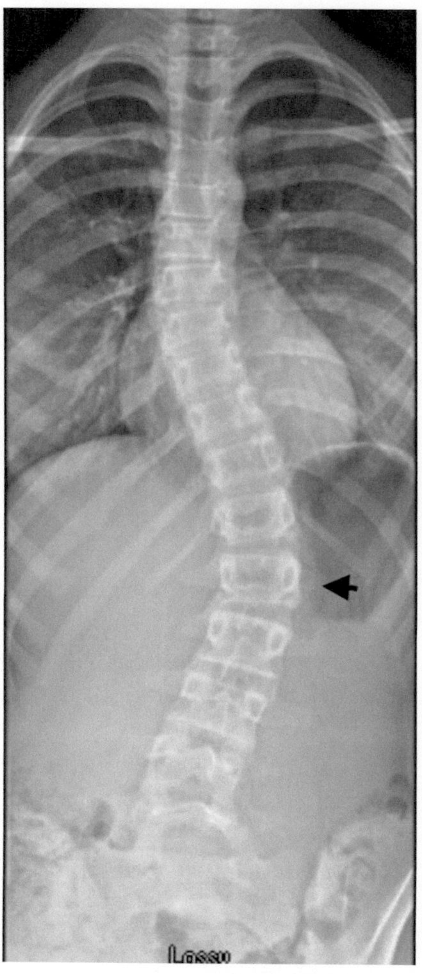

Fig. 3.1 In this adolescent with scoliosis, non-specific back pain would be expected to occur in the left lumbar region, along the apex of the curve (*arrow*), and where the prominence would be visible clinically

Fig. 3.2 This young child presented with thoracic back pain and a curve. Due to progressively worsening back pain, advanced imaging was obtained and showed an osteoid osteoma, demonstrating that back pain should not be attributed to a curve without assessing for causes of back pain that might also cause a curve

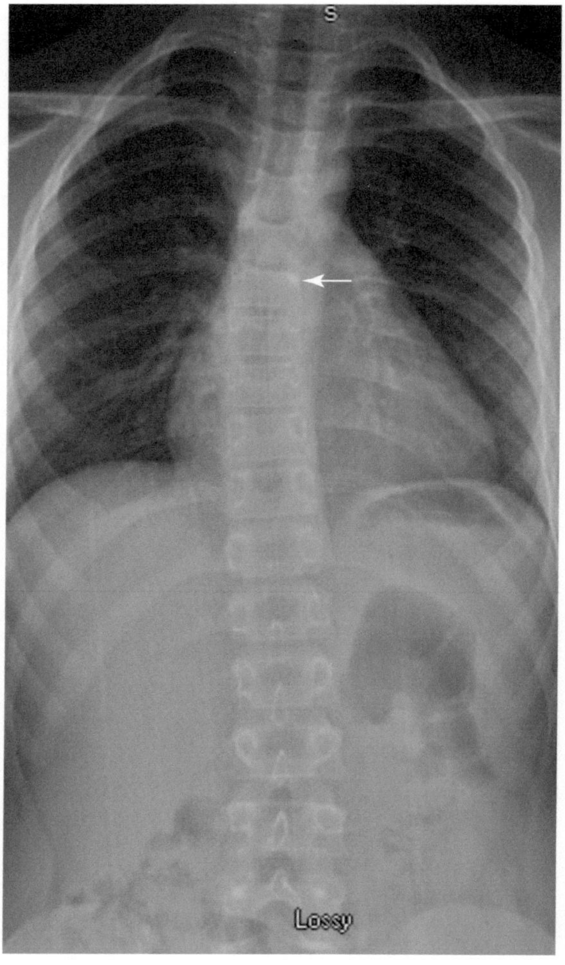

Back Pain in Children with Neuromuscular Disease

Patients with spina bifida, muscular dystrophy, and spinal muscular atrophy frequently experience back pain. Tethered cord syndrome is a consideration in children with spina bifida, and fractures may occur in children with muscular dystrophy and spinal muscular atrophy, but often imaging is negative, and the pain is non-specific [24, 25].

Muscle Strain and Spasm

While difficult to diagnose clinically, muscle strains present acutely and occur during activity with subsequent development of muscle spasm. Muscle strains consistently rate as one of the most common diagnoses for children presenting with low back pain but are best considered a diagnosis of exclusion since pain and muscle spasm occurs regularly in many pathologic causes of back pain, such as spondylolysis, insufficiency fracture, and malignancy. Radiographs prove helpful in identifying bony abnormalities, although plain x-rays may be negative in spondylolysis, so lack of improvement over a few days to weeks necessitates further work-up.

Spondylolysis/Spondylolisthesis

One of the most common causes of back pain in adolescents is spondylolysis. Spondylolysis involves a fracture through the pars interarticularis of the spine. Most cases involve the L5 pars interarticularis, but fractures do occur at other levels with decreasing frequency at higher lumbar vertebra. Usually the fracture happens as a result of repetitive stress or overuse with progressive or persistent low back pain, but occasionally an acute pars fracture occurs and presents with acute pain. Pain is often unilateral, although bilateral low back pain occurs due to bilateral spondylolysis or muscular pain on the side contralateral to the spondylolytic lesion. Spondylolisthesis most commonly develops from bilateral pars interarticularis fractures that allow for slippage of the vertebral body anteriorly. Other causes of spondylolisthesis include congenital abnormalities in vertebral development (dysplastic spondylolisthesis) and high energy trauma. Radicular symptoms rarely occur but may stem from a hematoma, edema around a fracture, disc herniation, or cyst development at the facet or the presence of spondylolisthesis [26]. Studies have failed to identify specific history or exam features of spondylolysis or spondylolisthesis other than a palpable step-off in the lumbar spine in the presence of severe spondylolisthesis. Accurate and timely diagnosis requires clinical suspicion and awareness of these disorders in children [27].

Spondylolysis constitutes the most common pathologic cause of low back pain in adolescents, but younger children can also sustain a fracture of the pars interarticularis [28]. Spondylolysis occurs more commonly in athletes than non-athletes, and while the most commonly implicated sports involve those with back extension, such as gymnastics, rowing, and football, athletes in almost any sport are at risk [29, 30]. Altered spinal mechanics due to imbalances in muscle activation, spinal mobility, tight hamstrings, or other structural issues are contributing factors [31].

Radiographs may demonstrate a lucency in the pars interarticularis. However, in some cases 2-view lumbar radiographs do not visualize the fracture (Fig. 3.3). Oblique radiographs have limited additional diagnostic benefit and expose patients to additional radiation [32]. CT and bone scans demonstrate high sensitivity in identifying spondylolysis, although both advanced imaging tests expose children to even higher amounts of ionizing radiation [33]. As a result, MRI has become a commonly used advanced imaging modality for detecting spondylolysis in children, with the added benefit of being able to detect stress reaction before a fracture has developed [34]. Spondylolisthesis is diagnosed using plain radiographs. The Meyerding classification is used to describe the degree of forward slip: I, 0–25%; II,

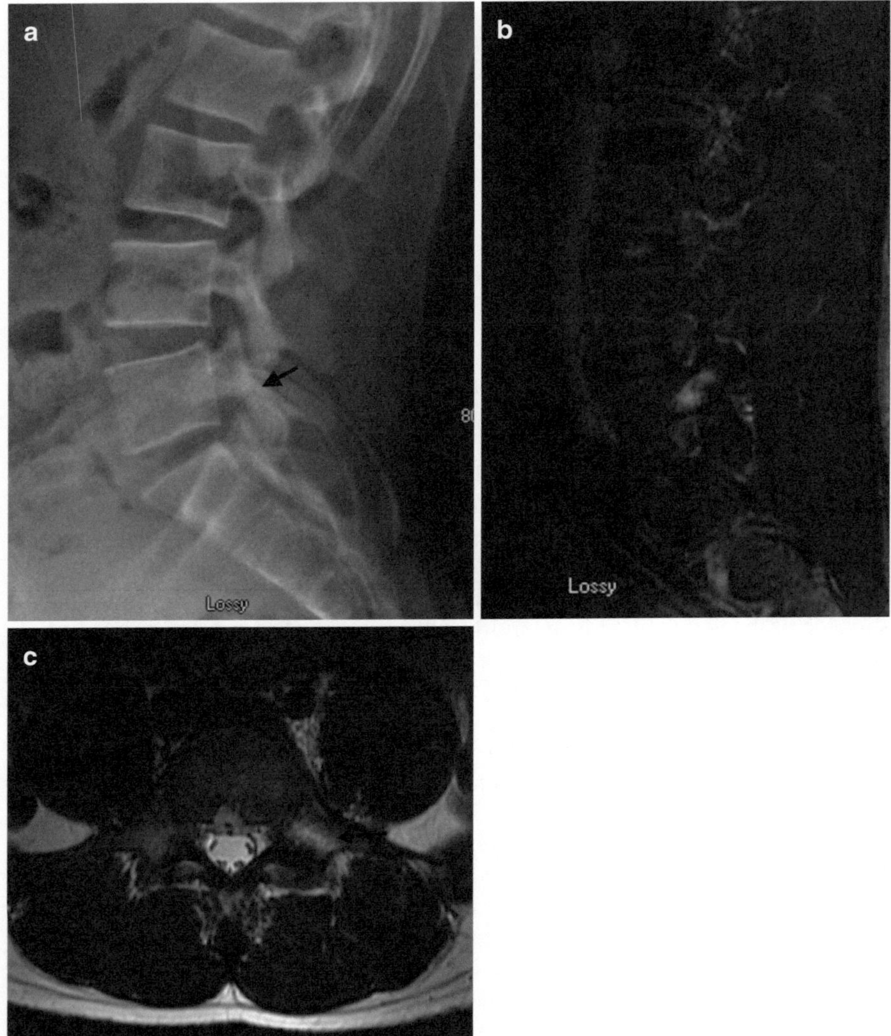

Fig. 3.3 This adolescent soccer player presented with left lower back pain. Plain radiographs (**a**) demonstrate a subtle lucency on the lateral view (*arrow*). Even with negative radiographs, spondylolysis would be high in the differential. Spondylolysis was confirmed on MRI as demonstrated by edema (white) on T2 images in the left pedicle and pars on sagittal (**b**) and axial (**c**) images

25–50%; III, 50–75%; and IV, 75–100% (Fig. 3.4). Spondyloptosis, also referred to as grade V, occurs when the vertebral body slides completely off of the one below it and becomes more distal in its location.

Treatment of spondylolysis involves rest until the pain resolves, followed by physical therapy to correct underlying biomechanical contributors, and gradual

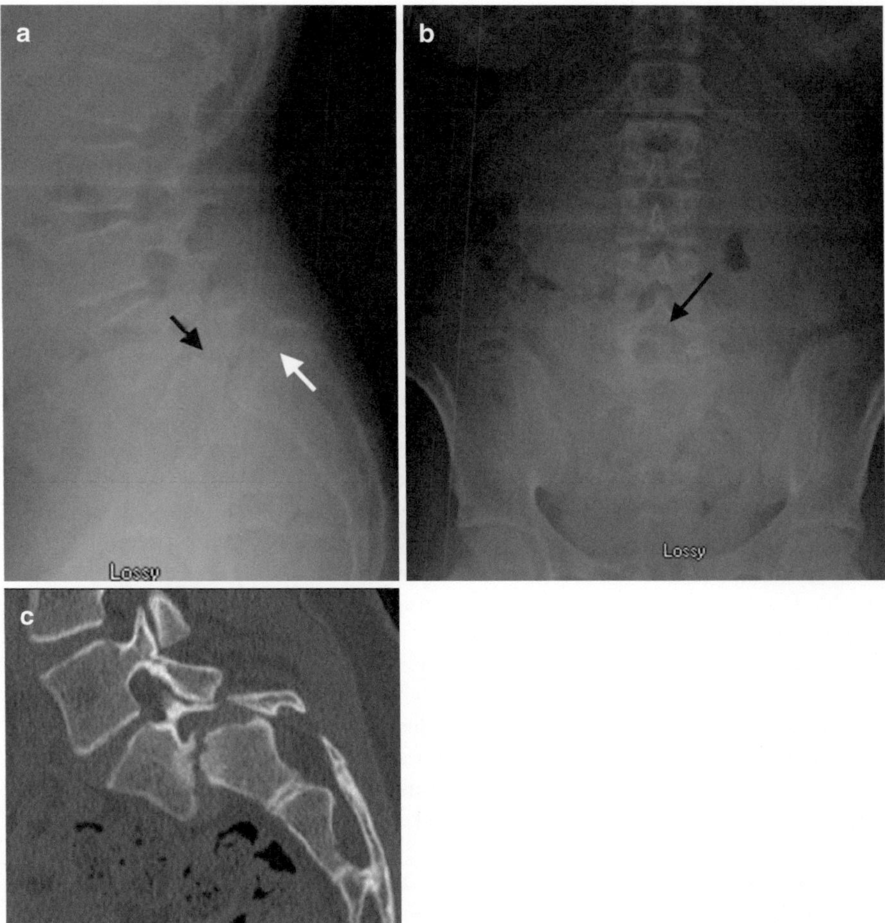

Fig. 3.4 Lateral radiograph (**a**) in an adolescent with low back pain and decreased flexion and extension of the spine demonstrate grade III spondylolisthesis with forward slip of L5 (*black arrow*) relative to S1 (*white arrow*). The posterior arch of L5 is visible on the AP view (**b**) (*arrow*). CT scan (**c**) better visualizes the listhesis and deformity of the endplates of L5 and S1

return to activities [35]. Bracing may be used to manage pain and restrict activities, using either semi-rigid lumbar corsets or rigid, anti-lordotic thoracolumbosacral (TLSO) or lumbosacral orthoses (LSO) [36]. Use of rigid bracing may improve bony healing in early lesions with high T2 signal on MRI, although up to 50% of individuals develop a pseudarthrosis [37, 38]. Bracing does not appear to significantly change long-term outcomes [37, 39], and approximately 70–80% of patients return to sport with conservative treatment, regardless of whether bony healing occurs. However, up to 50% of patients report recurrence of symptoms [36, 39, 40]. Since bilateral spondylolysis can result in spondylolisthesis, patients with bilateral spondylolysis, as well as spondylolisthesis, especially if dysplastic, should be followed radiographically every 6–12 months for progressive listhesis until skeletal maturity [37]. While lesser grades of slip (I and occasionally II) often remain asymptomatic once symptoms from spondylolysis resolve, higher grades (II–V) frequently cause persistent pain and may generate traction on the spinal nerve roots, causing radicular symptoms or even myelopathy. As a result, surgery is usually recommended for progressive slips of grade III or higher and may be an option in patients with spondylolysis with persistent pain.

Scheuermann Disease

Scheuermann disease is a disorder of unknown etiology that classically presents with rigid kyphosis and a gibbus deformity on forward bending in an adolescent. Parents often express concern about poor posture and an inability of their child to sit or stand up straight. Radiographs demonstrate >45 degrees of thoracic kyphosis and at least 3 consecutive thoracic vertebra with $\geq$5 degrees of anterior wedging, as well as irregularities of the endplates and narrowing of the disc spaces on lateral radiographs (Fig. 3.5). Schmorl nodes, representing eruptions of the intervertebral discs through the endplates, may also be seen.

Atypical, or lumbar, Scheuermann disease may present as a teenager with low back pain and decreased lumbar lordosis, with radiographs demonstrating loss of lordosis and Schmorl nodes, eruptions of the disc through the endplate, at one or multiple levels [41] (Fig. 3.6). Excessive thoracic kyphosis of >45 degrees, without evidence of Scheuermann disease, also causes back pain in some children. In these cases, evaluation for spinal cord syrinx or tethered cord as a cause may be warranted (see "Spinal Dysraphism").

Pain in Scheuermann disease may occur as a result of changes in mechanics due to the higher degrees of thoracic kyphosis and compensatory hyperlordosis of the lumbar spine in typical Scheuermann disease, hyperkyphosis at the thoracolumbar junction in lower thoracic disease, loss of lumbar lordosis in lumbar Scheuermann disease, and rigidity of the spine in all forms [42]. Long-term, patients do well and experience few limitations [43]. Neurologic complications are rare but may occur in cases of excessive kyphosis or disc protrusion [44].

Children presenting early in pubertal development may benefit from bracing to prevent progression of the kyphosis [45, 46]. Most patients, though, present late in adolescence, with parents attributing the kyphosis to poor posture and becoming concerned when it is not improving over time or when pain develops. Bracing at later ages, and in larger curves, may result in mild improvement but is often poorly tolerated so overall benefit is controversial [45, 47]. Physical therapy helps manage pain by addressing postural mechanics, spine flexibility, and activity modification [48]. Surgery is indicated for patients with pain refractory to therapy who have thoracic kyphosis >70–75 degrees to help restore alignment [49]. Rates of complications are higher in surgery for Scheuermann kyphosis than scoliosis, although patients become taller and leaner with surgery and experience improvement in self-image [49, 50].

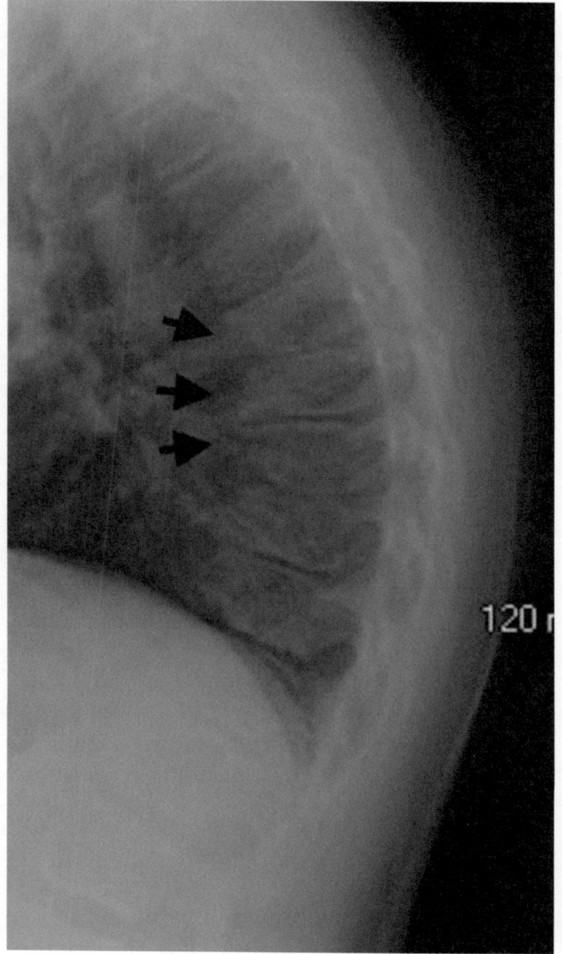

Fig. 3.5 Lateral x-ray of the thoracic spine demonstrates anterior wedging of three thoracic vertebral bodies (*arrows*) consistent with Scheuermann kyphosis

Degenerative Disease

Disc herniation in pediatric patients occurs infrequently, but when they do, patients experience back pain and often radiculopathy. In one study, the rate of disc disease or facet arthropathy in asymptomatic elite pediatric tennis players found on MRI exceeded 50%. Therefore, in this population, MRI is not helpful in identifying degenerative spine disease as a cause of pain but is beneficial in identifying causes of radiculopathy [51] (Fig. 3.7). An entity unique to children includes a vertebral endplate ring apophysis avulsion, which is best diagnosed by CT, visualizing the avulsed endplate [52]. Patients with herniated discs and ring apophyseal avulsion fractures benefit from physical therapy and modification of activities. Surgery is reserved for patients with neurologic deficits on presentation or pain refractory to conservative treatment for more than 6 weeks.

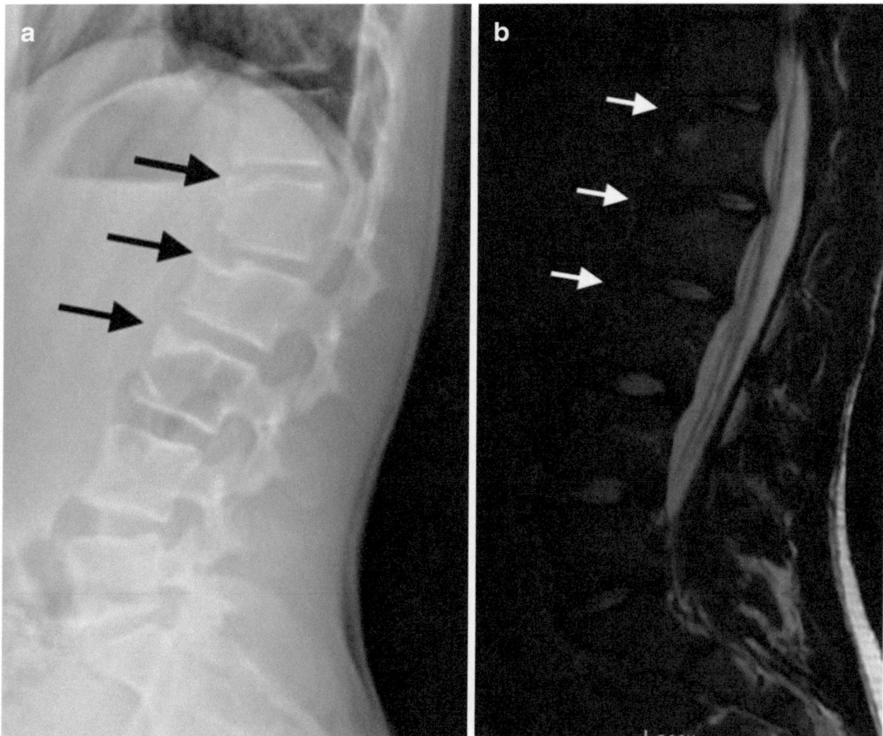

Fig. 3.6 Lateral x-ray (**a**) of the lumbar spine with decreased lumbar lordosis, kyphosis at the upper lumbar spine and anterior Schmorl nodes (*arrows*) consistent with lumbar, or atypical, Scheuermann disease. MRI (**b**) demonstrates the herniations (*arrows*) of the discs through the endplates

Bertolotti Syndrome

Bertolotti syndrome is the term for pain attributed to a transitional vertebra, either a partially sacralized lumbar vertebra or a partially lumbarized sacral vertebra (Fig. 3.8). In both cases, the transverse process on one side is enlarged and abuts the adjacent sacrum or ilium. On the partially sacralized side, there are increased T2 signal on MR and increased uptake on single-photon emission computed tomography (SPECT). Pain relief on injection of the involved area confirms the diagnosis of Bertolotti syndrome. Case reports involve primarily older adolescents and young to middle-aged adults [53]. Treatment is typically with physical therapy to adjust mechanics to decrease stress at the involved level and on the involved side. In rare cases, resection of the partially sacralized transverse process (if the disc is healthy) or fusion of the vertebral body to the sacrum (if that disc is narrow) may be a consideration for patients refractory to conservative treatment [54].

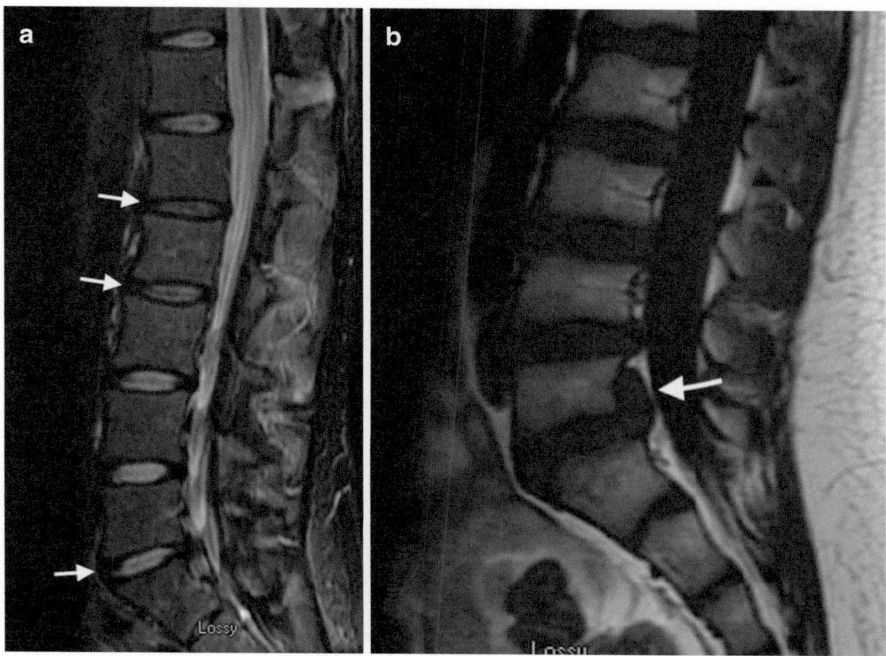

Fig. 3.7 MRI revealing disc desiccation (**a**), as evidenced by decreased brightness on T2 images (*arrows*), at multiple levels in an asymptomatic teenager. (**b**) Disc herniation posterior at L5-S1 (*arrow*) in a patient with acute onset of low back pain and radiculopathy

Fig. 3.8 AP lumbar x-ray displaying broad transverse processes at a transitional L5 vertebra, bilaterally (*arrows*)

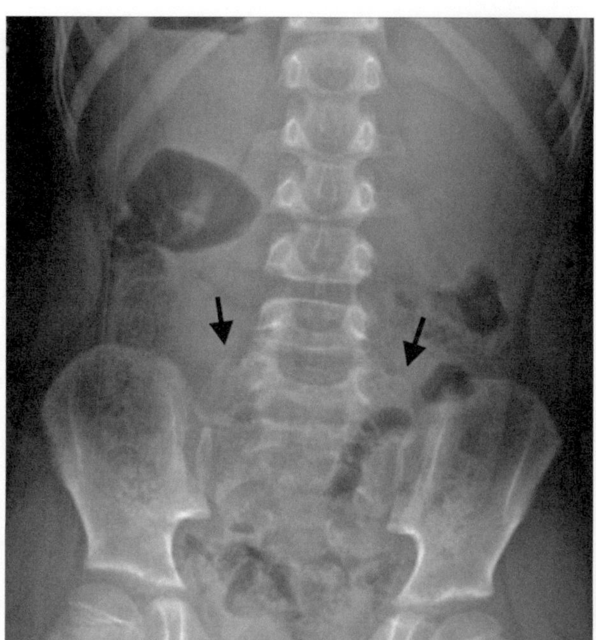

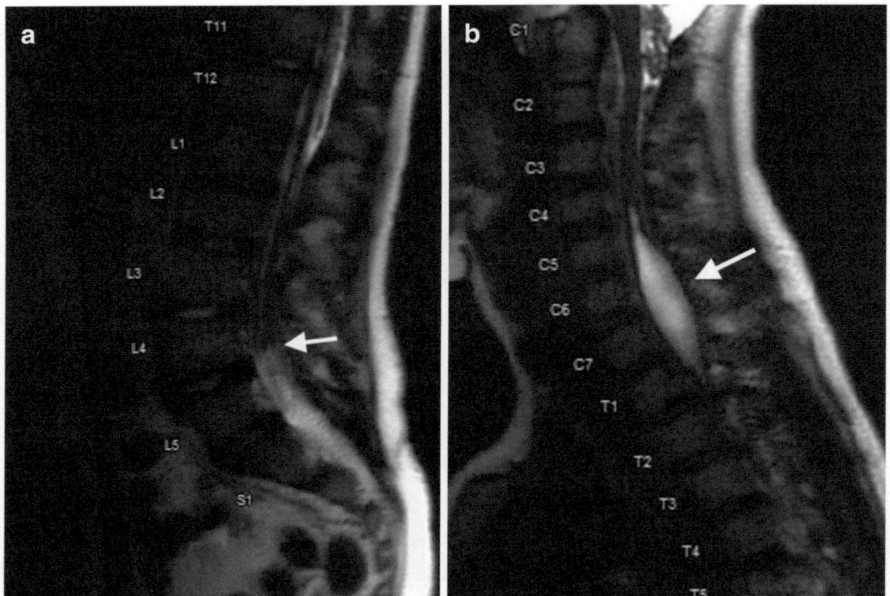

Fig. 3.9 MR images demonstrating (**a**) tethered cord (black vertical line) terminating at L4 (*white arrow*) and (**b**) spinal cord syrinx (*white arrow*) from C4 to T1

Spinal Dysraphism

Patients with a symptomatic tethered cord frequently present with low back pain with or without radiculopathy. Other physical exam findings further support concern for a tethered cord, such as a macular capillary hemangioma (previously known as a flammeus nevus) or a tuft of hair over the lumbar spine, gait abnormalities, muscle spasticity, cavus foot and/or clawing of the toes, incontinence of urine or stool or incomplete bladder emptying based on cystomyelogram, and/or spinal deformity (scoliosis, kyphosis, or scoliosis with kyphosis) [55, 56]. Detethering of the spinal cord may improve or prevent progression of symptoms, although some patients may experience worsening of symptoms after surgery [56, 57]. Retethering occurs commonly in children with spina bifida but only in a small number of children with idiopathic tethering. Scoliosis may progress after detethering, especially if the curve is >40 degrees or the child is very young [56, 58]. A spinal cord syrinx also may present with pain and may cause deformity of the spine (scoliosis, kyphosis, or scoliosis with kyphosis) [44, 59]. A tethered cord and a syrinx are best diagnosed by MRI (Fig. 3.9).

Benign but Locally Aggressive Tumors of the Spine

Osteoid Osteoma/Osteoblastoma

Osteoid osteoma is a <1 cm benign bone lesion of unknown etiology that always presents with pain and most commonly involves the pedicle or pars interarticularis in the spine. Patients typically experience progressively worsening back pain with the two classic characteristic signs of the pain – more severe pain at night and pain relieved by non-steroidal anti-inflammatory medications. Radiographs may or may not demonstrate the lesion although scoliosis and kyphosis are often present [60] (see Fig. 3.2). Due to the inflammatory nature of osteoid osteoma, osteoid osteoma may be seen on bone scan, but misdiagnosis as spondylolysis in lumbar lesions is not uncommon if advanced imaging is not obtained [61]. MRI typically demonstrates increased T2 signal around the lesion, but the central nidus may be difficult to identify, differentiating it from spondylolysis. CT scan best demonstrates the central nidus and confirms the diagnosis (Fig. 3.10). Some patients experience pain relief with use of NSAIDs, but for those who do not, or who have lesions increasing in size, treatment of osteoid osteoma and osteoblastoma of the spine is usually best done by excision of the lesion, which rarely results in instability of the spine. Radiofrequency ablation may also be effective for osteoid osteoma; however, this technique should not be used near the spinal cord or nerve roots [62, 63]. Osteoblastoma is a larger lesion than osteoid osteoma, >2 cm (Fig. 3.11), has similar characteristics in presentation, but due to its size may have neurologic symptoms, and on radiography and also is treated with resection [60].

Histiocytosis

Langerhans cell histiocytosis of the spine presents with back pain. The pain can be debilitating, causing difficulty sitting or walking. Some patients will refuse to walk. Systemic symptoms are rare. In the past the term "eosinophilic granuloma" was used to describe this lesion. Patients experience worsening pain with attempts at back flexion or extension and may have secondary scoliosis. Radiographs demonstrate collapse of the vertebral body with preservation of the surrounding intervertebral discs. The appearance of "vertebra plana" is highly suggestive for eosinophilic granuloma, although leukemia, Ewing sarcoma, and Tb may also cause flattening of the vertebral body (Fig. 3.12). MRI helps further evaluate the lesion. Laboratory analysis and sometimes a biopsy may be indicated to confirm or rule out the diagnosis [64].

Treatment of isolated histiocytosis of the vertebral body is usually conservative utilizing bracing for comfort and pain management. In some cases, chemotherapy, radiation, and/or local excision may be indicted [65]. With resolution of the pain, serial radiographs continue to demonstrate vertebra plana. In younger patients,

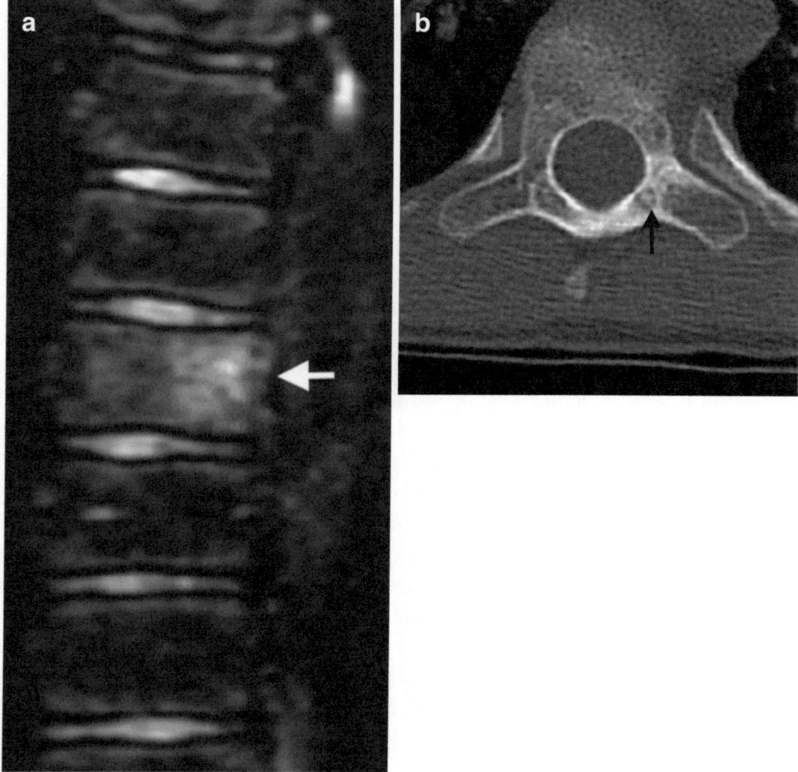

Fig. 3.10 Sagittal MRI (**a**) demonstrating edema extending into the left posterior vertebral body at T7 in the patient in Fig. 3.2. CT scan (**b**) revealing the central nidus typical of osteoid osteoma (same patient)

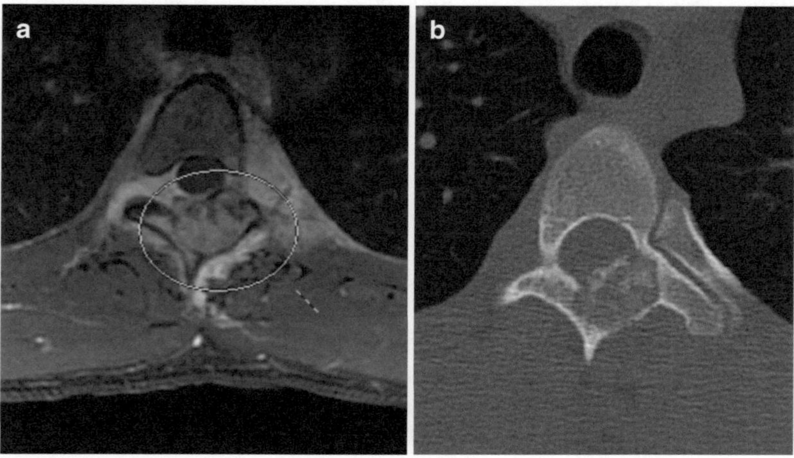

Fig. 3.11 MRI (**a**) and CT scan (**b**) demonstrating osteoblastoma of the lamina, pedicle and transverse process in a teenager presenting with thoracic back pain and a mild curve on plain radiographs

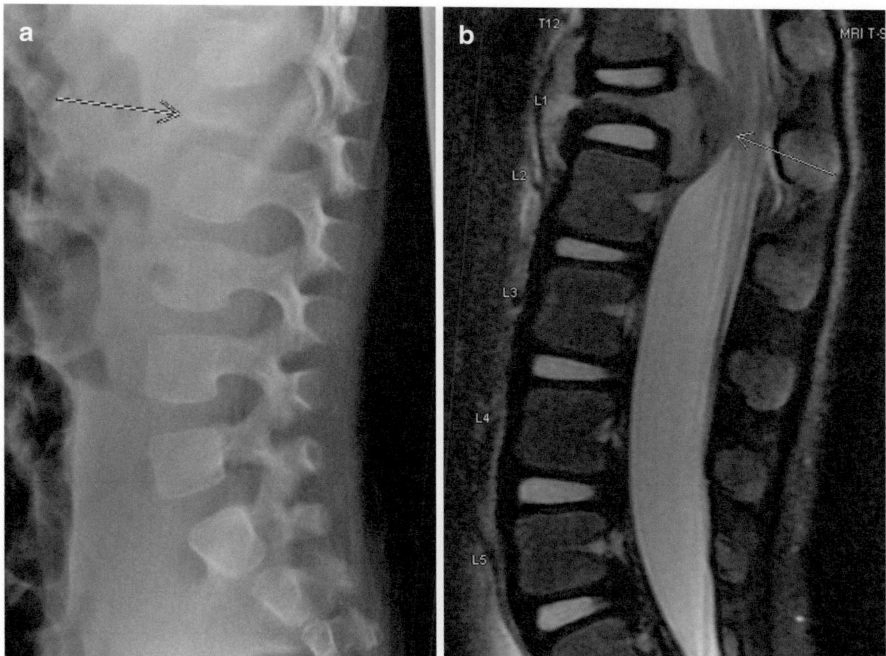

Fig. 3.12 Vertebra plana (*arrow*) on plain radiographs (**a**) in a 7-year-old who refused to walk. MRI (**b**) displaying a posterior mass (*arrow*) without soft tissue extension consistent with histiocytosis

ongoing growth of the vertebral body results in increased height of the vertebral body by skeletal maturity [66]. Other benign tumors that may present with back pain include aneurysmal bone cysts and spinal hemangiomas [67, 68].

Malignancy

Leukemia

Acute lymphocytic leukemia (ALL) is the most common malignancy of childhood; therefore, the differential diagnosis of back pain in a child should include ALL unless history, physical exam, and further work-up suggest otherwise. Back pain in patients with ALL is often worse at night and progressively worsens over time. Sometimes movement of the spine is limited, and patients appear more uncomfortable than anticipated for muscular/non-specific back pain. Other symptoms of leukemia, such as fever, lymphadenopathy, and hepatosplenomegaly, may not be present initially but typically develop over time. Radiographs may be unremarkable initially, but over time vertebral body collapse with anterior wedging may be seen at one, multiple, or nearly all levels, with progressive collapse [69, 70] (Fig. 3.13).

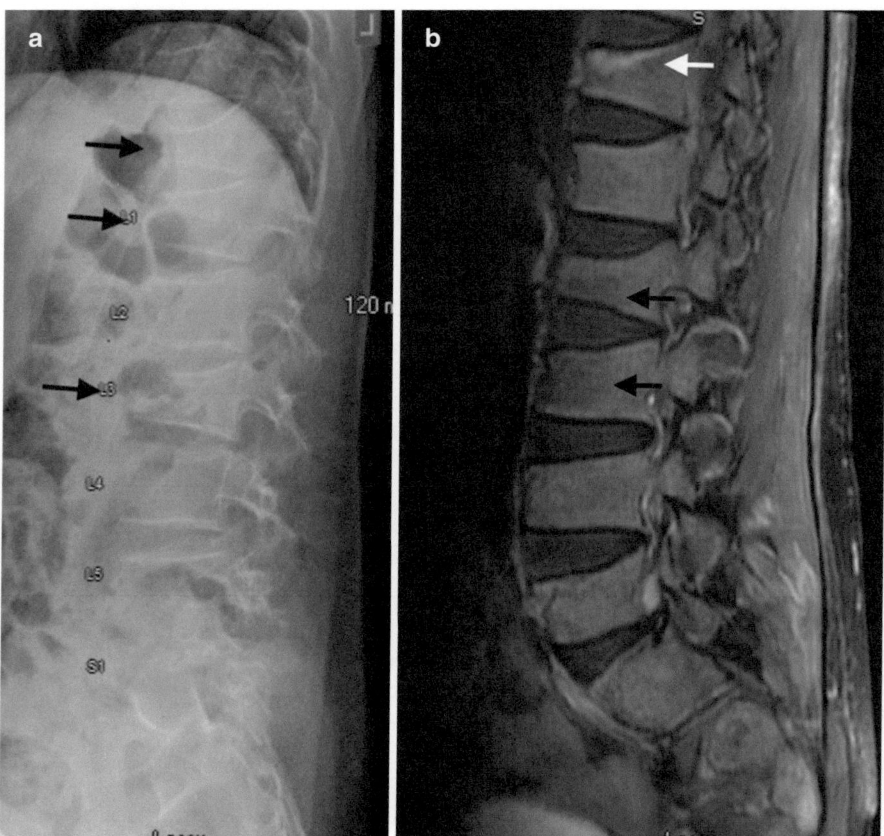

Fig. 3.13 (**a**) Multiple levels of vertebral body collapse (*arrows*) on plain radiographs in a patient with back pain and fever. (**b**) Mixed areas of hyper-intense (*white arrow*) and hypo-intense (*black arrows*) on T2-weighted MR imaging. The patient was diagnosed with acute lymphocytic leukemia

Unlike Scheuermann disease, endplate irregularities and Schmorl nodes are not present, and disc spaces are preserved.

On advanced imaging, leukemia has variable appearances. Bone scan may be "hot" or "cold" so close comparison to the appearance of other bones is important. On MRI, leukemia often appears as having mixed hypo- and hyper-intense signal on both T1 and T2 imaging, either at one or multiple levels (Fig. 3.13). Laboratory analysis may demonstrate typical high or low white blood cell count with neutropenia and the presence of blasts, anemia, and thrombocytopenia. In addition, the erythrocyte sedimentation rate, C-reactive protein, and lactate dehydrogenase may be elevated. However, laboratory values may be unremarkable early in the disease if the vertebral body is the initial area of involvement [71]. Vertebral compression fractures occur in over 25% of children receiving treatment for ALL over time, and diffuse osteoporosis may be seen [72].

Ewing Sarcoma

Ewing sarcoma, while rare, may present in the spine so remains in the differential of pediatric and adolescent back pain. Night pain and neurologic symptoms occur. The diagnosis is suspected when destructive lesions or vertebra plana are seen on plain radiographs. Laboratory studies may not demonstrate any significant abnormalities. MRI displays the characteristic findings of an associated soft tissue mass, and biopsy confirms the diagnosis. Treatment is with chemotherapy and/or radiation, although surgery may be used to decompress the spine when neurologic deficits are present [73].

Spinal Cord Tumor

Spinal cord tumors may present with or without neck or back pain. Most symptoms result from the mass effect of the tumor on the spinal cord or exiting spinal nerves. Symptoms may include changes in gait, scoliosis or torticollis, developmental delay, headache, or early handedness in an infant. Common radicular or myelopathic findings are changes in gait, loss of bowel or bladder control, radiating pain, weakness, numbness, and/or increased or decreased reflexes [74]. Frequently, children will have scoliosis, although the curve may appear atypical – left-sided; a short curve over just a few vertebral segments with abrupt angulation; a long, sweeping curve of the entire spine; concomitant kyphosis; and/or a spine that is out of balance (the head is not centered over the pelvis). Radiographs do not demonstrate destructive bony lesions. MRI identifies the lesion, often with mass effect on the spinal cord or nerve roots, consistent with the findings on neurologic exam; use of contrast is important in differentiating the grade of lesion [74].

The most common spinal cord tumors are gliomas, including astrocytomas and ependymomas. Glioblastoma and embryonal tumors also occur involving the spinal cord. Schwannomas are a benign tumor that surrounds the spinal nerve roots as they arise off the spinal cord, and neurofibromatosis may have tumor involvement around the spine. Treatment includes surgical resection with radiation and/or chemotherapy.

Infection

Discitis

Discitis is fairly unique to the pediatric population and may occur at any age [75]. Discitis results from hematogenous spread of bacteria to the vertebral endplate; osteomyelitis may occur as a sequelae of discitis. Children present with acute onset of back pain or the course may be more indolent. The average time to diagnosis in children with discitis is often weeks to months [75]. In acute presentations, fever is common, but these symptoms may not occur until late in the course in more indolent cases. Additional symptoms may include changes in gait, including refusal to walk, discomfort with flexion of the spine, and/or loss of lumbar lordosis [75]. Elevated white blood cell counts, erythrocyte sedimentation rate, and C-reactive protein are common [76].

Radiographs frequently demonstrate loss of the disc space in later stages of disease, as well as loss of lumbar lordosis or thoracic kyphosis, depending on the level of involvement. There may be changes in the appearance of the adjacent discs (Fig. 3.14a). MRI with contrast confirms loss of the disc height, inflammation of the adjacent vertebral endplates, and an adjacent soft tissue mass that may represent extrusion of the disc and/or abscess (Fig. 3.14b). Frequent infectious organisms include *Staphylococcus* and *Kingella kingae* (especially in younger children) [76]. Blood cultures should be obtained. In addition, ribosomal PCR is helpful and may reveal the infectious organism. The use of biopsy or aspiration of the involved area

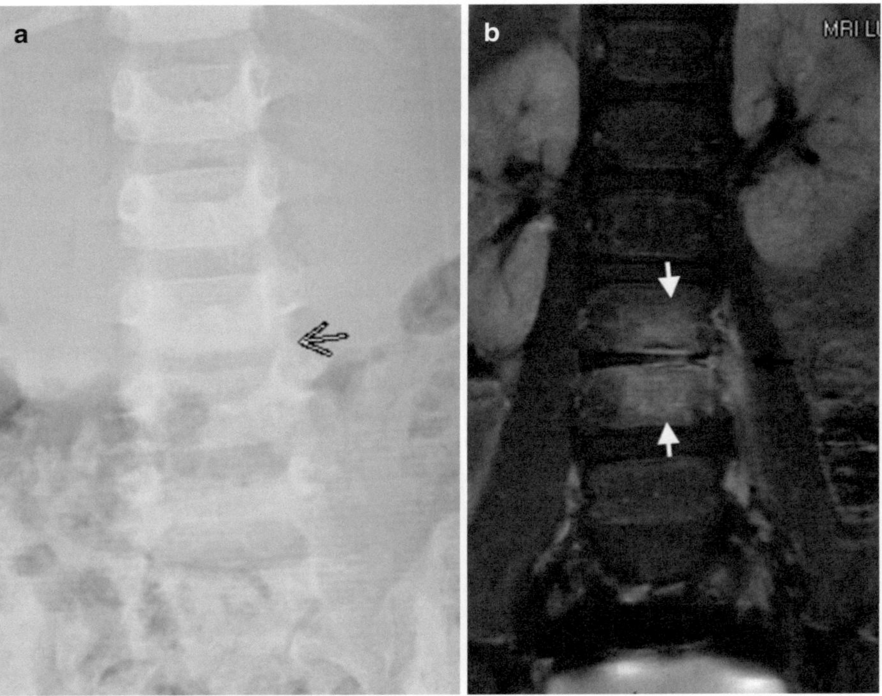

Fig. 3.14 (**a**) AP view plain radiograph of the lumbar spine demonstrating narrowing of the L3–4 disc space (*arrow*) in a 4-year-old with progressively worsening low back and hip pain, limp, and inability to flex or extend at his spine. (**b**) MRI reveals adjacent edema (*white arrows*) in the endplates of L3 and L4, narrowing of the disc space, and adjacent lateral mass (*black arrow*), consistent with discitis

to detect an organism is indicated for cases with unusual presentations, in cases refractory to initial antibiotic therapy, or if a tumor is suspected.

Treatment of discitis is often conservative. Spinal bracing with a TLSO provides comfort and may be sufficient alone in children with normal labs and no fever. However, appropriate antibiotics result in faster resolution of symptoms and decreased recurrence and are recommended in most cases [75, 77]. Surgical treatment of the infection is rarely needed. In some children the radiographic disc space remains decreased. In others the disc regenerates, while in others there may be auto-fusion of the two surrounding vertebral bodies [75]. Despite the radiographic findings, the long-term clinical prognosis is excellent.

Osteomyelitis

Isolated vertebral osteomyelitis is rare in children but may occur in those who are immunologically suppressed, have undergone spinal surgery or injection, or due to tuberculosis (also called Pott disease). The presentation may be acute or as gradually worsening back pain, usually without any history of obvious trauma. Fever, decreased spinal motion, and changes in gait or sitting may be reported. Examination often demonstrates painful movement, often with decreased range of motion; radicular symptoms may occur if vertebral body collapse is present.

Radiographs may be normal or demonstrate decreased height of the vertebral body due to bony collapse. Elevated white blood cell counts, erythrocyte sedimentation rate (ESR), and C-reactive protein are common. MRI, enhanced by the use of contrast, demonstrates the infiltrative infectious process often with surrounding destruction of bony architecture. Blood cultures often reveal the infectious organism. Biopsy or aspiration may be used to differentiate from other destructive processes, such as malignancy, or in an attempt to identify a causative organism. *Staphylococcus* is the primary causative organism, although tuberculosis should be suspected in children with risk factors [78]. Antibiotic treatment is the mainstay of therapy. Bracing with a thoracolumbosacral orthosis (TLSO) may be used to provide comfort. Osteomyelitis is often the sequelae of discitis.

Systemic Disease

Osteoporosis/Metabolic Bone Disease

Back pain from osteoporosis usually results from vertebral compression fractures in children on glucocorticoids for systemic disease or in children with metabolic bone diseases, such as hypophosphatasia, osteogenesis imperfecta, insufficiently treated hypophosphatemic rickets, nutritional deficiencies, and others. Development of vertebral fractures after use of glucocorticoids occurs commonly among children being treated for ALL and rheumatologic conditions [72, 79]. Patients with metabolic bone disease display other systemic findings, such as short stature, genu varum or valgum, and early tooth loss, as well as potentially a history of other fractures.

Radiographs of the spine demonstrate the insufficiency fractures, usually at multiple levels. Decreased mineralization may be evident (or increased mineralization in the case of osteopetrosis), although changes in mineralization may be difficult to detect in the spine due to overlying tissues or obscuration by other bony structures (Fig. 3.15). Additional radiographs may demonstrate changes of the underlying disease in the long bones of the skeleton. A skeletal survey is warranted if there is no history of confirmed metabolic bone disease, to identify other skeletal findings of an underlying systemic disorder, and to assess for other fractures if one suspects

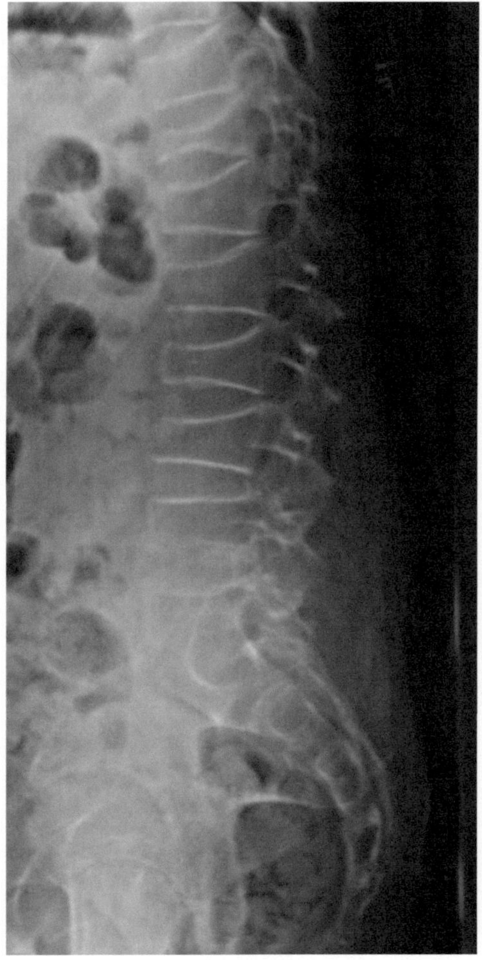

Fig. 3.15 Plain lateral lumbar spine radiograph demonstrating decreased height of all of the vertebral bodies and decreased mineralization in a pediatric patient with osteoporosis (dual-energy x-ray absorptiometry vertebral z-score was −4.0)

non-accidental trauma (which may also occur in the presence of underlying bone disease).

If the patient does not have a known diagnosis of an underlying bone disorder, additional laboratory testing may be beneficial in making the diagnosis including vitamin D (25-OH in most children and testing of 1,25-OH if there is concern for renal disease), parathyroid hormone (PTH), ionized calcium, phosphate, magnesium, and alkaline phosphatase. CBC with differential, ESR, and CRP can be obtained to assess for leukemia or infection. A urinalysis and a metabolic panel are obtained to assess for renal disease. A genetics consultation may be helpful [80]. Dual-energy x-ray absorptiometry assessing bone density and spine-specific density is important in determining future risk of fracture. Treatment of the primary disorder usually improves patient function and quality of life. In some cases bisphosphonates may be utilized.

Sickle Cell Disease

Sickle cell crises may present with back pain as a result of a bony crisis. Patients may display tenderness over the spine and limited range of motion [81]. Radiographs may not demonstrate any obvious abnormalities. White blood cell count may be elevated, making differentiation from infection difficult. MRI displays decreased signal centrally on both T1 and T2 imaging with surrounding T2 signal (Fig. 3.16). Treatment of sickle cell crisis involves oxygen and fluids, as well as pain management.

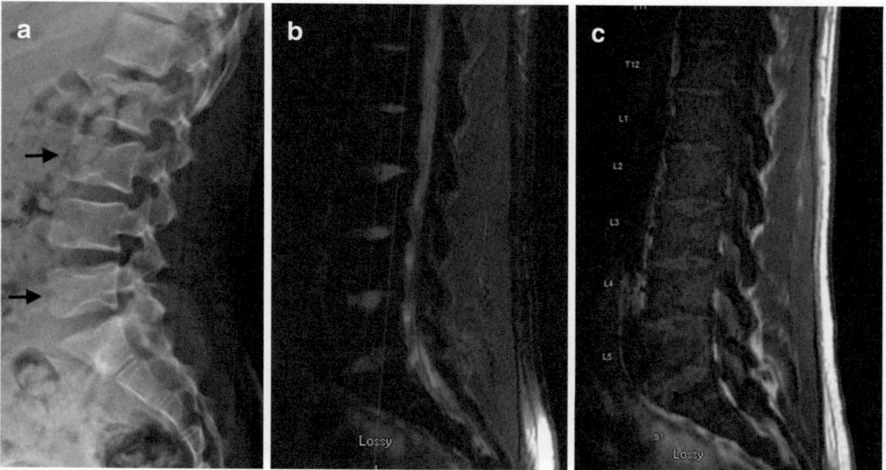

Fig. 3.16 (**a**) Plain lateral lumbar x-rays in a patient with sickle cell disease who has had multiple crises involving the lumbar spine and displays narrowing of multiple vertebral bodies (*arrows*). (**b**) Decreased vertebral body height is best seen on T2-weighted MRI, and (**c**) T1-weighted images reveal decreased signal throughout all vertebral bodies

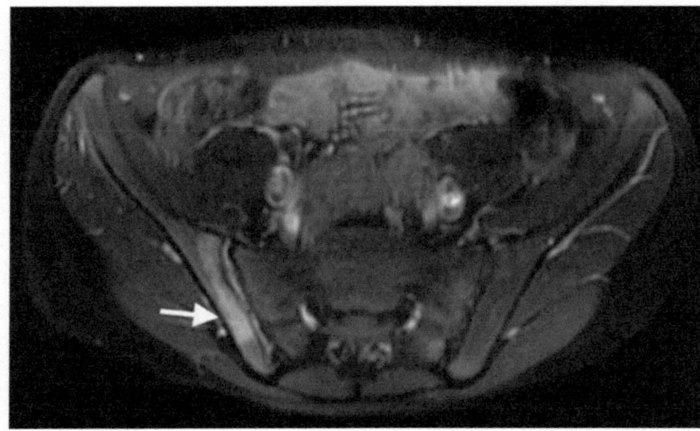

Fig. 3.17 MRI in a teenager with right low back pain and limp that was progressively worsening over 4 months demonstrating increased signal in the right sacroiliac region (*arrow*) on T2-weighted images consistent with spondyloarthropathy

Spondyloarthropathy

Spondyloarthropathy is an inflammatory arthritis involving the spine in enthesitis or psoriatic arthritis, primarily involving the sacroiliac (SI) joints. Tenderness over the SI joints and a positive FABER (flexion, abduction, external rotation) test raise suspicion regarding the diagnosis. Plain radiographs may demonstrate narrowing and sclerosis at the SI joints in advanced disease but appear normal early in the disease process. HLA-B27 may nor may not be positive [82]. MRI with and without contrast demonstrate increased T2 signal around the SI joint and enhancement with contrast (Fig. 3.17). Treatment involves systemic anti-inflammatories or disease-modifying agents. Injections of the SI joint are difficult but may be attempted in severe cases.

Extra-skeletal Causes of Back Pain

Urinary tract infection with renal involvement classically presents with flank pain, lateral to the spine at the lower portion of the rib cage. Fever may or may not be present. Percussion exacerbates the pain. Urinalysis further confirms the diagnosis when positive for leukocyte esterase and nitrites; urine microscopy and culture help determine the infectious organism. Back pain with shortness of breath suggests pneumothorax or pneumonia. Aortic dissection may present with back pain, although it is rare in children. Children at risk include those with connective tissue disorders, such as Marfan syndrome, Ehlers-Danlos syndrome, Loeys-Dietz syndrome, and other connective tissue disorders.

Editor Discussion

As this detailed chapter illustrates, all back pain does not stem from the spine. Multiple medical disorders can present with back pain. For example, the cause of back pain can be renal, urologic, pulmonary, gynecologic, or hematologic. The history and examination are the foundation of the back pain evaluation. Use imaging studies judiciously. Obtain laboratory analysis when concerned for infection, tumor, or inflammatory arthritis.

W. L. Hennrikus

The authors illustrate that back pain can be typical or atypical. Atypical frequently occurs in younger children, may be worse at night, and can be associated with stiffness and weakness or have neurological findings. On physical examination, measure height and weight as a baseline. Have the child move to test for stiffness and strength. Plain radiographs should be scrutinized for findings such as diffuse osteopenia, vertebral collapse, loss of disc height from discitis, soft tissue shadows from tumors, focal lesions as seen in vertebra plana, or increased sclerosis seen in osteoblastoma. Ideally view the radiograph yourself rather than accepting a normal report. Call the radiologist if you have any question about reported findings.

R. M. Schwend

References

1. Turner PG, Green JH, Galasko CS. Back pain in childhood. Spine. 1989;14(8):812–4.
2. Troussier B, Davoine P, de Gaudemaris R, Fauconnier J, Phelip X. Back pain in school children. A study among 1178 pupils. Scand J Rehabil Med. 1994;26(3):143–6.
3. Ramirez N, Flynn JM, Hill BW, Serrano JA, Calvo CE, Bredy R, et al. Evaluation of a systematic approach to pediatric back pain: the utility of magnetic resonance imaging. J Pediatr Orthop. 2015;35(1):28–32.
4. Bernstein RM, Cozen H. Evaluation of back pain in children and adolescents. Am Fam Physician. 2007;76(11):1669–76.
5. Dissing KB, Hestbaek L, Hartvigsen J, Williams C, Kamper S, Boyle E, et al. Spinal pain in Danish school children - how often and how long? The CHAMPS study-DK. BMC Musculoskelet Disord. 2017;18(1):67.
6. Kjaer P, Wedderkopp N, Korsholm L, Leboeuf-Yde C. Prevalence and tracking of back pain from childhood to adolescence. BMC Musculoskelet Disord. 2011;12:98.
7. Minghelli B, Oliveira R, Nunes C. Postural habits and weight of backpacks of Portuguese adolescents: Are they associated with scoliosis and low back pain? Work (Reading, Mass). 2016;54(1):197–208.
8. Meziat Filho N, Coutinho ES, Azevedo e Silva G. Association between home posture habits and low back pain in high school adolescents. Eur Spine J. 2015 Mar;24(3):425–33.
9. Dankaerts W, O'Sullivan P, Burnett A, Straker L. Altered patterns of superficial trunk muscle activation during sitting in nonspecific chronic low back pain patients: importance of subclassification. Spine. 2006;31(17):2017–23.
10. Szpalski M, Gunzburg R, Balague F, Nordin M, Melot C. A 2-year prospective longitudinal study on low back pain in primary school children. Eur Spine J. 2002;11(5):459–64.
11. Paulis WD, Silva S, Koes BW, van Middelkoop M. Overweight and obesity are associated with musculoskeletal complaints as early as childhood: a systematic review. Obes Rev. 2014;15(1):52–67.
12. Skaggs DL, Early SD, D'Ambra P, Tolo VT, Kay RM. Back pain and backpacks in school children. J Pediatr Orthop. 2006;26(3):358–63.

13. Shan Z, Deng G, Li J, Li Y, Zhang Y, Zhao Q. Correlational analysis of neck/shoulder pain and low back pain with the use of digital products, physical activity and psychological status among adolescents in Shanghai. PLoS One. 2013;8(10):e78109.
14. Moore MJ, White GL, Moore DL. Association of relative backpack weight with reported pain, pain sites, medical utilization, and lost school time in children and adolescents. J Sch Health. 2007;77(5):232–9.
15. Mackenzie WG, Sampath JS, Kruse RW, Sheir-Neiss GJ. Backpacks in children. Clin Orthop Relat Res. 2003;409:78–84.
16. Ahlqwist A, Hagman M, Kjellby-Wendt G, Beckung E. Physical therapy treatment of back complaints on children and adolescents. Spine. 2008;33(20):E721–7.
17. Calvo-Munoz I, Gomez-Conesa A, Sanchez-Meca J. Prevalence of low back pain in children and adolescents: a meta-analysis. BMC Pediatr. 2013;13:14.
18. Awwad AB, Hennrikus WL, Armstrong DG. Pediatric orthopaedic consults from chiropractic care. J Surg Orthop Adv. 2018;27:58–63.
19. Danielsson AJ, Nachemson AL. Back pain and function 22 years after brace treatment for adolescent idiopathic scoliosis: a case-control study-part I. Spine. 2003;28(18):2078–85; discussion 86
20. Danielsson AJ, Nachemson AL. Back pain and function 23 years after fusion for adolescent idiopathic scoliosis: a case-control study-part II. Spine. 2003;28(18):E373–83.
21. Sato T, Hirano T, Ito T, Morita O, Kikuchi R, Endo N, et al. Back pain in adolescents with idiopathic scoliosis: epidemiological study for 43,630 pupils in Niigata City, Japan. Eur Spine J. 2011;20(2):274–9.
22. Ramirez N, Johnston CE 2nd, Browne RH, Vazquez S. Back pain during orthotic treatment of idiopathic scoliosis. J Pediatr Orthop. 1999;19(2):198–201.
23. Zapata KA, Wang-Price SS, Sucato DJ. Six-month follow-up of supervised spinal stabilization exercises for low back pain in adolescent idiopathic scoliosis. Pediatr Phys Ther. 2017;29(1):62–6.
24. Lager C, Kroksmark AK. Pain in adolescents with spinal muscular atrophy and Duchenne and Becker muscular dystrophy. Eur J Paediatr Neurol. 2015;19(5):537–46.
25. Clancy CA, McGrath PJ, Oddson BE. Pain in children and adolescents with spina bifida. Dev Med Child Neurol. 2005;47(1):27–34.
26. Sairyo K, Sakai T, Amari R, Yasui N. Causes of radiculopathy in young athletes with spondylolysis. Am J Sports Med. 2010;38(2):357–62.
27. Grodahl LH, Fawcett L, Nazareth M, Smith R, Spencer S, Heneghan N, et al. Diagnostic utility of patient history and physical examination data to detect spondylolysis and spondylolisthesis in athletes with low back pain: a systematic review. Man Ther. 2016;24:7–17.
28. Nielsen E, Andras LM, Skaggs DL. Diagnosis of spondylolysis and spondylolisthesis is delayed six months after seeing nonorthopedic providers. Spine Deform. 2018;6(3):263–6.
29. Soler T, Calderon C. The prevalence of spondylolysis in the Spanish elite athlete. Am J Sports Med. 2000;28(1):57–62.
30. Ladenhauf HN, Fabricant PD, Grossman E, Widmann RF, Green DW. Athletic participation in children with symptomatic spondylolysis in the New York area. Med Sci Sports Exerc. 2013;45(10):1971–4.
31. Ichikawa N, Ohara Y, Morishita T, Taniguichi Y, Koshikawa A, Matsukura N. An aetiological study on spondylolysis from a biomechanical aspect. Br J Sports Med. 1982;16(3):135–41.
32. Beck NA, Miller R, Baldwin K, Zhu X, Spiegel D, Drummond D, et al. Do oblique views add value in the diagnosis of spondylolysis in adolescents? J Bone Joint Surg Am. 2013;95(10):e65.
33. Miller R, Beck NA, Sampson NR, Zhu X, Flynn JM, Drummond D. Imaging modalities for low back pain in children: a review of spondylolysis and undiagnosed mechanical back pain. J Pediatr Orthop. 2013;33(3):282–8.
34. Rush JK, Astur N, Scott S, Kelly DM, Sawyer JR, Warner WC Jr. Use of magnetic resonance imaging in the evaluation of spondylolysis. J Pediatr Orthop. 2015;35(3):271–5.

35. El Rassi G, Takemitsu M, Glutting J, Shah SA. Effect of sports modification on clinical outcome in children and adolescent athletes with symptomatic lumbar spondylolysis. Am J Phys Med Rehabil. 2013;92(12):1070–4.
36. Steiner ME, Micheli LJ. Treatment of symptomatic spondylolysis and spondylolisthesis with the modified Boston brace. Spine. 1985;10(10):937–43.
37. Fujii K, Katoh S, Sairyo K, Ikata T, Yasui N. Union of defects in the pars interarticularis of the lumbar spine in children and adolescents. The radiological outcome after conservative treatment. J Bone Joint Surg Br. 2004;86(2):225–31.
38. Sairyo K, Sakai T, Yasui N, Dezawa A. Conservative treatment for pediatric lumbar spondylolysis to achieve bone healing using a hard brace: what type and how long?: clinical article. J Neurosurg Spine. 2012;16(6):610–4.
39. Sousa T, Skaggs DL, Chan P, Yamaguchi KT Jr, Borgella J, Lee C, et al. Benign natural history of spondylolysis in adolescence with midterm follow-up. Spine Deform. 2017;5(2):134–8.
40. Selhorst M, Fischer A, Graft K, Ravindran R, Peters E, Rodenberg R, et al. Long-term clinical outcomes and factors that predict poor prognosis in athletes after a diagnosis of acute spondylolysis: a retrospective review with telephone follow-up. J Orthop Sports Phys Ther. 2016;46(12):1029–36.
41. Blumenthal SL, Roach J, Herring JA. Lumbar Scheuermann. A clinical series and classification. Spine. 1987;12(9):929–32.
42. Lonner B, Yoo A, Terran JS, Sponseller P, Samdani A, Betz R, et al. Effect of spinal deformity on adolescent quality of life: comparison of operative scheuermann kyphosis, adolescent idiopathic scoliosis, and normal controls. Spine. 2013;38(12):1049–55.
43. Murray PM, Weinstein SL, Spratt KF. The natural history and long-term follow-up of Scheuermann kyphosis. J Bone Joint Surg Am. 1993;75(2):236–48.
44. Lonner BS, Toombs CS, Mechlin M, Ciavarra G, Shah SA, Samdani AF, et al. MRI screening in operative Scheuermann Kyphosis: is it necessary? Spine Deform. 2017;5(2):124–33.
45. Weiss HR, Turnbull D, Bohr S. Brace treatment for patients with Scheuermann disease – a review of the literature and first experiences with a new brace design. Scoliosis. 2009;4:22.
46. Sachs B, Bradford D, Winter R, Lonstein J, Moe J, Willson S. Scheuermann kyphosis. Follow-up of Milwaukee-brace treatment. J Bone Joint Surg Am. 1987;69(1):50–7.
47. Montgomery SP, Erwin WE. Scheuermann kyphosis--long-term results of Milwaukee braces treatment. Spine. 1981;6(1):5–8.
48. Weiss HR, Dieckmann J, Gerner HJ. Effect of intensive rehabilitation on pain in patients with Scheuermann disease. Stud Health Technol Inform. 2002;88:254–7.
49. Lonner BS, Toombs CS, Guss M, Braaksma B, Shah SA, Samdani A, et al. Complications in operative Scheuermann kyphosis: do the pitfalls differ from operative adolescent idiopathic scoliosis? Spine. 2015;40(5):305–11.
50. Toombs C, Lonner B, Shah S, Samdani A, Cahill P, Shufflebarger H, et al. Quality of life improvement following surgery in adolescent spinal deformity patients: a comparison between Scheuermann Kyphosis and adolescent idiopathic scoliosis. Spine Deform. 2018;6(6):676–83.
51. Alyas F, Turner M, Connell D. MRI findings in the lumbar spines of asymptomatic, adolescent, elite tennis players. Br J Sports Med. 2007;41(11):836–41; discussion 41.
52. Chang CH, Lee ZL, Chen WJ, Tan CF, Chen LH. Clinical significance of ring apophysis fracture in adolescent lumbar disc herniation. Spine. 2008;33(16):1750–4.
53. Quinlan JF, Duke D, Eustace S. Bertolotti's syndrome. A cause of back pain in young people. J Bone Joint Surg Br. 2006;88(9):1183–6.
54. Santavirta S, Tallroth K, Ylinen P, Suoranta H. Surgical treatment of Bertolotti's syndrome. Follow-up of 16 patients. Arch Orthop Trauma Surg. 1993;112(2):82–7.
55. McGirt MJ, Mehta V, Garces-Ambrossi G, Gottfried O, Solakoglu C, Gokaslan ZL, et al. Pediatric tethered cord syndrome: response of scoliosis to untethering procedures. Clinical article. J Neurosurg Pediatr. 2009;4(3):270–4.
56. Ostling LR, Bierbrauer KS, Kuntz C. Outcome, reoperation, and complications in 99 consecutive children operated for tight or fatty filum. World Neurosurg. 2012;77(1):187–91.

57. Tseng JH, Kuo MF, Kwang Tu Y, Tseng MY. Outcome of untethering for symptomatic spina bifida occulta with lumbosacral spinal cord tethering in 31 patients: analysis of preoperative prognostic factors. Spine J. 2008;8(4):630–8.
58. Geyik M, Alptekin M, Erkutlu I, Geyik S, Erbas C, Pusat S, et al. Tethered cord syndrome in children: a single-center experience with 162 patients. Childs Nerv Syst. 2015;31(9):1559–63.
59. Rodriguez A, Kuhn EN, Somasundaram A, Couture DE. Management of idiopathic pediatric syringohydromyelia. J Neurosurg Pediatr. 2015;16(4):452–7.
60. Burn SC, Ansorge O, Zeller R, Drake JM. Management of osteoblastoma and osteoid osteoma of the spine in childhood. J Neurosurg Pediatr. 2009;4(5):434–8.
61. Ono T, Sakamoto A, Jono O, Shimizu A. Osteoid osteoma can occur at the pars interarticularis of the lumbar spine, leading to misdiagnosis of lumbar Spondylolysis. Am J Case Rep. 2018;19:207–13.
62. Faddoul J, Faddoul Y, Kobaiter-Maarrawi S, Moussa R, Rizk T, Nohra G, et al. Radiofrequency ablation of spinal osteoid osteoma: a prospective study. J Neurosurg Spine. 2017;26(3):313–8.
63. Kadhim M, Binitie O, O'Toole P, Grigoriou E, De Mattos CB, Dormans JP. Surgical resection of osteoid osteoma and osteoblastoma of the spine. J Pediatr Orthop B. 2017;26(4):362–9.
64. Huang WD, Yang XH, Wu ZP, Huang Q, Xiao JR, Yang MS, et al. Langerhans cell histiocytosis of spine: a comparative study of clinical, imaging features, and diagnosis in children, adolescents, and adults. Spine J. 2013;13(9):1108–17.
65. Greenlee JD, Fenoy AJ, Donovan KA, Menezes AH. Eosinophilic granuloma in the pediatric spine. Pediatr Neurosurg. 2007;43(4):285–92.
66. Raab P, Hohmann F, Kuhl J, Krauspe R. Vertebral remodeling in eosinophilic granuloma of the spine. A long-term follow-up. Spine. 1998;23(12):1351–4.
67. Lim JB, Sharma H, Reid R, Reece AT. Aneurysmal bone cysts of the vertebrae. J Orthop Surg (Hong Kong). 2012;20(2):201–4.
68. Pretell-Mazzini J, Chikwava KR, Dormans JP. Low back pain in a child associated with acute onset cauda equina syndrome: a rare presentation of an aggressive vertebral hemangioma: a case report. J Pediatr Orthop. 2012;32(3):271–6.
69. Liu B, Gwal K, Servaes S, Zhuang H. Acute lymphocytic leukemia presented as back pain and revealed by bone scintigraphy. Clin Nucl Med. 2013;38(8):649–51.
70. Santangelo JR, Thomson JD. Childhood leukemia presenting with back pain and vertebral compression fractures. Am J Orthop (Belle Mead NJ). 1999;28(4):257–60.
71. Kayser R, Mahlfeld K, Nebelung W, Grasshoff H. Vertebral collapse and normal peripheral blood cell count at the onset of acute lymphatic leukemia in childhood. J Pediatr Orthop. 2000;9(1):55–7.
72. Cummings EA, Ma J, Fernandez CV, Halton J, Alos N, Miettunen PM, et al. Incident vertebral fractures in children with leukemia during the four years following diagnosis. J Clin Endocrinol Metab. 2015;100(9):3408–17.
73. Grubb MR, Currier BL, Pritchard DJ, Ebersold MJ. Primary Ewing's sarcoma of the spine. Spine. 1994;19(3):309–13.
74. Crawford JR, Zaninovic A, Santi M, Rushing EJ, Olsen CH, Keating RF, et al. Primary spinal cord tumors of childhood: effects of clinical presentation, radiographic features, and pathology on survival. J Neuro-Oncol. 2009;95(2):259–69.
75. Brown R, Hussain M, McHugh K, Novelli V, Jones D. Discitis in young children. J Bone Joint Surg Br. 2001;83(1):106–11.
76. Dayer R, Alzahrani MM, Saran N, Ouellet JA, Journeau P, Tabard-Fougere A, et al. Spinal infections in children: a multicentre retrospective study. Bone Joint J. 2018;100-B(4):542–8.
77. Ring D, Johnston CE 2nd, Wenger DR. Pyogenic infectious spondylitis in children: the convergence of discitis and vertebral osteomyelitis. J Pediatr Orthop. 1995;15(5):652–60.
78. Mete B, Kurt C, Yilmaz MH, Ertan G, Ozaras R, Mert A, et al. Vertebral osteomyelitis: eight years' experience of 100 cases. Rheumatol Int. 2012;32(11):3591–7.

79. Huber AM, Gaboury I, Cabral DA, Lang B, Ni A, Stephure D, et al. Prevalent vertebral fractures among children initiating glucocorticoid therapy for the treatment of rheumatic disorders. Arthritis Care Res. 2010;62(4):516–26.
80. Ward LM, Konji VN, Ma J. The management of osteoporosis in children. Osteoporos Int. 2016;27(7):2147–79.
81. Roger E, Letts M. Sickle cell disease of the spine in children. Can J Surg. 1999;42(4):289–92.
82. Weiss PF, Xiao R, Biko DM, Chauvin NA. Assessment of sacroiliitis at diagnosis of juvenile spondyloarthritis by radiography, magnetic resonance imaging, and clinical examination. Arthritis Care Res (Hoboken). 2016;68(2):187–94.

Chapter 4
History Evaluation of the Child or Adolescent with Back Pain Including Ten Red Flags

Surya N. Mundluru and Norman Y. Otsuka

Introduction

Back pain in the child or adolescent patient is one of the most common reasons for physician assessment and referral. Back pain prevalence in the teenage years has been purported in the literature as high as 35% [1]. Although the majority of time it is musculoskeletal in nature and self-remitting, it still necessitates a thorough evaluation to rule out disorders that can result in significant disability, such as infection or tumor. Back pain itself should not be construed as a diagnosis, but rather a symptom of some underlying process. The physician should be able to take a thorough and detailed history to help direct for further diagnostic modalities as part of the workup. Activity modifications, exercises, rehabilitation, and management of emotional stressors can prevent recurrent episodes for most cases of musculoskeletal back pain. However, in cases of severe and persistent back pain, a thorough history combined with a detailed physical exam and appropriate imaging studies is necessary to determine if serious underlying pathology is to blame.

The evaluation and treatment of back pain in the pediatric and adolescent patient are challenging. A thorough history is key. In many cases, back pain is a symptom of an underlying disorder. Typically, the etiology is musculoskeletal and can be managed by exercise, stretching, and rehabilitation. In a few cases, back pain is a symptom of a nefarious and potentially life-threatening diagnosis. A systematic approach to obtaining the patient and parental history is the best approach to avoid missing the underlying diagnosis [2].

S. N. Mundluru (✉)
Department of Pediatric Orthopaedic Surgery, University of Texas McGovern School of Medicine, Houston, TX, USA
e-mail: Surya.N.Mundluru@uth.tmc.edu

N. Y. Otsuka
Division of Orthopaedic Surgery, Southern Illinois University School of Medicine, Springfield, IL, USA

© Springer Nature Switzerland AG 2021
R. M. Schwend, W. L. Hennrikus (eds.), *Back Pain in the Young Child and Adolescent*, https://doi.org/10.1007/978-3-030-50758-9_4

The author's preferred systematic evaluation starts with a consistent dialogue with the patient and parent. If the child is younger than 10 years of age, the parent will most likely provide the majority of the history; however, if older than 10, the patient can provide the history, and the parent can add additional information. Leave questions as open-ended as possible, allowing the child and family members the opportunity to fully express their concerns. A written checklist of questions about back pain is helpful so that important findings are not missed [3].

Guidelines for History Taking Related to Back Pain in the Child and Adolescent
11 Key Questions

1. How old is the child?
2. What is the nature of the back pain?

   - Duration?
   - Frequency?
   - Relationship to activity?
   - Alleviating and aggravating factors/medications?

3. History of trauma?
4. Any radiating symptoms in the legs? Pain with walking?
5. Incontinence or enuresis?
6. Signs of chronic disease or illness?
7. Issues with birth and development?
8. Family history of back conditions or disc?

   - Herniations?

9. Family history of spinal deformity? Family history of spinal surgical procedures?
10. Any emotional or social stressors and behavioral or mood concerns?
11. What are the child's or family's thoughts as to the cause of the pain?

11 Standard Questions

1. *What is the child's age?*

   This is most important to understand the various conditions, pain perception, and response to the pain. Younger patients have an entirely different set of diagnostic possibilities compared to the adolescent.
2. *What is the nature of the back pain?*

   Ask about the nature of symptoms such as duration, frequency, location, temporal relationship to activity, and alleviating and aggravating factors. Acute onset of back pain with no other associated symptoms infers that the pain is likely musculoskeletal in nature. However, chronic pain that is insidious in onset with associated symptoms suggests a more serious underlying condition. Alleviating or aggravating factors play in important role in helping to focus the differential diagnoses. For example, pain with hyperextension activities during sports that localizes to the lower back could indicate acute or chronic spondylolysis [4, 5]. Pain in the abdomen and retroperitoneum could be referred from the back. Prescribed medications, over-the-counter medications, and supplements are important historical findings. For example, night pain that resolves with NSAIDs could indicate an osteoid osteoma or osteoblastoma in the posterior elements of the spine (Fig. 4.1).

3. *Was there a history of trauma? Was it a high-energy injury or low energy? Were there any other associated injuries that occurred?*

   Establishing details related to the mechanism of injury is very important. Few children younger than 10 years of age sustain significant traumatic injuries of the spinal column. However, in children older than 10 years, back trauma can result in fractures, ligamentous injury, or neurological injury (Fig. 4.2). Also, consider child abuse in an infant with a spine injury if the mechanism is not well explained.

4. *Is there any radiation of pain/numbness spreading down to the lower extremities or saddle anesthesia? Does the pain affect the patient's ability to walk, and if so, how long has the walking been affected?*

   Radiating symptoms, saddle anesthesia, and new-onset ambulatory issues are red flags. These symptoms could suggest a space-occupying lesion or compression within the spinal canal within the lumbar region causing a cauda equina syndrome. Establishing the duration of the symptoms is important as early intervention favors better outcomes. Examples of disorders that lead to red flag symptoms include intraspinal tumors, primary bone tumors with mass effect, lumbar stenosis, acute disc herniations (Fig. 4.3), or a fractured vertebral endplate. Red flag symptoms warrant a thorough physical exam and urgent advance imaging [6–8].

5. *Are there any new-onset incontinence or enuresis?*

   Incontinence and enuresis are red flags. Establishing the duration of the symptoms is paramount. Bowel and bladder dysfunction occur due to compression or injury of the sacral nerve roots. The sacral micturition center is located at S2–S4. The internal anal sphincter is controlled by parasympathetic stimulation from S1 to S3. Disorders that cause injury at this level include a tethered cord or a space-occupying or space-narrowing lesions.

6. *Does the child have any symptoms of chronic illness, such as fevers, weight loss, increasing fatigue, and pain in other joints or extremities?*

   Fever is a red flag indicating possible infection such as acute discitis or an epidural abscess. CBC, ESR, and CRP are indicated. Many chronic or systemic illnesses can affect the spinal column. Malignancy including leukemia and primary or secondary bone tumors can present with back pain or referred limb pain [9]. Rheumatologic conditions such as ankylosing spondylitis can present with back pain and fatigue [10].

   After obtaining a history related to the patient's back pain, also obtain a detailed past medical, family, and social history.

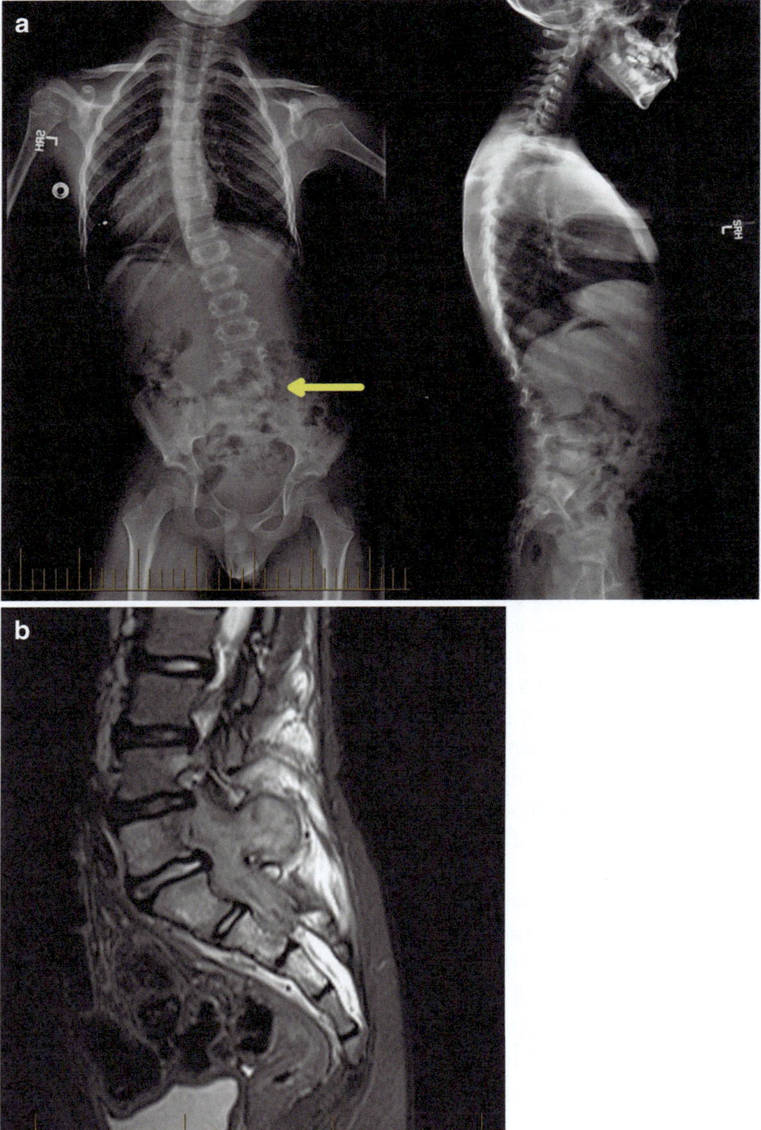

Fig. 4.1 (**a**) Posteroanterior (PA) and lateral standing spine images of a 9-year-old boy with 6-month history of chronic low back pain, which was worse at night. The pain radiated to his left leg and foot, and he was tripping over that foot. Examination confirmed a left foot drop. Initial plain radiographs were read as "left thoracic scoliosis, mild 25 degrees." However, notice that the pedicles at L5 are absent on the AP image and the lateral image shows expanded L5 posterior elements. When the pain was not relieved with a brace, an MRI was obtained (**b**). The MRI was suggestive of malignancy, which greatly worried the parents and the primary care physician. CT was then ordered (**c**) which showed the expanded posterior elements, consistent with osteoblastoma. The correct sequence should have been plain radiograph to suggest the diagnosis and then CT to confirm the diagnosis, with MRI done for preoperative planning

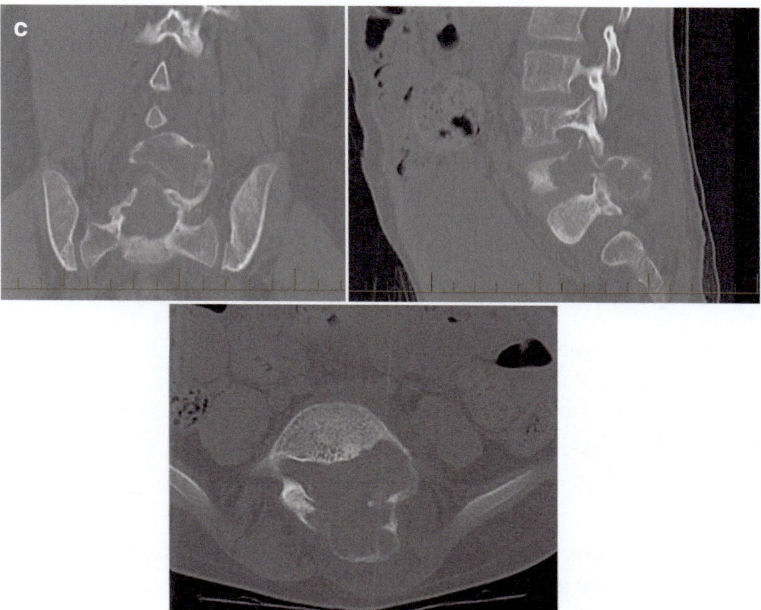

Fig. 4.1 (continued)

Fig. 4.2 An 8-year-old girl was injured when a car ran her over. When initially evaluated, she was paraplegic. Plain radiographs were read as normal. Because of the paraplegia, an MRI was obtained. This showed a ligamentous injury at C6–C7 (*arrow*) and anterior wedging of the vertebra with signal change from T1 to T8 (*arrow*). In children, ligamentous and bony injury can occur over multiple levels, for which the spinal cord does not tolerate. She was treated with a brace and made full recovery

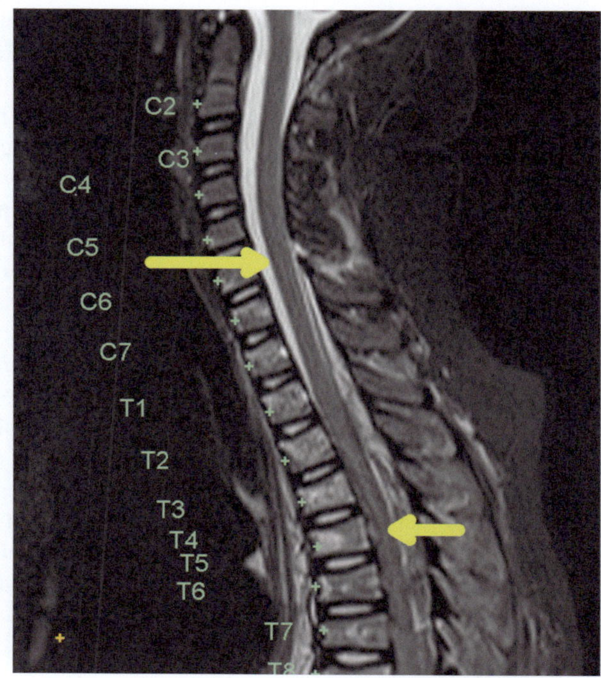

> **Red Flags: Findings During History That Should Raise Your Concern for a More Serious Underlying Pathology**
> - History of high-energy trauma
> - Significant amounts of pain with restriction of motion and motor weakness
> - Systemic illness, fever, or night sweats
> - Unintentional weight loss
> - Inability to walk
> - Enuresis or incontinence and saddle anesthesia
> - Night pain
> - History of malignancy or immunosuppression
> - New structural deformity
> - Inflammatory disorder, multiple joint involvement, iritis, rashes, colitis, urethral discharge, and morning stiffness

7. *Any significant issues at birth or during development? If so, what interventions or treatments were undertaken?*

   Obtaining a birth and developmental history is necessary when treating children and can be helpful in the workup of back pain. For example, a patient with developmental delays may raise your suspicions for neurological or genetic conditions. If the child has had normal development but has recently demonstrated difficulty walking and enuresis, this could suggest cord tethering.

8. *Family history of back conditions or disc herniations? Any past medical history of significance?*

   Sometimes just asking the patient or patient family if there is any history of spine problems or disc herniations can very helpful in the workup. A family history of multiple disc herniations requiring surgery could suggest an increased risk for the patient as well. A family history of spinal stenosis could raise the suspicion of congenital stenosis in the patient. If the patient has a history of spina bifida, there is an increased concern for tethering of the cord. A medical history of malignancy or immunosuppressive illnesses or steroid use could be related to back pain.

9. *History or family history of spinal deformity requiring treatment such as bracing or surgery?*

   Spinal deformity can be associated with back pain. It is important to determine if the child has previously been diagnosed or treated for scoliosis or kyphosis. For example, Scheuermann's kyphosis can lead to significant back pain. Historically, scoliosis has not been associated with back pain, but recent literature supports an association [11, 12]. Spinal deformities have some degree of familial inheritance, so determining if any first-degree relatives have had a spinal deformity is important.

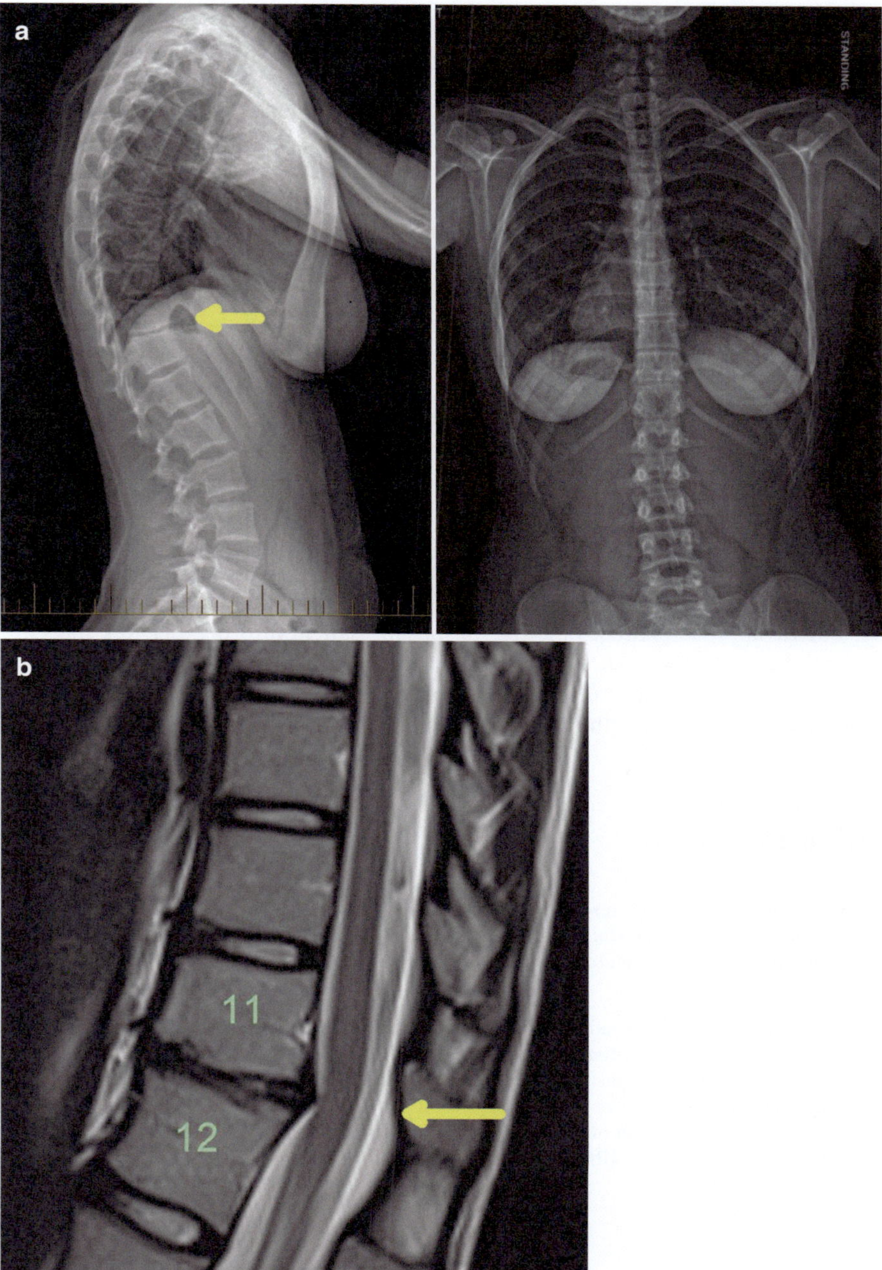

Fig. 4.3 A 15-year-old girl had chronic lower thoracic back pain for 6 months, stiffness, but without neurological symptoms. Plain radiographs showed focal kyphosis and disc narrowing at T11–T12 disc (**a**). Because the pain was intense and did not resolve with conservative treatment (rest, PT, brace, medication), an MRI was obtained showing abnormal disc with protrusion into the spinal canal (**b**). The pain resolved temporarily with Marcaine injection into the disc and then permanently with removal of the disc and fusion of the T11–T12 vertebral bodies

10. *Does the child have any ongoing current social stressors and behavioral or mood concerns?*

    Obtaining a social history is very important and often an overlooked aspect of history taking. In school-age children, multiple reports in the literature have shown an association between book bag weight and back pain in children and adolescents. Psychosocial stressors and depression have been linked to back pain in children and adolescents. Getting a sense of the patient's daily routine, mental health, and well-being can be helpful part of the workup [13–17].

11. *Finally, always ask the child or the caretaker if they have any other concerns, what their thoughts are, what they feel is the major contributor to the pain, and what they hope to gain from the visit today.* The goal of the history is to determine relevant information, allow the child and the family to express their concerns, and give the physician insight about red flags. Based on the history, a directed physical exam can be performed and imaging studies obtained.

Summary

Back pain in the child or adolescent is common. A detailed history is key. Using a systematic approach reduces the risk of missing salient information. Red flags are findings in the history that may indicate a more serious underlying condition. The overall goal of the history is to develop an accurate patient story in the physician's mind that will help guide the physical exam and laboratory and imaging studies.

Editor Discussion

Back pain is a common presenting complaint associated with a wide variety of acute and chronic medical and surgical conditions. It is important that a thorough history is obtained to identify any red flags indicating that a patient requires further diagnostic investigations.

W.L. Hennrikus

As the child becomes an adolescent, lifestyle becomes more relevant to the underlying explanation for back pain compared to the younger child. This includes excessive time with electronic devises, poor posture, family or personal stress, sleep hours and sleep quality, weight and nutrition, over or under physical activity, backpacks, core strengthening activities, and excessive amount of time at work. But as the case examples illustrate, still be vigilant to night pain, spine stiffness, neurological findings, or pain that does not have clear underlying diagnosis.

R.M. Schwend

References

1. Joergensen AC, Hestbaek L, Andersen PK, Nybo Andersen AM. Epidemiology of spinal pain in children: a study within the Danish National Birth Cohort. Eur J Pediatr. 2019;178(5):695–706.
2. Junge T, Wedderkopp N, Boyle E, Kjaer P. The natural course of low back pain from childhood to young adulthood – a systematic review. Chiropr Man Therap. 2019;27:10.
3. Calvo-Muñoz I, Kovacs FM, Roqué M, Gago Fernández I, Calvo J. Risk factors for low back pain in childhood and adolescence: a systematic review. Clin J Pain. 2018;34(5):468–84.
4. Berger RG, Doyle SM. Spondylolysis 2019 update. Curr Opin Pediatr. 2019;31(1):61–8.
5. Mataliotakis GI, Tsirikos AI. Spondylolysis and spondylolisthesis in children and adolescents: current concepts and treatment. Orthop Trauma. 2017;31(6):395–401.
6. Fuglkjaer S, Vach W, Hartvigsen J, Wedderkopp N, Junge T, Hestbæk L. Does lower extremity pain precede spinal pain? A longitudinal study. Eur J Pediatr. 2018;177(12):1803–10.
7. Biagiarelli FS, Piga S, Reale A, Parisi P, et al. Management of children presenting with low back pain to emergency department. Am J Emerg Med. 2019;37(4):672–9.
8. Xu X, Han S, Jiang L, Yang S, et al. Clinical features and treatment outcomes of Langerhans cell histiocytosis of the spine. Spine J. 2018;18(10):1755–62.
9. Dho YS, Kim H, Wang KC, Kim SK, et al. Pediatric spinal epidural lymphoma presenting with compressive myelopathy: a distinct pattern of disease presentation. World Neurosurg. 2018;114:e689–97.
10. Brayda-Bruno M, Albano D, Cannella G, Galbusera F, Zerbi A. Endplate lesions in the lumbar spine: a novel MRI-based classification scheme and epidemiology in low back pain patients. Eur Spine J. 2018;27(11):2854–61.
11. Calloni SF, Huisman TA, Poretti A, Soares BP. Back pain and scoliosis in children: when to image, what to consider. Neuroradiol J. 2017;30(5):393–404.
12. Teles AR, Ocay DD, Bin Shebreen A, Tice A, Saran N, Ouellet JA, Ferland CE. Evidence of impaired pain modulation in adolescents with idiopathic scoliosis and chronic back pain. Spine J. 2019;19(4):677–86.
13. Akbar F, AlBesharah M, Al-Baghli J, Bulbul F, Mohammad D, Qadoura B, Al-Taiar A. Prevalence of low Back pain among adolescents in relation to the weight of school bags. BMC Musculoskelet Disord. 2019;20(1):37.
14. Batley S, Aartun E, Boyle E, Hartvigsen J, Stern PJ, Hestbæk L. The association between psychological and social factors and spinal pain in adolescents. Eur J Pediatr. 2019;178(3):275–86.
15. Dissing KB, Hestbæk L, Hartvigsen J, Williams C, Kamper S, Boyle E, Wedderkopp N. Spinal pain in Danish school children – how often and how long? The CHAMPS Study-DK. BMC Musculoskelet Disord. 2017;18(1):67.
16. Yamato TP, Maher CG, Traeger AC, Wiliams CM, Kamper SJ. Do schoolbags cause back pain in children and adolescents? A systematic review. Br J Sports Med. 2018;52(19):1241–5.
17. Szita J, Boja S, Szilagyi A, Somhegyi A, Varga PP, Lazary A. Risk factors of non-specific spinal pain in childhood. Eur Spine J. 2018;27(5):1119–26.

Chapter 5
Physical Examination of the Child or Adolescent with Back Pain

Howard R. Epps

A careful, detailed history is an essential prerequisite to the physical examination and guides the focus of the examination [1, 2]. The onset, location, duration, severity, frequency, and exacerbating or relieving factors of the pain should be documented. A story of trauma should be noted. A history of fever, night pain, or weight loss should be ascertained, as these can indicate a more serious problem. Morning stiffness suggests an inflammatory problem. The history suggests a short differential diagnosis. The physical examination helps to further refine the list of causes or potentially confirm the diagnosis. After these two critical parts of the evaluation are completed, the physician can determine if investigation with additional imaging modalities is needed. The best initial imaging test is usually a posteroanterior (PA) and lateral plain radiograph of the area of the spine causing pain. Advanced imaging studies such as an MRI scan are ordered on a case by case basis in collaboration with the specialist physician.

Evaluation of the child with back pain starts with the overall condition of the child. Obtain height, weight, and temperature if infection is suspected. If the child is excessively short with a spine deformity, suspect a skeletal dysplasia. Compare weight to previous weight to determine if there has been a marked change. Is the child well or sick? Note the maturity status, nutrition, overall appearance, presence of generalized laxity, or unusual stiffness.

Spine examination starts with inspection of standing posture and gait. Is the child comfortable and well balanced, off to the side, or pitched forward? Limping should be noted or the inability in a younger child to walk. The child should be given adequate space for proper assessment of the gait cycle, typically outside the examination room in the hallway. A heel-toe gait pattern suggests normal function of the L4 and S1 nerve roots [1]. A waddling Trendelenburg gait indicates weakness of the gluteal muscles, often from hip pathology, but could be from L5 or S1 weakness due to spinal pathology.

H. R. Epps (✉)
Private Practice, Houston, TX, USA

© Springer Nature Switzerland AG 2021
R. M. Schwend, W. L. Hennrikus (eds.), *Back Pain in the Young Child and Adolescent,* https://doi.org/10.1007/978-3-030-50758-9_5

"""

For inspection, the child should wear a gown with the opening in the back. The child should wear underpants or shorts for complete evaluation of the lower back and extremities. The examiner looks for skin lesions such as the café au lait spots of neurofibromatosis, hairy patches, lipomas, or birth marks as these can indicate an underlying neurologic or bone problem [3] (Fig. 5.1). The child should stand with

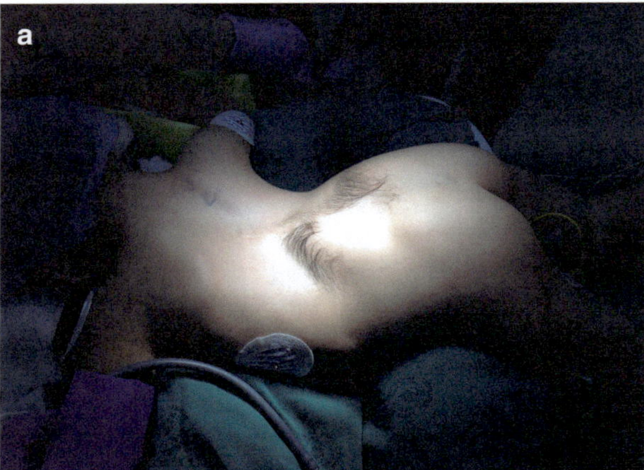

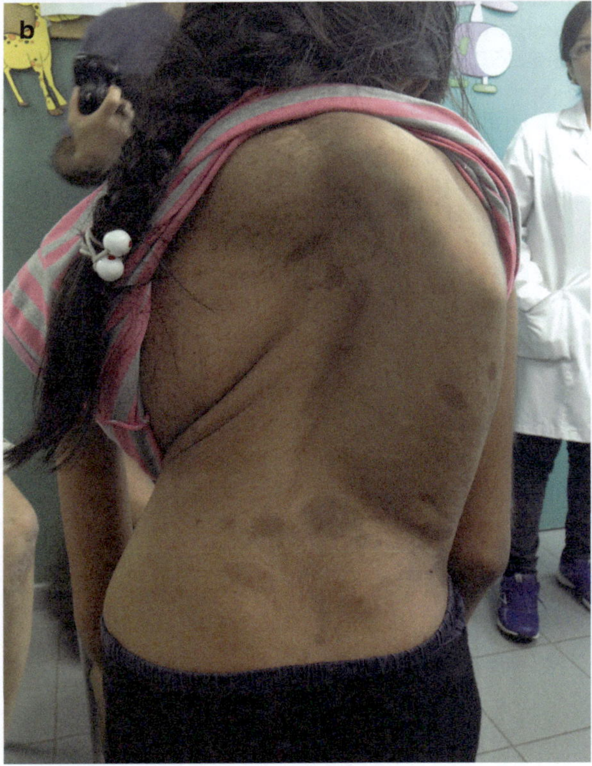

Fig. 5.1 (**a**) A photograph of the skin of the lumbar spine with a hairy patch. (**b**) A 12-year-old girl with neurofibromatosis type 1. Notice the numerous large café au lait marks and upper right thoracic dystrophic scoliosis. There is also a cervical-thoracic plexiform neurofibroma with previous biopsy incision in the upper thoracic spine

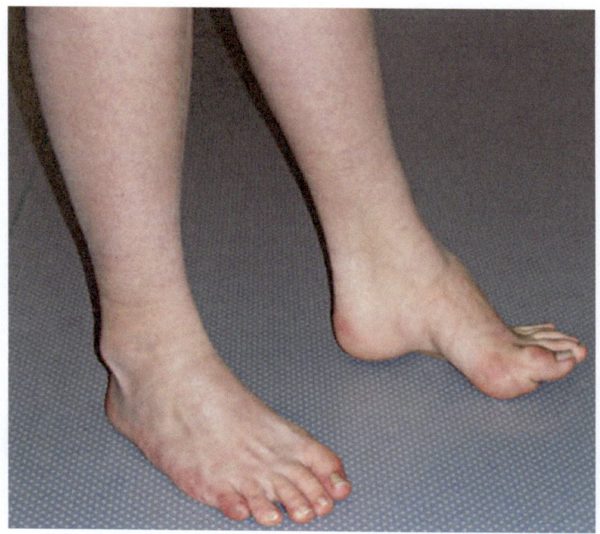

Fig. 5.2 Photograph of a high-arched or cavus foot. (From Dreher et al. [8]. Reprinted with permission from Springer Nature)

knees straight to identify any pelvic obliquity, which could represent a possible limb length discrepancy. The spine is inspected for obvious curvature, which can be confirmed by palpation. The examiner should look for symmetry of the shoulder blades and of the waist or difference in shoulder heights. The head should rest centered above the pelvis, and a truncal shift suggests an abnormal curvature of the spine.

The contour of the trunk should be inspected from the front, behind, and sides. Looking from the side, the examiner should note the presence or absence of the normal cervical lordosis, thoracic kyphosis, and lumbar lordosis. Inspection should always include the feet, as a high-arched or cavus foot could indicate intraspinal pathology (Fig. 5.2).

Palpation starts with the posterior elements in the midline. The examiner feels for areas of tenderness, deviation, or a step-off. The paraspinal muscles and the facet joints are palpated for tenderness. The sacroiliac joints and the iliac crests are also palpated [2].

Range of motion should be assessed, with forward flexion to touch the floor expected (Fig. 5.3). Inability to do so could reflect anterior spine column pathology or hamstring tightness. Back extension may cause pain coming from the posterior elements of the spine. To assess rotation, the examiner stabilizes the pelvis with both hands while the patient rotates in each direction. Lateral bending to each side completes the range of motion assessment.

A careful, detailed neurologic examination comprises the next portion of the exam. Strength, sensation, proprioception, and reflexes are tested. It can be helpful to try to do the exam by the neurologic levels of function [3]. A focused exam can be achieved by asking the patient to walk on the heels, toes (gastrocnemius), and outsides of the feet (tibialis anterior), squat down, and rise up from squatting position (quadriceps and hamstrings and gluteus maximus). The Gower maneuver is

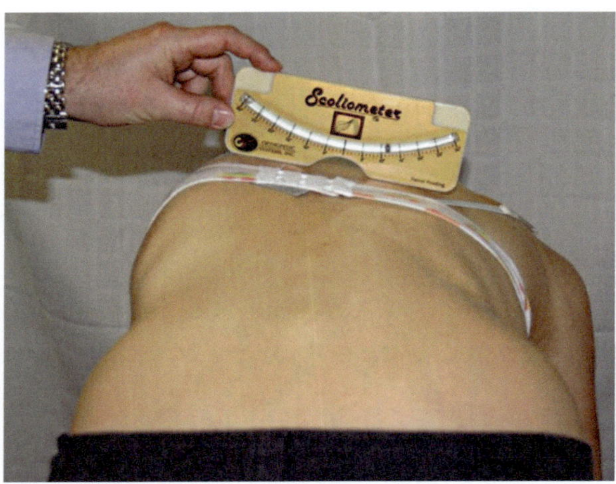

Fig. 5.3 A patient doing the Adams forward bend test with a scoliometer

done by asking the child to sit on the floor and then to stand up. Proximal weakness, such as seen in Duchenne muscular dystrophy (DMD) or other muscle diseases, will be evident if the hands are needed to assist in becoming upright. If the examiner personally does these maneuvers and asks the patient to do them as well, it can be perceived as a game with younger children. Since so many children have chronic lifestyle-related weakness of their core muscles associated with their back pain, in this context, consider specifically testing their trunk and hip core muscle strength. Ask the child to do ten well-executed push-ups, five deep squats, and ten sit-ups. Stressing the body a little can help bring out weakness that would not be apparent with just static testing.

The sensory dermatomes are delineated as follows:

L1. The sensory distribution of the L1 root is anterior hip in the inguinal area.
L2. The dermatome for L2 resides on the anterior thigh.
L3. Sensory distribution of the L3 root covers the anterior aspect of the knee.
L4. L4 sensory distribution is the anteromedial aspect of the lower leg.
L5. The L5 dermatome is the anterolateral aspect of the lower leg.
S1. The S1 dermatome includes the perineum and the posterior aspect of the leg extending to the lateral two toes.

Motor strength is tested by neurologic level, as outlined in Table 5.1. Deep tendon reflexes like the knee jerk and ankle jerk should be tested as well as the plantar response, looking for a Babinski sign. With the patient supine, abdominal reflexes should be tested. Each quadrant of the abdomen should be stroked diagonally toward the umbilicus to elicit a response (Fig. 5.4). Asymmetry or absence of abdominal reflexes can indicate spinal cord pathology, most commonly syringomyelia [4].

Special testing can provide focused information. The flexion, abduction, and external rotation (FABER) test is used for the sacroiliac joints. One leg is placed in figure four position with the foot crossed at the knee. Pressure on the inside of the

Table 5.1   Motor function by neurologic level

Motor test	Nerve root(s)	Nerve
Hip abduction	L5	Superior gluteal
Hip adduction	L2–L4	Obturator
Hip flexion	T12–L3	Nerves from T12 to L3
Hip extension	S1	Inferior gluteal n.
Knee extension	L2–L4	Femoral n.
Foot dorsiflexion, inversion	L4	Deep peroneal n.
Great toe extension	L5	Deep peroneal n.
Foot eversion	S1	Superficial peroneal n.

Data from Hoppenfeld [3]

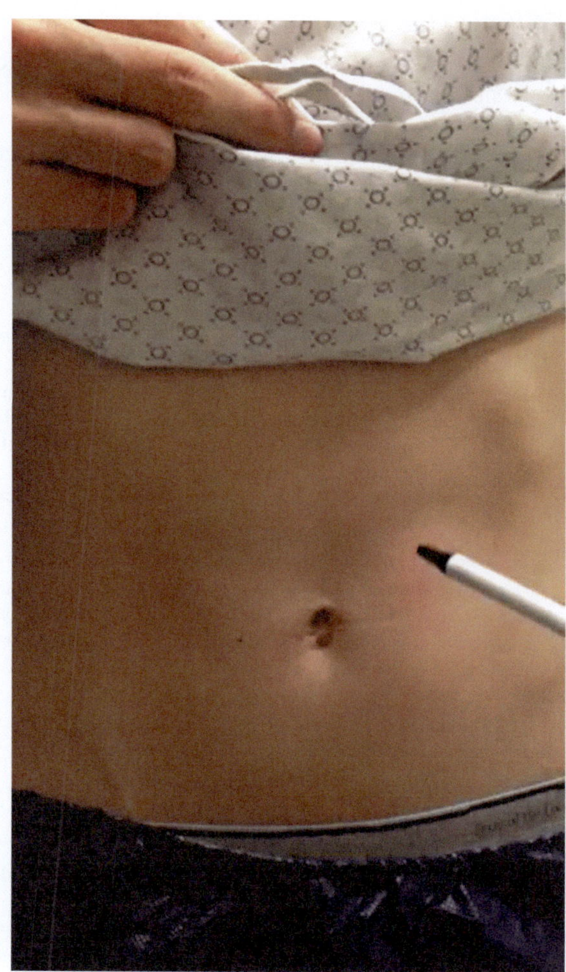

Fig. 5.4   Photograph of the umbilical reflex

flexed knee and the contralateral iliac crest elicits back pain if there is sacroiliac joint pathology [5]. The single leg extension or "stork" test isolates unilateral posterior element pathology [1]. The patient stands on one leg, and the back is gently extended. Straight leg raising in the supine position assesses hamstring tightness or lower back pathology.

One challenge is differentiating between organic back pain and nonorganic or functional pain. Traditionally, several signs known as Waddell signs – symptom magnification, pain with axial compression or rotation, diffuse tenderness, nonanatomic sensory distribution, and changing exam with distraction – were consistent with a nonorganic cause [6]. Another author, however, suggests that Waddell signs do not adequately discriminate between organic and nonorganic causes of pain [7].

Pearls
- The child with such stiffness that it is painful to touch the knees or is very slow to touch the knees may have painful enough back pain to warrant further evaluation.
- If the child can bend so far forward that they can touch the floor with their palms, they likely have ligamentous laxity.

Editor Discussion

For the young child under 5 years of age with back pain, one should always think about discitis as an etiology. Always assess their temperature, although it may not be elevated. For more chronic discitis, appetite may be affected and weight loss is possible. Finally, the child with discitis may walk a little slower than usual, have a mild limp, and be reluctant or slow to bend forward to touch the floor.

For video on how I perform the 2 minute screening examination of the child's spine, visit POSNAcademy.org.

R.M. Schwend

The physical exam and the history are the foundation in the workup of a child with back pain. Simple findings on a focused physical exam such as a cavus foot, tight hamstrings, kyphosis, a hair patch at the bottom of the spine, or a fever can alert the physician as to the need for complementary imaging and laboratory tests.

W.L. Hennrikus

References

1. Haus BM, Micheli LJ. Back pain in the pediatric and adolescent athlete. Clin Sports Med. 2012;31(3):423–40.
2. Taxter AJ, Chauvin NA, Weiss PF. Diagnosis and treatment of low back pain in the pediatric population. Phys Sportsmed. 2014;42(1):94–104.

3. Hoppenfeld S. Physical examination of the spine and extremities. East Norwalk: Appleton-Century-Crofts; 1976.
4. Armstrong A, Hubbard M, editors. Essentials of musculoskeletal care 5. Rosemont: American Academy of Orthopaedic Surgeons; 2016.
5. MacDonald J, Stuart E, Rodenberg R. Musculoskeletal low back pain in school-aged children: a review. JAMA Pediatr. 2017;171(3):280–7.
6. Waddell G, McCulloch J, Kummel E. Nonorganic physical signs in low-back pain. Spine. 1980;55:117–25.
7. Fishbain D, et al. A structured evidence-based review on the meaning of nonorganic physical signs: Waddell signs. Pain Med. 2003;4:141–54.
8. Dreher T, Beckmann NA, Wenz W. Surgical treatment of severe cavovarus foot deformity in Charcot-Marie-tooth disease. JBJS Essent Surg Tech. 2015;5(2):e11.

Chapter 6
Radiologic Imaging and Laboratory Evaluation of Back Pain in Children and Adolescents

Brian A. Shaw and Nicholas E. Arlas

Introduction

Most children and adolescents presenting with back pain for the first time to their physician will not need radiographic imaging or laboratory studies. While back pain is increasingly common in childhood, reports have shown that pain resolves in roughly 90% spontaneously and is typically due to sprains, strains, and "nonspecific" etiologies [1]. Back pain becomes more common with older age, and it is more likely that a serious underlying condition will be identified under age 10 years than near skeletal maturity, at which time nearly 100% of the population reports at least one episode of back pain [2–4]. Imaging and/or laboratory studies are indicated if there are red flags as discussed in Chaps. 4 and 5, deformity, or persistent/recurrent pain unresponsive to conservative measures such as time (generally over 6-week duration), relative rest, physical therapy, and over-the-counter nonsteroidal anti-inflammatory drugs (NSAIDs). Red flags include radicular pain, numbness or subjective weakness, night pain, bowel or bladder incontinence, fever, unexplained weight loss, and abnormal neurologic findings on physical examination such as gait deviation, reflex asymmetry, atrophy, altered or lost sensation, limited straight leg raise, marked stiffness, and objective weakness on manual motor testing.

B. A. Shaw (✉) · N. E. Arlas
Department of Orthopedic Surgery, University of Colorado – School of Medicine, Colorado Springs, CO, USA

© Springer Nature Switzerland AG 2021
R. M. Schwend, W. L. Hennrikus (eds.), *Back Pain in the Young Child and Adolescent.* https://doi.org/10.1007/978-3-030-50758-9_6

Imaging

Role of Plain Radiography

When red flags, deformity, or persistent/recurrent pain are encountered, plain radiography is indicated. As a general principle for all musculoskeletal disorders in children, plain radiography is *always* performed prior to advanced imaging. For thoracic pain, standard two-view orthogonal (anterior to posterior (AP) and lateral) images are ordered. For lumbar pain, standard two-view orthogonal AP and lateral images are also ordered. In the past, *oblique views* of the lumbar spine were ordered to visualize spondylolysis, but recent studies have shown that the addition of oblique views does not improve the diagnostic yield, and therefore, these are rarely indicated today [5]. If more detailed imaging of very specific anatomic levels is desired, AP and lateral "Spot Films" of the thoracic, lumbar, and lumbosacral spine can be ordered.

When *deformity* such as scoliosis, lordosis, or kyphosis is the major finding, then the standard radiologic study to order is a two-view (posterior to anterior (PA) and lateral) standing full-spine film (Fig. 6.1). The film is shot PA rather than AP because of the slightly lower radiation exposure to the thyroid and vital organs compared with AP exposure and also because deformity surgeons typically view the films in the same manner they would clinically examine a patient's back: posterior to anterior. Exceptions are when the child is unable to stand due to young age or neuromuscular condition, in which case an AP film is taken either sitting or supine. It is critically important that the entire spine is visualized on these initial deformity films in order to properly assess overall spinal balance, determine pattern and type of curve, measure deformity severity using the Cobb method (see Chap. 13), and determine the presence or absence of congenital, infectious, or neoplastic lesions which may be incidental or causative. If an inadequate film is initially obtained, then the patient may require another film resulting in additional cost and radiation exposure. In addition to examining the spine itself, it is important to evaluate the soft tissue structures, looking for findings such as pulmonary nodules, kidney stones, and ingested foreign bodies. These non-spinal findings may be clues to the cause for the child's back pain or may be incidental findings with little or great importance. Finally, for known neuromuscular conditions, it is helpful to include the pelvis and hips in the initial images because pelvic obliquity with hip subluxation or dislocation can cause pain (Fig. 6.2).

In infants and young or disabled children with spinal *deformity*, it may be impossible to obtain standing films, and either sitting or supine films may be substituted. These films should be marked by the technologist as such for later comparison to follow-up films, which may be done standing. If the examiner is screening for scoliosis, a generally accepted scoliometer reading of 7 degrees or greater on the forward bend test indicates that radiography should be performed [6].

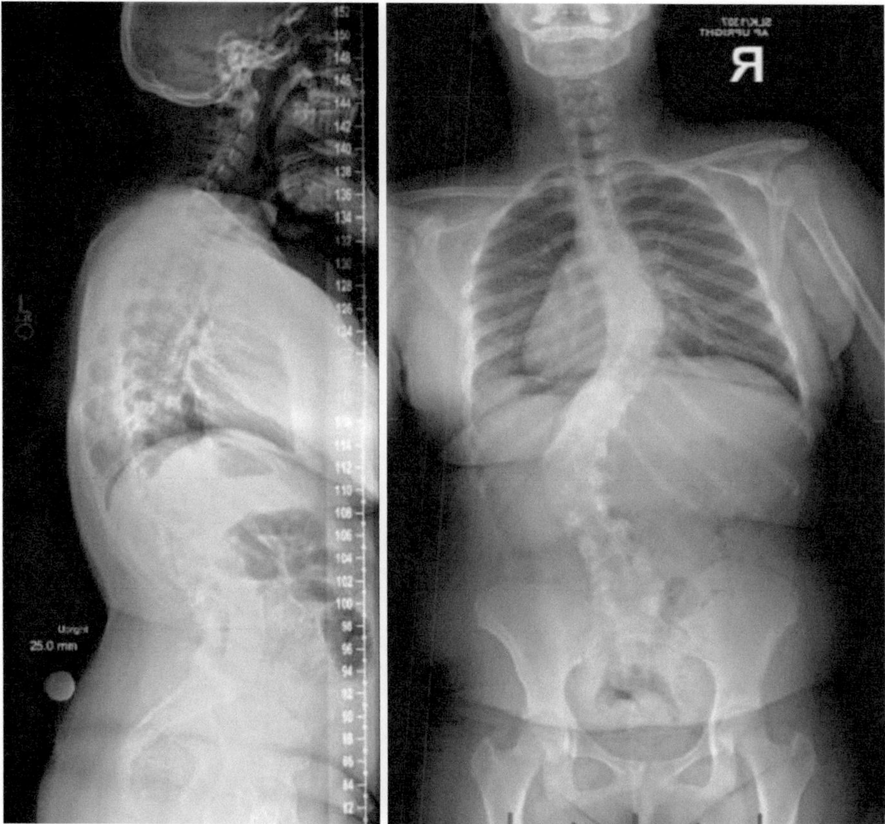

Fig. 6.1 PA and lateral standing radiograph of a teenager with adolescent idiopathic scoliosis. Note that the entire spine and pelvis are included on this initial PA film

Radiation Exposure

With modern digital radiologic technique, the radiation exposure to children and adolescents undergoing standard imaging studies is minimal. While there is no truly safe dose of radiation, exposure should rarely be a consideration when ordering indicated plain radiographic studies. The principles of as low as reasonably achievable (ALARA) and the Image Gently campaign (Society of Pediatric Radiology and others) should be applied to all ionizing imaging studies (https://www.imagegently. org/). This area does remain an area of active research, and the clinician should note changes in guidelines as they evolve [7, 8].

Fig. 6.2 An AP supine radiograph of a child with spina bifida. Note the importance of including the hips and pelvis which show dysplastic subluxated hips. The circle indicates inter-pedicular widening of the lumbar vertebrae with lack of posterior elements, characteristic of spina bifida

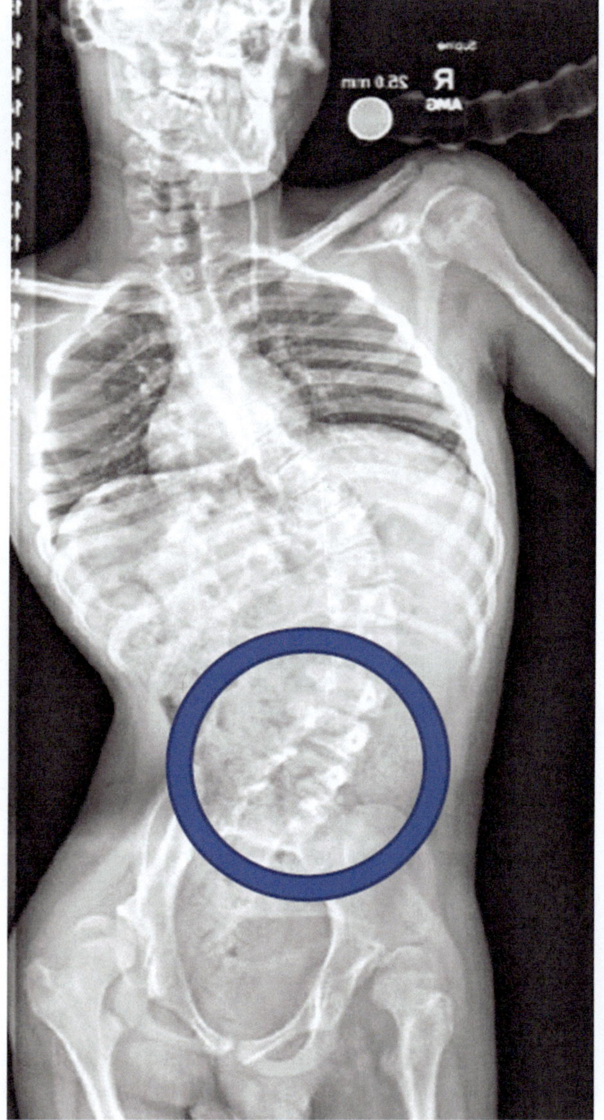

Special Views

In addition to the standard radiologic views noted above, other views may be obtained, but these should generally be ordered by the treating orthopedic surgeon. These include flexion/extension lateral lumbosacral images for spondylolisthesis, left and right lateral bending films for scoliosis, and thoracic extension films over a bolster for kyphosis. The reason for deferring these special studies to the treating physician is that they are usually not diagnostic but instead help determine the treatment plan. They also may require special standardized equipment and techniques not readily available in all radiology departments.

Role of Computerized Tomography (CT Scan)

Computerized tomography (CT) has largely been supplanted by MRI because of associated radiation exposure but still has a role in the evaluation of pediatric back pain. CT technology has developed to become much faster and deliver less radiation than in the past. A full rotation of the CT scanner takes less than 0.5 seconds, and the technology builds a complete reconstruction based on that rotation in tenths of a second [8]. A typical CT scan will deliver radiation doses of between 3 and 9 millisieverts (mSv) (background US radiation is 3.1 mSv/year) [9]. Specific indications for CT scanning in the pediatric age group are evaluation of vertebral cortical integrity and 3-D modelling of the spine. CT is better than MRI at demonstrating bony cortical detail and spondylosis and may be used to demonstrate fractures or cortical tumors such as osteoid osteomas (Fig. 6.3). The relative value of CT versus MRI depends on the quality of local technology and the expertise of the technicians operating the scanner and the radiologists/specialists interpreting the study.

A frequent question is whether it is better to use a CT or MRI for diagnosis of early spondylolysis; the MRI (Fig. 6.4) will show bony edema and "pre-lysis" edema better than CT, but the CT will show whether there is an established cortical fracture line. Often it is best to consult with your institutional radiologist or orthopedic surgeon to determine the better study for a particular indication. As a general rule, it is wise to consult with the appropriate specialist whenever ordering an advanced study beyond initial radiography or defer to that specialist to order the study.

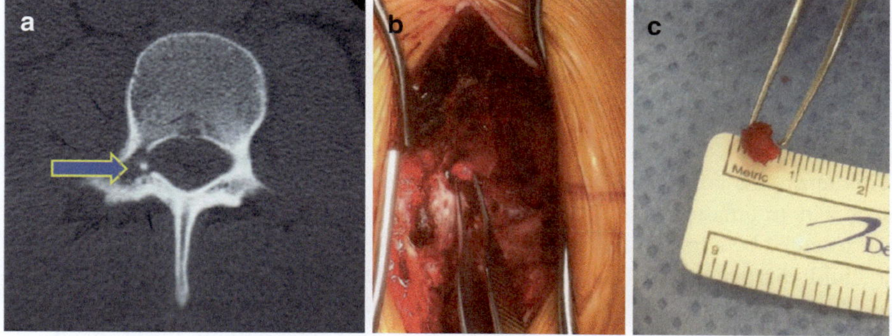

Fig. 6.3 Fine-cut CT scan showing a pea-sized osteoid osteoma of a vertebral pedicle. (**a**) CT of spine showing osteoid osteoma (*arrow*). (**b**) Surgical removal of osteoid osteoma from the spine. (**c**) Osteoid osteoma specimen

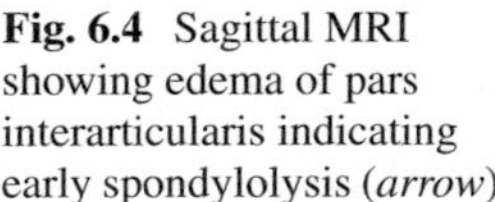

Fig. 6.4 Sagittal MRI showing edema of pars interarticularis indicating early spondylolysis (*arrow*)

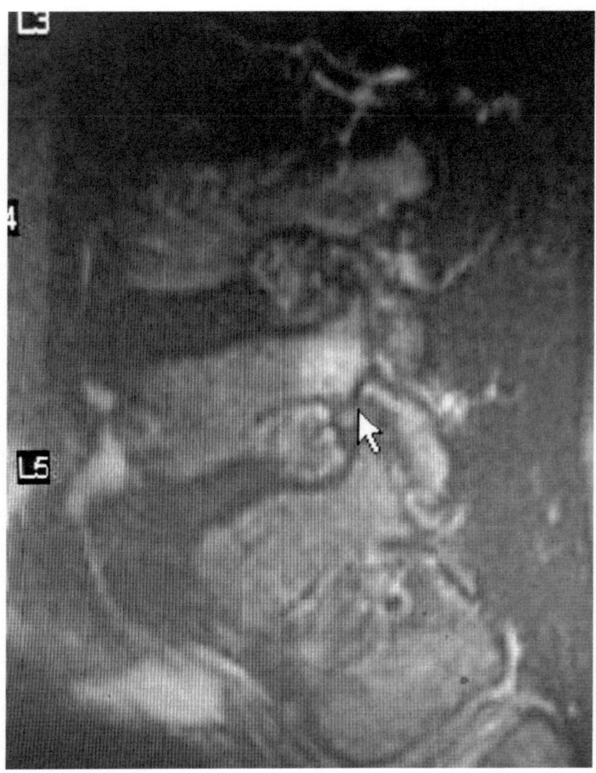

Finally, CT may be used as a first-line study in the evaluation of the multi-trauma patient and will readily demonstrate vertebral fractures and dislocations. However, CT and plain radiography will by definition miss Spinal Cord Injury Without Radiographic Abnormality (SCIWORA) injuries, which only MRI can detect.

Spinal Cord Injury Without Radiographic Abnormality (SCIWORA)

This term was coined in 1982 to describe circumstances in which children were seen with traumatic spinal cord injuries but their radiographs were normal [10]. This is explained by a much larger percentage of non-bony elements of the spine present in children versus adults (cartilaginous end plates, discs, and facet joints) and the much greater flexibility of the pediatric versus adult spinal column. If a fracture through non-bony tissue is non-displaced or if the spinal column flexes, bends, or extends excessively even without fracturing, the much less flexible spinal cord may be damaged, with no acute changes observed on plain radiography or even CT. The immature spinal column can stretch 5 cm before disruption, but the spinal cord can only stretch 6 mm. There may be injuries to the spinal column without spinal neurologic injury which will be apparent only on MRI.

Technetium Nuclear Bone Scan

Like CT, technetium nuclear bone scanning of the spine and other anatomic regions is becoming less frequently performed because MRI can show much more detail and without any radiation exposure. The best current use of a nuclear bone scan is in patients who present with concerning but vague symptoms (Fig. 6.5). Rather than

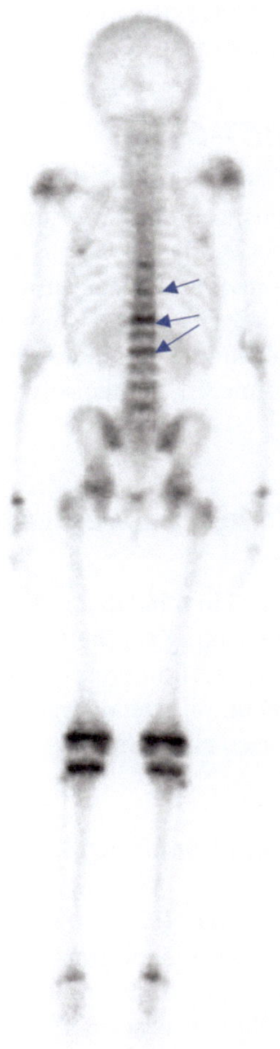

Fig. 6.5 Example of total body nuclear bone scan showing increased uptake in several vertebral bodies with disseminated neoplasm (*arrows*)

order a CT or MRI of an entire spinal region, the nuclear bone scan can image the entire spine and identify a specific anatomic site for further detailed investigation by CT or MRI. The nuclear bone scan works by intravenously injecting radioactive Technetium-99m methylene diphosphonate (MDP) which is taken up by the bone undergoing abnormally high metabolic activity and to areas of increased blood flow [11]. Areas such as growth plates which are metabolically active due to high bone turnover typically exhibit intense uptake in the pediatric population. Bone scan is sensitive but nonspecific in the detection of infection and tumors but may be falsely negative or "cold" in the setting of low bone turnover such as in eosinophilic granuloma and chronic Brodie's abscess. A more advanced form of nuclear bone scanning is single-photon emission computed tomography, or SPECT.

A common indication for nuclear bone scanning is seeking disseminated bone lesions such as metastases in patients with known cancers including neuroblastoma, Ewing's sarcoma, and osteosarcoma and in patients with suspected multifocal osteomyelitis.

PET-CT

Positron emission tomography-CT (PET-CT) is mentioned here for completeness but is ordered only as a tertiary study by a surgical or oncologic specialist in staging a neoplasm, measuring response to therapy, or performing surveillance for metastatic disease. It is not typically ordered for the initial evaluation of back pain. The technique combines the injection of a radiopharmaceutical with conventional anatomic CT to precisely identify areas of abnormal metabolic activity.

Imaging Findings on Plain Radiography

Keep in mind that radiography is not indicated for the majority of children and teens presenting for the first time with back pain unless red flags or deformity are noted. This section presents typical abnormal plain radiographic findings and their interpretation. Details regarding each clinical condition are described in Part II, case-based chapters.

Initial Approach to Reading Plain Radiographs of the Spine

Note carefully the name of the patient and the date the film was taken. Are there earlier or later films for comparison? Is left or right clearly marked? By convention, scoliosis films are taken and examined *posterior to anterior* (PA) so the patient's right side is seen on the right side of the screen; this can be confusing for most physicians who view chest films as anterior to posterior in dimension. Is the film marked to indicate whether the film was taken standing, supine, or with any special positioning? Are the hips visible? Examine the soft tissues and margins of the film for incidental findings which may be obscure or otherwise overlooked. Then, focus on the spine itself. Note the maturity of the patient from the appearance of the triradiate cartilage and the iliac crest ossification.

Disc Disease and Schmorl's Nodes

Loss of disc height is easily appreciated by comparing adjacent levels. This could indicate traumatic injury, infection (spondylodiscitis), congenital anomaly, or tumor. Disc disease increases with age and is therefore much more common in adults than in children and teens. After about age 30 years, discs desiccate and start to lose their elasticity and "shock absorber" effect (Fig. 6.6).

Plain films may also show a *vertebral end plate fracture,* also known as *apophyseal ring fracture* or "hard disc" which is a unique pediatric form of disc pathology in which the posterior margin of a vertebral end plate and attached annulus break off and may then impinge on the spinal canal or nerve roots (Fig. 6.7). There will be a history of acute traumatic injury with immediate symptoms of severe pain and possible nerve root or cauda equina irritation. These children clinically present in a similar manner to adults with acute disc herniations, but by contrast, adult disc herniations are herniations of the nucleus pulposis through the annulus, rather than the annulus and end plate themselves.

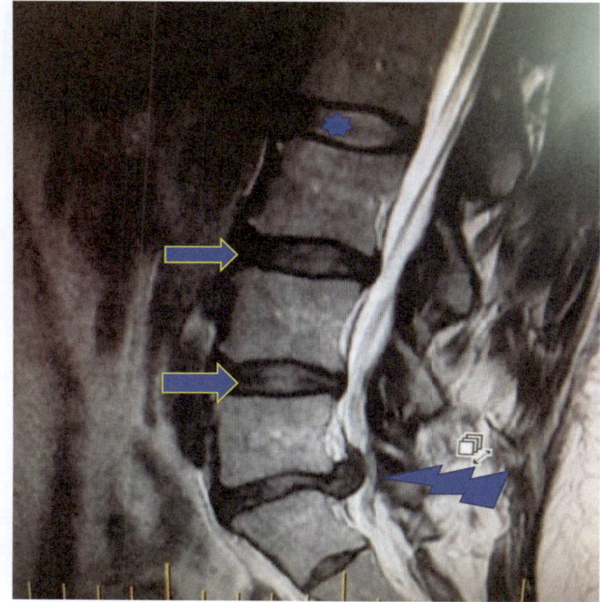

Fig. 6.6 MRI of lumbar spine showing dark discs which indicate loss of normal hydration and herniated L5/S1 nucleus pulposis (star = normal disc, large arrows = dehydrated "black" discs with posterior bulging, and jagged arrow = frankly herniated disc)

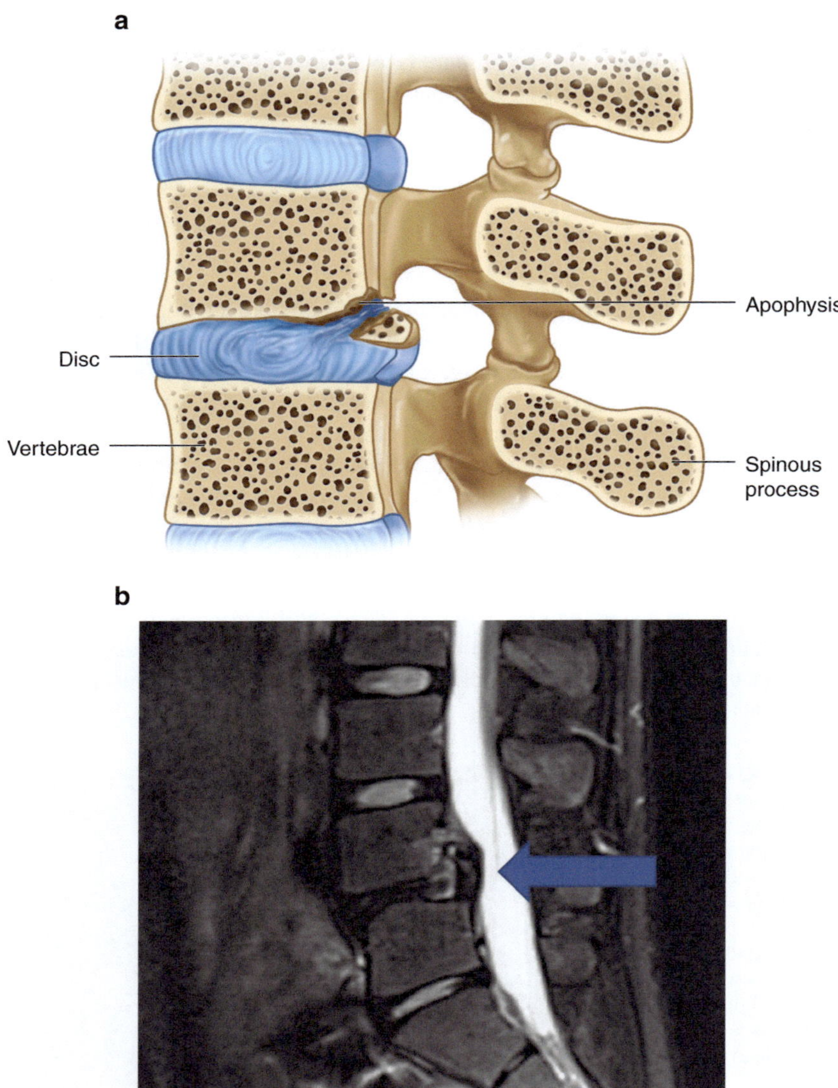

Fig. 6.7 (**a**) Illustration of vertebral end plate fracture also known as apophyseal ring fracture or "hard disc." (**b**) MRI of apophyseal ring fracture with extrusion of annulus into spinal canal (*arrow*)

Schmorl's nodes are developmental irregularities of the end plates of immature vertebrae (Fig. 6.8). They represent herniations of the disc into the adjacent vertebral end plates, not to be confused with disc herniations into the spinal canal or neural foramen. Schmorl's nodes are usually seen in the preteen and teen years and are *often incidental findings*. However, if they are prominent and at several levels,

Fig. 6.8 Schmorl's nodes involving several lumbar vertebral body end plates (*triple arrow*). Single arrow shows normal disc space with normal vertebral end plates

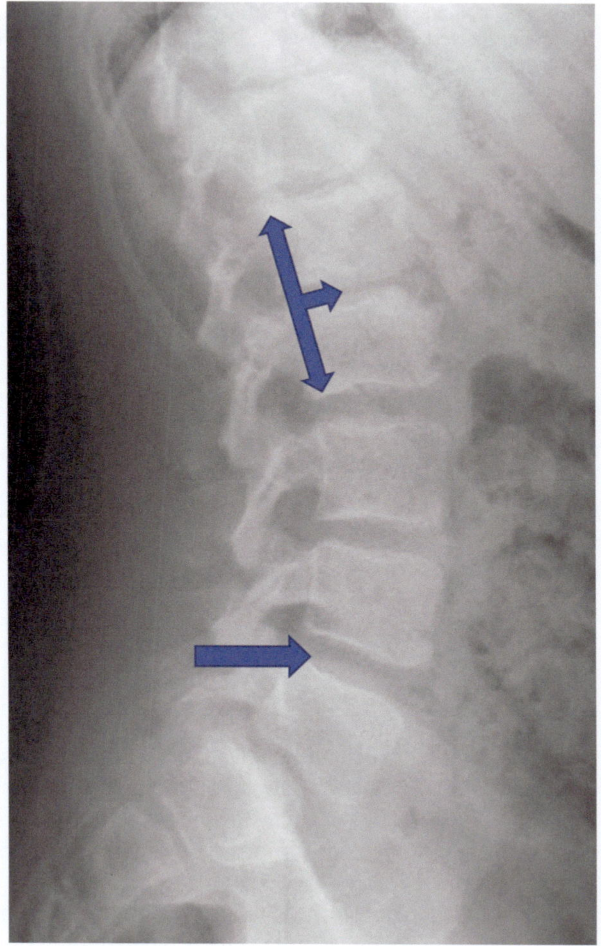

they may become symptomatic, causing "discogenic" pain; this is pain localized to the back without nerve root irritation (sciatica). In most cases, pain gradually resolves over time, and treatment is symptomatic –not surgical. No advanced imaging is required unless other pain etiology is suspected.

Fracture or Dislocation

Fracture or dislocation of any part of the thoracic or lumbar spine is usually appreciated by a loss in the normal contour and alignment of the visualized spinal column. Adjacent levels are easily compared. Step-offs in the anterior or posterior vertebral body lines and perched, jumped, or fractured facets can be seen. One form of pediatric injury is the *Chance fracture*, most commonly caused by acute spinal flexion

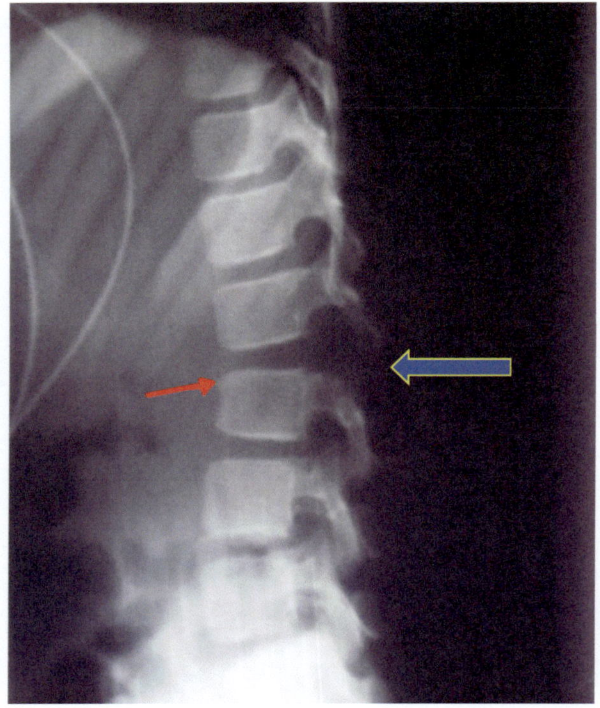

Fig. 6.9 A compression fracture of the vertebral body (anterior column, small arrow) combined with distraction injury (ligamentous or bony rupture, large arrow) of the posterior column is a variant of Chance fracture, seen most commonly with use of a lap belt without shoulder harness

as in the use of a lap belt without a shoulder harness; this causes compression injury of the anterior column and distraction of the posterior column (Fig. 6.9). The lateral film shows a gap between adjacent spinous processes (torn soft tissues) and various degrees of anterior column injury (compression or burst fracture) which together may cause spinal cord or cauda equina injury.

A generally benign type of spinal fracture seen commonly in the pediatric age group is a *compression fracture* (Fig. 6.10). Compression fractures occur with axial force to the spine such as when jumping from a height and landing on both feet or buttocks, often with a flexion moment. Isolated compression fractures are stable injuries that do not cause neurologic impairment, are more common in children than adults because of less dense pediatric bone, and generally heal without sequelae. It is not unusual to see two or three contiguous vertebral compression fractures or even more on MRI or CT imaging.

Scheuermann's Kyphosis

Scheuermann's kyphosis is a developmental disorder of unknown etiology which may affect either the thoracic or lumbar spine. Radiographs are typically ordered because a teen presents with a painful rigid kyphosis, and the diagnosis is readily made on the lateral film. Classically, the diagnosis is confirmed by three contiguous vertebrae wedged 5 degrees or more (Fig. 6.11). Advanced imaging is not usually indicated, and

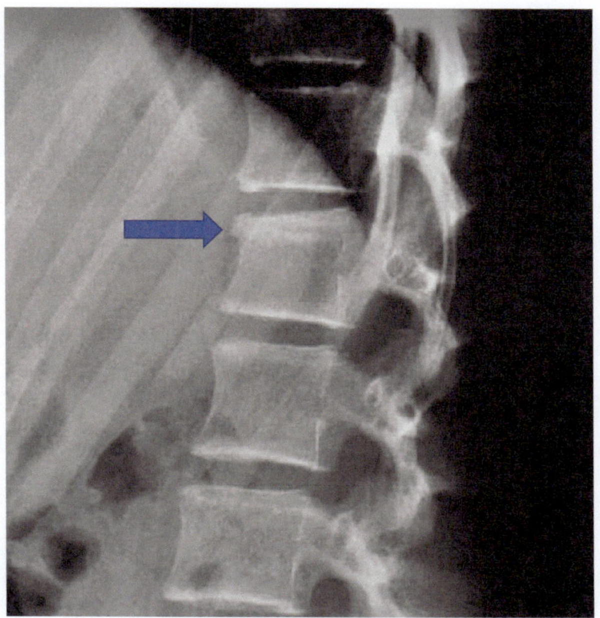

Fig. 6.10 Vertebral body compression fracture in 16-year-old girl (*arrow*)

treatment starts with physical therapy and possibly bracing, reserving surgery for more severe cases, such as when thoracic kyphosis exceeds 80 degrees. Any degree of lumbar kyphosis may be an indication for surgery, especially if there is pain.

Some experts consider Scheuermann kyphosis to be an extreme form of Schmorl's nodes; others do not. The mere presence of Schmorl's nodes does not lead to Scheuermann's kyphosis.

Transitional Vertebra

A transitional vertebrae occurs at the lumbosacral junction and may have combined features of either a lumbar or sacral vertebra. Sometimes there is an extra vertebra at the lumbosacral junction, and on one side, it may appear to be an extra lumbar vertebra and on the other an extra sacral vertebra. This is usually an incidental finding and rarely a cause for back pain. No additional imaging is required, and surgery is rarely indicated. A very large L5 transverse process that impinges onto the iliac wing or the sacrum can be painful and is termed Bertolotti syndrome

Spina Bifida Occulta

Like transitional vertebrae, *spina bifida occulta* is usually an incidental finding and not symptomatic. It is a small midline defect in the spinous process, usually of L5 and S1, occurs in about 6% of the population, and may be associated with an

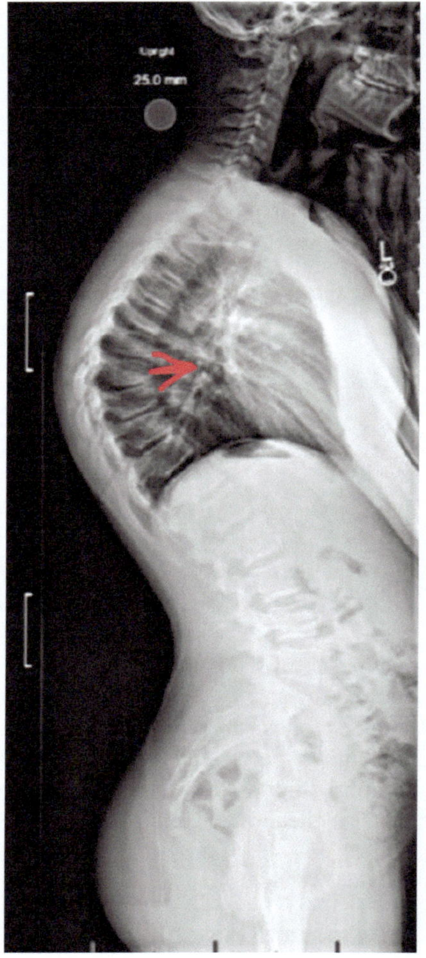

Fig. 6.11 Scheuermann's kyphosis is a developmental kyphotic deformity which may occur in the thoracic, thoracolumbar, or lumbar spine associated with anterior wedging of the apical vertebrae (*three red lines*)

increased risk of spondylolysis. Therefore, if it is seen in the setting of low back pain, consider spondylolysis as the possible etiology. An isolated radiographic finding of spina bifida occulta does not cause back pain and does not require further imaging.

Spondylolysis and Spondylolisthesis

Spondylolysis is by far the most common identifiable cause of back pain in the pediatric age group. It is a stress fracture of the pars interarticularis of a lumbar vertebra, usually L4 or L5 (Fig. 6.12). These typically occur in athletes for which

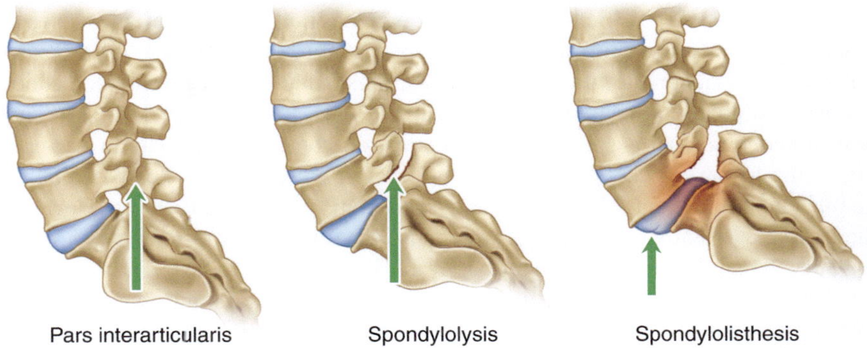

Fig. 6.12 Spondylolysis and spondylolisthesis. *Spondylolysis* is a non-displaced developmental, traumatic, or degenerative fracture through the pars interarticularis that may lead to *spondylolisthesis* which is a slippage of one vertebra over the subjacent vertebra

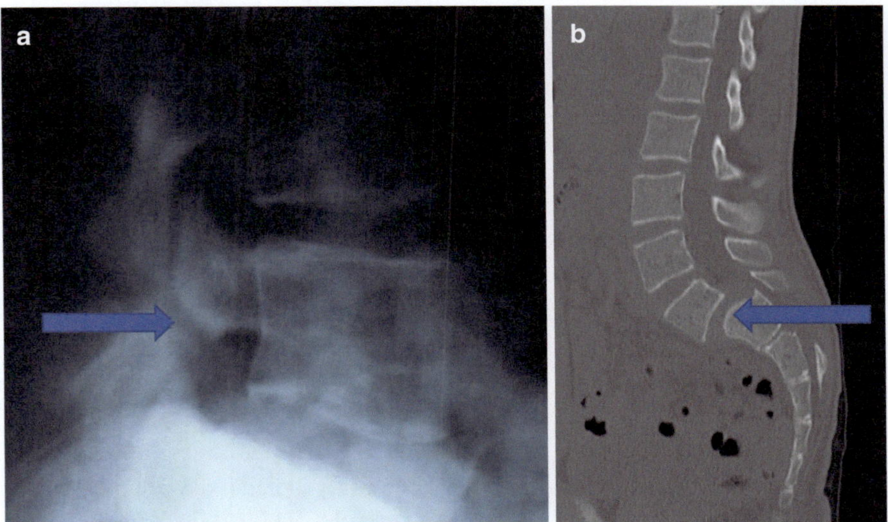

Fig. 6.13 (**a**) L5 spondylolysis in a 14-year-old gymnast (*arrow*). (**b**) An unstable high-grade L5/S1 developmental spondylolisthesis in a 13-year-old boy (*arrow*)

their sport requires repetitive lumbar extension such as dance, gymnastics, and football line positions. However, there is also a developmental component, and spondylolysis can be seen in any athlete or nonathlete. Spina bifida occulta is an associated radiographic finding and may be a predisposing factor.

Plain AP and lateral lumbar radiographs may show an established spondylolysis (Fig. 6.13a). In the past, oblique views were taken to look for the so-called "scotty dog" sign, but these have been shown to be no more sensitive than the standard AP and lateral views [12, 13]. However, plain radiography may not reveal an early-stage spondylolysis in which a complete fracture has not yet occurred; in such cases where spondylolysis is clinically suspected by a history of low back pain associated with sport activity and tightness of the hamstrings, an MRI may reveal bone edema localized to unilateral or bilateral pars (see Fig. 6.4). In this early stage, complete cessation of aggravating sport, physical therapy, and bracing may result in true healing of the lesion. In later stages, once the fracture (also called a "pars defect") is visible on plain radiography, it will not heal without surgical intervention. However, the usual treatment is symptomatic and nonsurgical because most athletes are able to return to sport without complete bony healing of their defect. The symptoms resolve despite nonunion of the fracture. There is still a role for a limited-cut CT in assessing a defect which is suspected but not seen on plain film or MRI and for assessing healing potential (sclerotic borders unlikely to heal) or response to treatment. These are best ordered by the specialist physician.

In contrast to spondylolysis, *spondylolisthesis* is a slippage of one vertebra with respect to its adjacent vertebra (Fig. 6.12). Slippage requires an initial spondylolysis defect, after which the disc and anterior column structures become deficient, allowing one vertebra to slip forward over the one below it. In pediatrics, there are two basic types of spondylolisthesis: traumatic and developmental (Fig. 6.13b). The developmental type is much more common and can be further subdivided into stable and unstable variants [14]. Unstable slips may progress from low grade to high grade and even to complete *spondyloptosis* in which L5 slips completely over S1 and falls into the pelvis. It is critical to note that typical sports-related spondylolysis does not progress to significant spondylolisthesis, and therefore, surgery is not performed for most pediatric patients with spondylolysis. On the other hand, high-grade (more than 50% slipped forward) symptomatic unstable developmental or traumatic spondylolisthesis is usually surgically stabilized.

Spinal Deformity

As noted previously, radiography for spinal deformity includes the complete spine, PA and lateral, and standing if possible (see Fig. 6.1). Scoliosis, kyphosis, and lordosis are measured using the Cobb method (see Chap. 13). Generally, kyphosis greater than 60 degrees and scoliosis greater than 15 degrees are considered abnormal and reasons for orthopedic referral. Do not be fooled by *apparent scoliosis*: this occurs when there is a limb length inequality causing a pelvic tilt which then causes the spine to curve but without the rotational deformity typically seen in true idiopathic scoliosis (Fig. 6.14). The pelvic tilt (or pelvic obliquity) is readily seen on the standing film. Another film can be taken with an appropriate-sized block underneath the shorter limb, which levels the pelvis and lessens the scoliosis.

Scoliosis, kyphosis, and lordosis are descriptive terms and not diagnoses. An accurate diagnosis is made only after performance of a detailed general physical examination and appropriate imaging. The *neurologic* examination may reveal

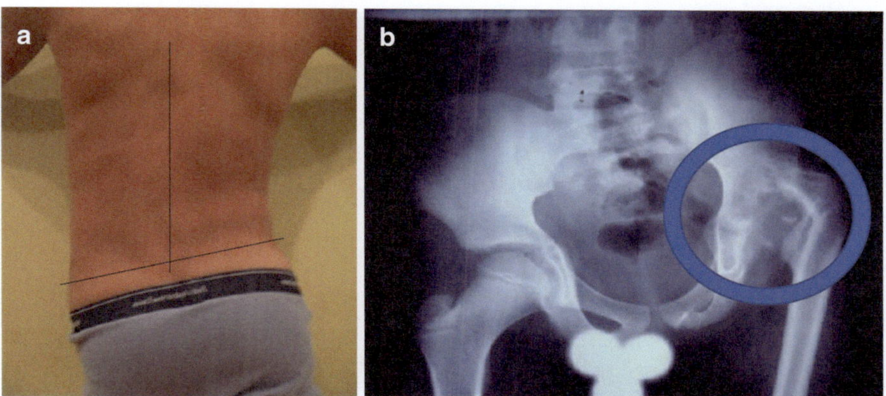

Fig. 6.14 (**a**) Apparent, but not true, scoliosis due to a limb length difference causing pelvic obliquity while standing. (**b**) In this case, the limb length difference is caused by a dislocated hip (*circled*)

asymmetric reflexes, spasticity, weakness, or gait disturbance, all indicating a neuromuscular etiology. The *skin* examination may reveal findings indicating a *syndromic* etiology such as multiple café au lait spots and axillary freckling typical of neurofibromatosis type 1 or hyperelasticity with multiple prominent scars characteristic of Ehlers-Danlos syndrome. The *musculoskeletal* examination may reveal long fingers and toes or painful foot deformity suggestive of Marfan's syndrome. A unilateral foot deformity such as cavus or equinus, along with a midline hair patch or dimple above the gluteal crease, may indicate a tethered spinal cord (see also Chap. 5: Physical Examination).

Adolescent idiopathic scoliosis is the most common type of scoliosis and typically occurs in otherwise healthy adolescent girls. The exact pathophysiology is unknown, but there is a definite genetic component. On PA imaging, there is not only a lateral spinal curvature (deformity in the coronal plane) but also a rotational component which accounts for the rib hump seen on physical examination and also a lordotic component creating a loss of normal thoracic kyphosis. The rotation is seen on PA imaging as asymmetry of the pedicles, and the loss of thoracic kyphosis is evident on the lateral film (Fig. 6.15). Indications for MR imaging for idiopathic scoliosis is controversial, with some orthopedic surgeons imaging every case of scoliosis and others reserving MRI for suspected non-idiopathic forms such apex left thoracic curves which occasionally are associated with Chiari malformations and syringomyelia. MRI may also be obtained before scoliosis surgery.

Besides *adolescent idiopathic scoliosis*, there are neuromuscular, syndromic, neoplastic, and developmental etiologies of scoliosis. Clues about etiology found on plain films include a short sharp curve associated with a hemivertebra or fused ribs as seen in *congenital scoliosis*, in which one or more vertebrae are malformed at birth. These patients should be evaluated with cardiac and renal ultrasound imaging because these organs develop in utero at the same time as the spine and are often

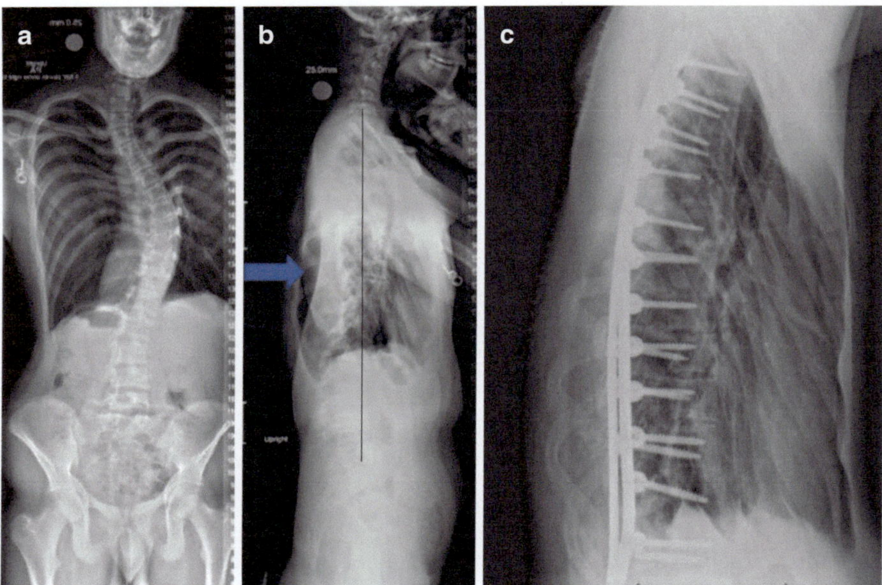

Fig. 6.15 (**a**) The PA image shows scoliosis with vertebral rotation (arrow points to prominent ribs resulting from the vertebral rotation and causing paraspinal prominence or "rib hump" seen on the Adams forward bend test). (**b**) The lateral film shows the thoracic hypokyphosis or lordosis commonly associated with idiopathic scoliosis (*vertical line*). (**c**) Postoperative film showing partial correction of thoracic lordosis

also malformed approximately 20% of the time. A long sweeping thoracic and lumbar scoliosis without rotational component can indicate a neurogenic disorder, such as cerebral palsy or chronic cervical spinal cord injury. It is important to examine the hips in these cases for subluxation or dislocation. Seating imbalance may aggravate the curve and lead to increased pain and decubitus ulcer formation.

Advanced imaging for spinal deformity is best determined by the treating physician. Usually, this will be an MRI of the *entire spinal axis* including the brain stem, looking for Chiari malformation, syringomyelia, intradural or extradural neoplasm, diastematomyelia, and spinal cord tethering. MRI is more likely to find an underlying etiology for *early-onset scoliosis* (those presenting under age 10 years) rather than *adolescent idiopathic scoliosis*. Young children, typically less than 8 years of age, will require sedation or general anesthesia for this study.

Vertebra Plana

Vertebra plana (flat vertebra) is seen on both AP and lateral images and may occur at any level. Classically, it represents an eosinophilic granuloma (Langerhans cell histiocytosis) which has weakened the vertebral body to a point of collapse but may be caused by any destructive process including infection such as tuberculosis,

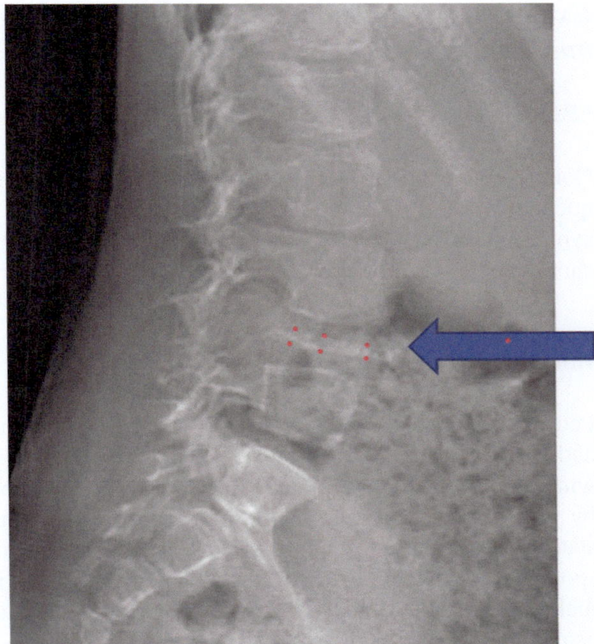

Fig. 6.16 Vertebral plana in a young child caused by vascular malformation weakening the bone (arrow points to flattened remnant of vertebral body, also outlined in red dots)

Ewing's sarcoma, and hemangioma (Fig. 6.16). Advanced imaging (MRI) and referral are always indicated, with biopsy depending upon clinical, laboratory, and MRI results.

MRI

MRI is never the first choice in spinal imaging: plain radiography is always done first because it is simple, readily available, inexpensive, and often diagnostic. The radiation exposure of plain films using modern radiologic equipment is minimal. Further, MRI in the absence of legitimate indications risks discovering clinically unimportant findings which may generate parental/patient/physician anxiety and further invasive unnecessary diagnostic and therapeutic tests which carry their own inherent risks.

In general, MRI following radiography is ordered for back pain associated with red flag signs, including pain that does not resolve within a reasonable amount of time (6 weeks), does not respond to usual conservative measures such as cessation from sport, occurs in child under age 10 years, has no apparent explanation, interferes with normal sleep, or is associated with fever, chills, weight loss, neurologic complaint, or impairment.

MRI is sometimes done with intravenous contrast: this decision is dependent upon the differential diagnosis and specifications of the equipment being used and therefore best left to the discretion of your informed radiologist.

Examples of Commonly Encountered Pediatric Variations and Abnormalities

"Bulging Discs"

Commonly reported "bulging discs" are normal variants with no clinical consequence. These are best thought of as incidental findings which do not correlate with symptoms of back pain. They are not disc herniations or "pre-herniations" and should be ignored.

Infection

Pediatric spinal infections are usually hematogenous and involve both the vertebra and adjacent disc space(s) – hence the name *spondylodiscitis*. Infection is suspected with nontraumatic onset of back pain and sometimes abdominal pain accompanied by fever, malaise, and in later stages neurologic findings secondary to epidural space encroachment. Infection may be acute as in acute staphylococcal bacterial spondylodiscitis or may be chronic and indolent as seen in fungal or AFB infections including coccidioidomycosis (valley fever) and tuberculosis. MRI for infection is usually done urgently (same or next day) but may be emergent if the child is very ill or demonstrating neurologic impairment (Fig. 6.17).

A condition which is often confused with bacterial or fungal spondylodiscitis is chronic recurrent multifocal osteomyelitis, or CRMO. This mysterious condition causes painful inflammatory bone changes often with elevation in serologic inflammatory markers and can occur in the long bones, pelvis, and spine. No etiologic infectious organism has been identified, and treatment is therefore symptomatic. Imaging clues are a mixture of new and healing lesions, typical multifocal pattern, and lack of abscess formation or sinus tracts [15].

Tumor

Many types of tumors and tumorlike conditions may affect the spinal column. Examples of the more common entities are provided here.

- Osteoid osteoma and its closely related larger cousin osteoblastoma

  - These benign neoplasms typically occur in the posterior spinal elements of teens and young adults and classically cause night pain without associated illness or neurologic symptoms. The pain responds to aspirin and NSAID medication quite dramatically, which is a reliable diagnostic clue. Histologically, these lesions are identical, but grossly osteoid osteomas are tiny pea-sized tumors (<1 cm), which may not be visible on plain films (see Fig. 6.3). Osteoblastomas are larger (>2 cm) and often visible as bone-forming lesions in the posterior elements on plain radiography (Fig. 6.18). Osteoid

Fig. 6.17 Spondylodiscitis. Acute bacterial infection causing adjacent vertebral body edema (*star*), disc deformation, and abscess between vertebral bodies and anterior longitudinal ligament (*arrow*)

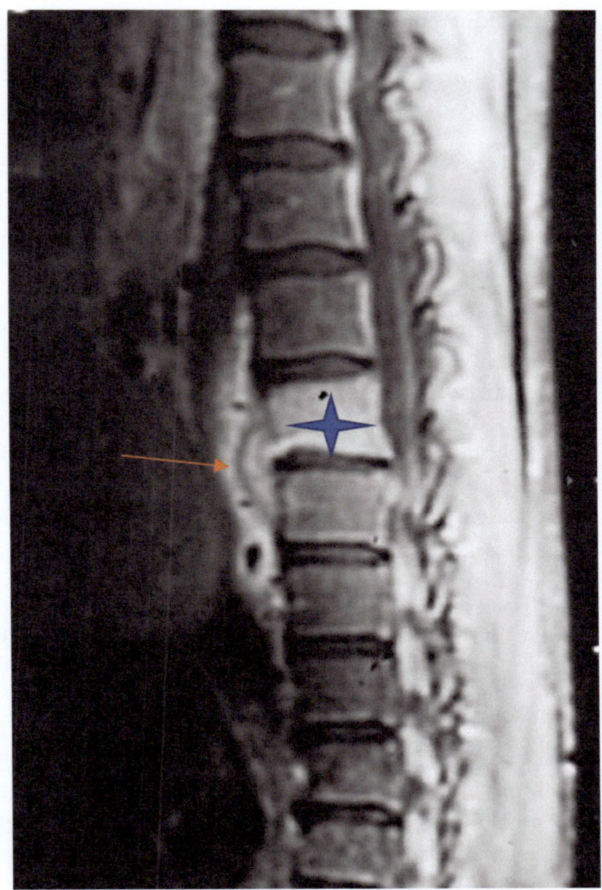

Fig. 6.18 CT scan of osteoblastoma (star indicates lytic expansile lesion in posterior elements of vertebrae)

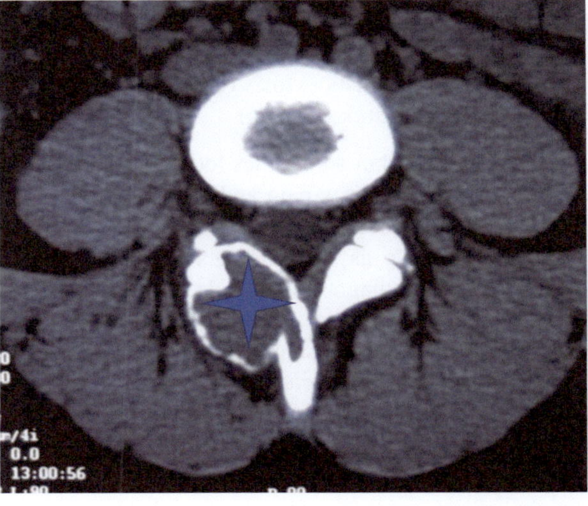

osteomas are very painful due to high production of inflammatory prostaglandins, hence the dramatic pain relief with NSAIDS. If not readily seen on MRI, a SPECT technetium bone scan may be useful in locating the lesion, and CT can be done for confirmation and preoperative planning.

- Ewing's sarcoma and osteosarcoma

  - These are the two most common pediatric primary malignancies of the pediatric spine and are often symptomatic for months before diagnosis. This is because the lesions may be initially slow-growing and symptoms vague, combined with the extremely low incidence compared with benign back pain, thus lessening clinical suspicion. Clues are night pain, pain not improved with rest, relentlessly progressive pain, and, in late cases, neurologic deficit and systemic symptoms. Plain radiographs may initially be negative, but MRI is usually diagnostic. Sometimes it can be difficult to differentiate infection from neoplasm until a biopsy with cultures is obtained. As part of tumor staging, imaging of the entire spine and skeleton is done with MRI, PET-CT, and/or nuclear bone scan, looking for metastatic or skip lesions.

- Metastatic neuroblastoma

  - The spine is a common site for pediatric metastatic neuroblastoma. Lytic lesions may be visible on plain radiography, but advanced imaging is required for staging.

- Leukemia

  - About 20% of children with leukemia present with musculoskeletal symptoms, including back pain. Depending upon duration of symptoms, plain imaging may show characteristic "banding" of the vertebral bodies, along with diffuse osteopenia and multiple compression fractures (Fig. 6.19). A young child with leukemia may not explicitly complain of back pain, but parents will often observe decreased activity and inability to pick objects off the floor. Think of leukemia when faced with a young child with back pain or dysfunction who also appears ill.

- Langerhans cell histiocytosis (unifocal LCH, previously known as eosinophilic granuloma or histiocytosis X)

  - This benign but sometimes locally aggressive lesion can present with vague complaints of back pain and dysfunction but rarely progresses to neurologic sequelae. Discussed above, the plain films may show a wafer-thin vertebral body, known as "vertebra plana" (see Fig. 6.16). MRI is usually done to confirm the diagnosis and rule out mimics such as malignancy or infection; sometimes a biopsy is required. The systemic or multifocal forms of LCH have several confusing names including Letterer-Siwe disease and Hand-Schuller-Christian triad which may be aggressive and fatal [16]. Therefore, it is important to thoroughly evaluate a vertebra plana lesion and to consider referral to a pediatric oncologist to rule out systemic involvement. Of note, skeletal LCH may be "cold" on nuclear bone scan. LCH is still one of the rare

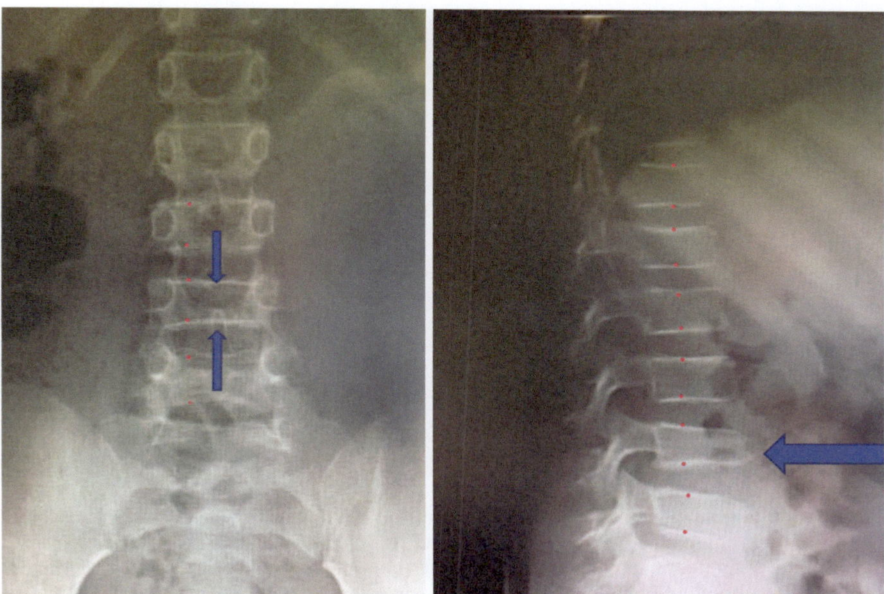

Fig. 6.19 AP and lateral radiographs of a 5-year-old girl with several weeks of back pain showing prominent vertebral end plates also known as "banding" (*red dots*), diffuse osteopenia, and compression fracture of L4 (*vertical arrows*). Her WBC count and differential were *normal*, but bone marrow aspirate showed leukemia

conditions for which a *skeletal survey* may be indicated. A skeletal survey consists of diagnostic plain films of the entire skeleton, including the skull, looking for lytic lesions.

- Aneurysmal bone cyst (ABC)

  - ABC is a misnomer; it looks like a cyst but is a true neoplasm. ABCs do not metastasize but may be fast growing and locally destructive. A patient with a spinal ABC typically presents with rapid onset of progressive back pain, cessation of sport activity, deformity, and possible neurologic impairment. MRI is almost always diagnostic showing local bone destruction and cystic fluid levels within the lesion (Fig. 6.20). Mimics are telangiectatic osteosarcoma and infection. Treatment is surgical, and recurrence is common.

Congenital

Arnold Chiari type 1 malformation and *syringomyelia* are closely related findings that may cause headaches, back pain, spinal deformity, and neurologic impairment (Fig. 6.21). They are the most commonly detected imaging abnormalities in the setting of scoliosis which may initially be thought of as idiopathic but for which MRI is ordered routinely or for suspicion of non-idiopathic (termed *atypical*) type. After

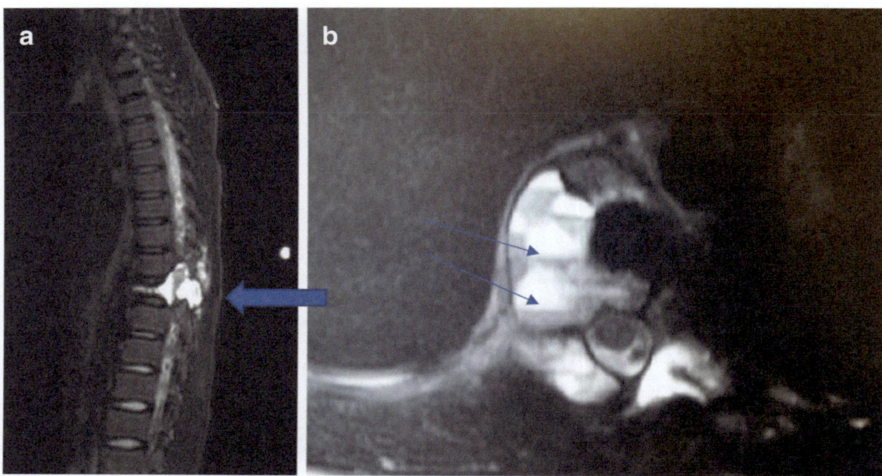

Fig. 6.20 (**a**) Aneurysmal bone cyst (ABC) presenting with rapid onset of back pain and disability in a 10-year-old boy. MR sagittal image shows vertebral collapse with high signal lesion replacing the vertebral body and occupying extradural space (*arrow*). (**b**) Transverse (axial) image shows cystic cavities with fluid levels (*small arrows*) characteristic of ABC

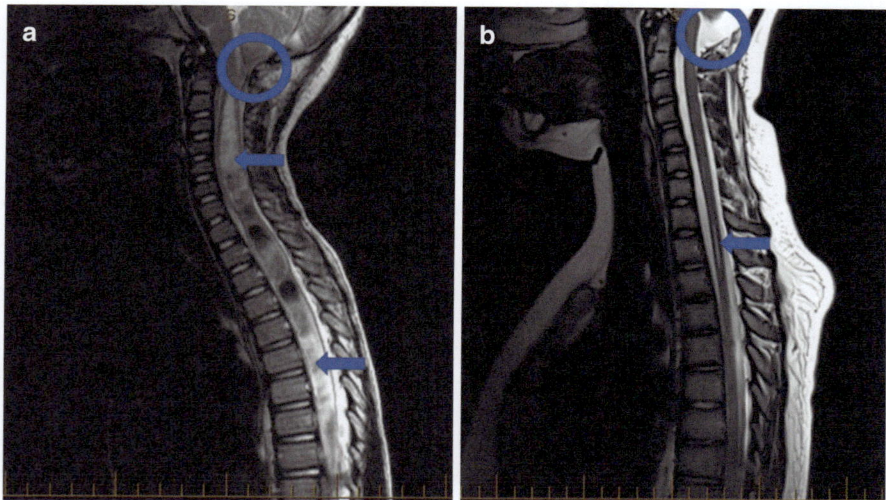

Fig. 6.21 (**a**) A 4 yo with early-onset thoracic scoliosis measuring 30 degrees. An asymmetric abdominal reflex was also noted. MRI showed a Chiari type 1 malformation (*circle*) and large syrinx extending the length of her cervical and thoracic spine (*arrows*). She underwent decompression of the Chiari malformation. (**b**) MRI at age 15 years showed resolution of the Chiari lesion (*circle*) and with only a small residual syrinx (*arrow*). Her scoliosis remained stable and never needed surgical treatment

neurosurgical consultation, the Chiari malformation is often decompressed. Rarely, the syrinx requires surgical shunt.

A *diastematomyelia* is a bone spur which runs anterior to posterior through the spinal canal, thus splitting the spinal cord or cauda equina (Fig. 6.22). As the child grows, this may create a tethering of the spinal cord or nerves and neurologic impairment. MRI will show it, but CT can be used to better define the bony anatomy preoperatively. Treatment is excision.

A more common form of *tethered cord* occurs in the filum terminale in which scar tissue from a spina bifida lesion or lipomeningocele prevents longitudinal growth as the child grows, resulting in neurologic deficits involving bowel, bladder, and lower extremities. This is best evaluated with serial MRI and neurosurgical release indicated for progressive impairment. Local clinical signs of tethered spinal cord are overlying spina bifida closure scar, nontender fatty soft tissue mass, midline dimple, or hair patch above the gluteal crease [17] (Fig. 6.23).

Congenital scoliosis is a spinal column defect present at birth, but which may not clinically or radiographically manifest until later growth and development (Fig. 6.24). There are different varieties of congenital spinal deformity described

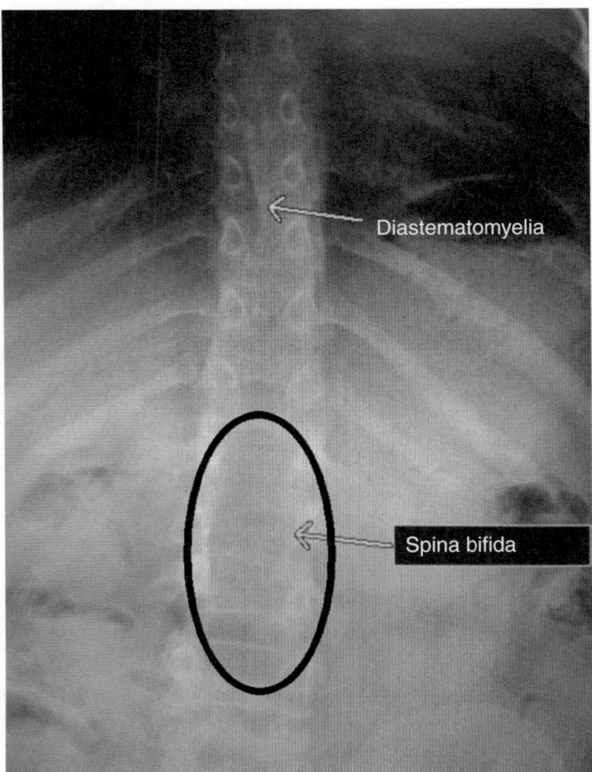

Fig. 6.22 Diastematomyelia (*arrow*). In this case, it is associated with spina bifida occulta; the circle indicates missing posterior elements in several spinal segments

Fig. 6.23 Midline hair patch in same patient as shown in Fig. 6.22

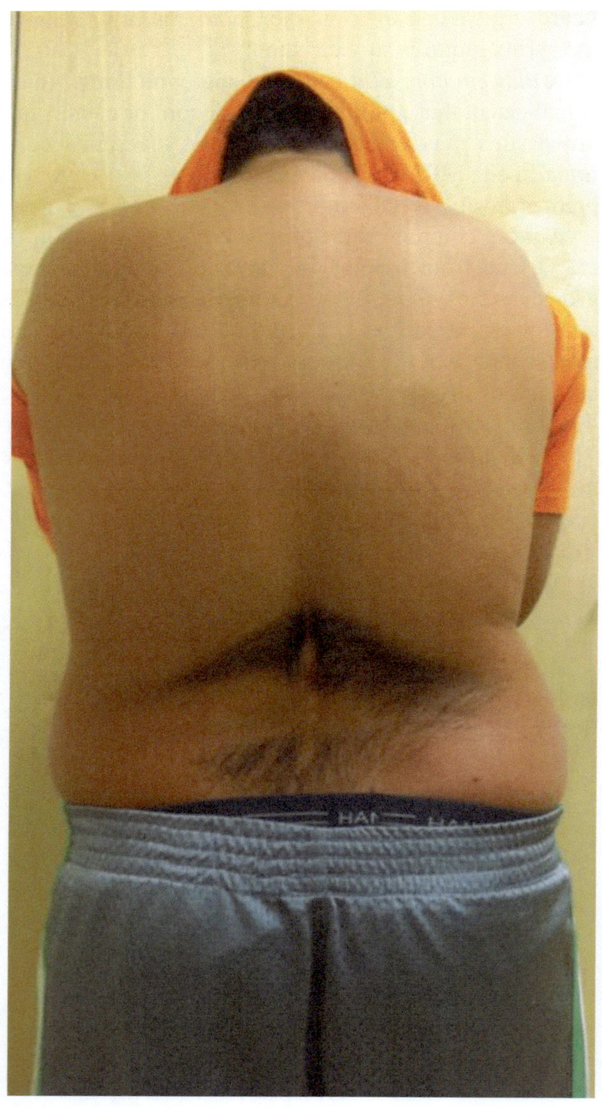

by the shape of the malformed vertebrae such as hemivertebra, butterfly vertebra, block vertebra, and bar (unilateral fused vertebrae). Fused ribs seen on chest radiography may be a clue to the presence of congenital scoliosis. Because the heart and kidneys are forming at the same embryonic time as the spine, the finding of a congenital scoliosis requires further imaging (usually ultrasound) of the heart and kidneys.

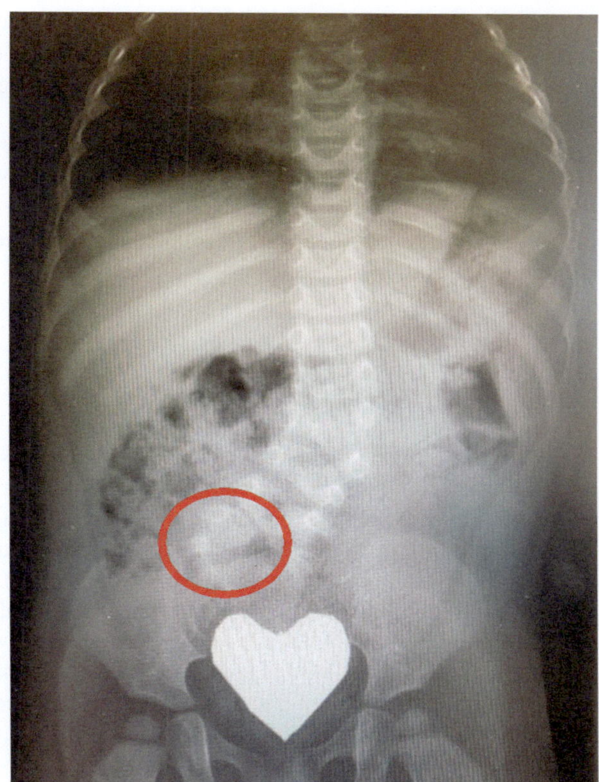

Fig. 6.24 Congenital scoliosis caused by a hemivertebra at the lumbosacral junction (*circle*) resulting in a markedly unbalanced spine

Laboratory Evaluation of Back Pain in Children and Adolescents

The initial laboratory evaluation of back pain in children and adolescents is straightforward. Laboratory studies will be normal for mechanical back pain and may be abnormal for inflammatory causes of back pain. Inflammatory causes are infectious, rheumatologic, and some neoplastic. The basic first-order studies are white blood cell (WBC), count with differential, erythrocyte sedimentation rate (ESR), and C-reactive protein (CRP). ESR and CRP are considered "acute phase reactants" which are general indicators of inflammation anywhere in the body and are therefore completely nonspecific. However, they are fairly sensitive, and it is important to know that the CRP will rise earlier than ESR in response to inflammation and will decline faster in response to treatment. Normative values depend on your hospital laboratory guidelines.

The WBC count with differential is not sensitive and therefore should not be relied upon to diagnose spinal infection or inflammatory tumor such as Ewing's sarcoma. It is useful when elevated but not useful when normal. Also, the WBC count with differential may be perfectly normal in early cases of leukemia and even later when there are bony changes visible on plain radiographs. Do not be misled by a normal WBC count.

If infection is suspected, then routine blood cultures should be obtained, if feasible, before treating with antibiotics and may need to be repeated if initially negative. Serologic studies such as coccidioidomycosis titers and Lyme disease testing may be performed for patients with unusual exposures or those who live in endemic areas.

Rheumatologic Testing

Rheumatologic testing for spinal disease in children is usually not indicated initially except for testing for HLA-B27 antigen when ankylosing spondylitis is suspected. Ankylosing spondylitis may present in a teen or young adult with morning pain and stiffness, relieved with gentle activity and tenderness around the sacroiliac joints. The flexion, abduction, and external rotation (FABER) test (see Chap. 5) may be positive for pain in the low back and sacroiliac region. Plain films may show sclerosis of the SI joints, and MRI is useful in early stages when SI joints may appear normal on plain films. If MRI is considered for suspicion of ankylosing spondylitis, first speak with your radiologist because special sequences are required to detect early imaging findings [18].

> **Pearls for Imaging Studies**
> - Be especially suspicious of children less than age 10 years and especially those less than 5 years with back pain as having an underlying etiology.
> - Plain radiographs should be obtained to *confirm* your clinical suspicion. If you suspect that a child with back pain does not have a serious condition (i.e., the out of shape teen with several week history of mechanical back pain), plain films may be delayed.
> - When obtaining plain radiographs, always obtain two views (usually PA and lateral). Be careful of excessive shielding since the film may need to be repeated if a key area of concern is hidden. Make sure your institution adheres to principles of as low as reasonably achievable (ALARA).
> - Be cautious about accepting a "normal" radiographic reading if you are suspicious of an underlying condition. Read the radiograph yourself, or go over the findings with the radiologist or orthopedic surgeon.

Editor Discussion

Ideally you will have a close working relationship with an orthopedic surgeon in your community who you can consult with for children who have more than the routine type of back pain. Although you may decide to order your own advanced imaging (CT or MRI) studies for children, there are many very distinct advantages to deferring to your orthopedic surgeon:

- For these atypical cases, you may want the specialist to see the child in consultation, so you can defer to the specialist to order the advanced imaging, if it is needed or not.
- It is not always clear what type of study is needed.
- If there are insurance precertification issues, then you will not have to deal with that.
- If the consulting orthopedic surgeon will be the treating specialist, it is often better for them to order the MRI or CT how they prefer it to be done.
- There are many decisions to be made in ordering advanced imaging: How much of the spine to image, i.e., entire cervical, thoracic, lumbar, and sacral spine? With anesthesia sedation or not? What to do with implants and other body metal? IV contrast or no contrast? Size of magnet needed? Special sequences needed? What to do with the abnormal findings? What to do with unexpected normal variations or incidental findings?
- It creates more work to have to follow up on normal MRI results and a LOT more work to follow up with the family on serious findings. The worse is to find out from the radiologist who is reading the study that you ordered that there is a spinal malignancy or infection on Friday evening, when all your staff are gone and you must talk with the family throughout the weekend.
- Often, the specialist, from her/his experience, can convince the family that MRI imaging is not needed or can be deferred to a later age, and parents will agree.

   R.M. Schwend

Imaging and lab tests compliment the history and physical exam in the evaluation of a child with back pain. This well written, comprehensive chapter helps guide the primary care physician about what study to order for suspected causes of back pain. Two-view, AP and Lateral, plain x-ray films of the area in question is always the best initial imaging study. The pediatric orthopedic surgeon or neurosurgeon may be better prepared to order advanced imaging, and leaving the decision to her about the specifics of the advanced imaging test to order is prudent. Lastly, remember that all back pain does not come from the spine, and abdominal, renal, gynecological, and hematological etiologies should be considered.

   W.L. Hennrikus

References

1. Yang S, Werner BC, Singla A, Abel MF. Low back pain in adolescents: a 1-year analysis of eventual diagnoses. J Pediatr Orthop. 2017;37(5):344–7.
2. Kjaer P, Wedderkopp N, Korsholm L, Leboeuf-Yde C. Prevalence and tracking of back pain from childhood to adolescence. BMC Musculoskelet Disord. 2011;12(1):98.
3. Smith DR, Leggat PA. Back pain in the young: a review of studies conducted among school children and university students. Curr Pediatr Rev. 2007;3(1):69–77.

4. Jones GT, MacFarlane GJ. Epidemiology of low back pain in children and adolescents. Arch Dis Child. 2005;90(3):312–6.
5. Beck NA, Miller R, Baldwin K, Zhu X, Spiegel D, Drummond D, Sankar WN, Flynn JM. Do oblique views add value in the diagnosis of spondylolysis in adolescents? J Bone Joint Surg Am. 2013;95(10):e65.
6. Korovessis PG, Stamatakis MV. Prediction of scoliotic cobb angle with the use of the scoliometer. Spine (Phila Pa 1976). 1996;21(14):1661–6.
7. Mulvihill DJ, Jhawar S, Kostis JB, Goyal S. Diagnostic medical imaging in pediatric patients and subsequent cancer risk. Acad Radiol. 2017;24(11):1456–62.
8. Pauwels EK, Bourguignon MH. Radiation dose features and solid cancer induction in pediatric computed tomography. Med Princ Pract. 2012;21(6):508–15.
9. Haaga JR, Boll D. Computed tomography & magnetic resonance imaging of the whole body E-book. Amsterdam, Edinburgh, Oxford, London, New York, Philadelphia, and St. Louis: Elsevier Health Sciences; 2016.
10. Pang D, Wilberger JE. Spinal cord injury without radiographic abnormalities in children. J Neurosurg. 1982;57(1):114–29.
11. Drubach LA. Nuclear medicine techniques in pediatric bone imaging. In seminars in nuclear medicine 2017 May 1 (Vol. 47, No. 3, pp. 190–203). WB Saunders.
12. Al-Tawil K, Lopez D, Blackman M, Suresh S. Oblique "Scotty dog" versus antero-posterior (AP) views in performing x-ray guided facet joint injections. J Clin Orthop Trauma. 2018;9:S145–8.
13. Libson E, Bloom RA, Dinari G. Symptomatic and asymptomatic spondylolysis and spondylolisthesis in young adults. Int Orthop. 1983;6(4):259–61.
14. Hresko MT, Labelle H, Roussouly P, Berthonnaud E. Classification of high-grade spondylolistheses based on pelvic version and spine balance: possible rationale for reduction. Spine. 2007;32(20):2208–13.
15. Koplas MC, Simonelli PS, Bauer TW, Joyce MJ, Sundaram M. Your diagnosis? Chronic recurrent multifocal osteomyelitis. Orthopedics. 2010;33(4):218.
16. Allen CE, Merad M, McClain KL. Langerhans-cell histiocytosis. New Eng J Med. 2018;379(9):856–68.
17. Dias MS. Innocent pits and dermal sinus tracts: an oft-misdiagnosed distinction [Internet]. AAP Gateway. American Academy of Pediatrics; 2010 [cited 2019Mar10]. Available from: https://www.aappublications.org/content/31/7/39.
18. Mease PJ. Diagnosis and management of ankylosing spondylitis: key concepts for the non-rheumatologist [Internet]. PeerView. Penn State College of Medicine and PVI, PeerView Institute for Medical Education, Novartis Pharmaceuticals Corporation; 2018 [cited 2019Mar10]. Available from: http://www.peerview.com/p/index.html?collection=150204919&presentation=150204919-p1&SpecialtyID=180&ProfessionID=18&AOMID=32&Promocode=900#screen1.

Chapter 7
Putting It All Together: What to Keep and What to Refer?

Richard M. Schwend

> *"Back pain in a nutshell- what is the child's growth (age and maturity) and what is the underlying diagnosis?"*
>
> Richard Schwend
>
> *"Young children are all about activity, teenagers about appearance, adults about comfort."*
>
> Colin Mosely

Practice Gap

Twenty to thirty percent of office visits may be for musculoskeletal-related disorders, but only about 2% of time in pediatric residency training is spent on musculoskeletal medicine [1]. Many pediatricians in training and practice describe a deficiency in knowledge, competency, confidence, and performance in the evaluation of a child with a musculoskeletal condition.

Change of Practice

Perform a focused history and physical examination on all children with back pain, and when appropriate, obtain plain radiographs and laboratory tests. Make an accurate diagnosis, appropriate treatment, or timely referral.

Electronic Supplementary Material The online version of this chapter (https://doi.org/10.1007/978-3-030-50758-9_7) contains supplementary material, which is available to authorized users.

R. M. Schwend (✉)
Department of Orthopaedic Surgery, Children's Mercy Hospital, Kansas City, MO, USA
e-mail: rmschwend@cmh.edu

© Springer Nature Switzerland AG 2021
R. M. Schwend, W. L. Hennrikus (eds.), *Back Pain in the Young Child and Adolescent*, https://doi.org/10.1007/978-3-030-50758-9_7

> **Learning Objectives**
> - Perform a focused, practical back examination including a neurological exam.
> - Understand ten history and ten physical red flags associated with back pain. These will be emphasized in the case studies in Chaps. 8–32.
> - Understand when to treat and follow a patient yourself and when to refer.

Epidemiology

Back pain is very common in children and even more common in adults. Although at any given time fewer than 10% of children have back pain, approximately a third of adolescents presenting to a pediatric sports practice report having had back pain in the past year [2]. As with pain in general, back pain is a nonspecific complaint that is more prevalent in older children, females, those with a greater BMI, backpack wearers, and those who participate in sports [2]. Many cases of back pain should be considered as a normal life experience, and for some children, no treatment is needed. Surgery is rarely indicated, so it should be unusual to refer a child with "back pain" and no underlying diagnosis to a surgeon. Despite this, nonspecific back pain is a very common reason for a referral to an orthopedic surgeon from a pediatrician office [3].

The actual prevalence of an underlying diagnosis depends on the population and referral pattern. In a subspecialty pediatric spine practice, a cause for the back pain was found in 85% of cases [4]. However, more recent studies from emergency room and office settings reported the reverse to be the case. Brooks et al., in a review of pediatric emergency department cases, found a non-pathologic diagnosis in 77% of back pain visits. Brooks reported that the pain was due to mechanical back pain or muscle strain in most cases [5]. Only 2.3% of visits had an underlying pathologic diagnosis, with plain radiographs rather than MRI, CT, or laboratory studies helping to make the diagnosis. Another emergency room study about back pain found the following diagnoses: direct trauma (25%), muscle strain (24%), sickle cell crisis (13%), idiopathic (13%), urinary tract infection (5%), and viral (4%) [6]. Feldman et al. in Toronto evaluated a wide age range of children with disabling back pain presenting to a pediatric orthopedic office using SPECT scan [7]. The study population included young children (range 2.7–17 years old) and children having severe pain. In 78% of cases, there was no obvious etiology. Spondylolysis was found in 7%, tumor in 4.6%, and "other" in 10% (infection, Scheuermann kyphosis, herniated disc, kidney disease, facet arthritis, disc disease, congenital anomalies, and tethered spinal cord) [7]. Miller likewise reported that 78% of children 10–19 years of age presenting with back pain had mechanical low back pain [8].

Risk Factors

Some risk factors may be preventable: high BMI, smoking, sport specialization with overuse, excessive muscle tightness, working excessive hours, and backpack use [9]. Backpacks may cause short-term pain. More pain occurs if the backpack is of a large weight or if not worn properly. One author reports that backpacks can cause an acute loss of disc height on MRI [10]. Sports specialization in soccer, basketball and lacrosse, baseball, tennis, and football can lead to back pain and spondylolysis even in the fittest of athletes [11].

Natural History

A history of back pain in childhood is the best predictor of back pain as an adult [12]. A large Danish twin study confirmed this association of low back pain in childhood and adolescence and low back pain in adults [13]. While one-half of adolescents entering adulthood continue to have a low prevalence of back pain, up to 10–33% will have either an increase or persistently high prevalence of low back pain as adults [14, 15]. Feldman et al. found that for children with disabling pain, 71% continued to have pain years later [7].

Difference Between a Younger and Older Child

Postnatal growth is greatest during infancy. Young children are very active, and some have pain by the end of the day. The pain can be nonspecific (growing pains) and poorly localized. Very young children with significant back pain may present with abdominal pain, pelvic pain, or reluctance to walk. As the child becomes older, pain localization becomes easier, but the common locations of pain can change. For example, in a cross-sectional study of children in Denmark, thoracic back pain was most common in childhood; lumbar and thoracic pain was equally common in adolescents. Neck pain or pain in more than one location was unusual [16].

General Principles of Back Pain in Children

- Back pain is a symptom not a diagnosis, so always seek the underlying diagnosis.
- Under age 10 years, think of inflammation and the pitfall diagnoses to avoid missing tumors and infections. Inflammation = stiffness. This inflammation can show up as night pain, limp, or refusal to walk.

- For the child older than age 10 years, think of mechanical etiology, spondylolysis, spondylolisthesis, or Scheuermann kyphosis, but don't forget the pitfall diagnoses.
- Some conditions are seen in all ages: infection, injury, osteochondromas, osteoid osteoma, and mechanical back pain.
- Pitfall diagnoses don't always present with significant back pain.
- Always examine the patient distally for signs of neurological dysfunction. Inquire about bowel or bladder dysfunction. Also ask about limb pain, spasticity, weakness, numbness or other symptoms, and difficulty walking or running.
- Always examine the feet when evaluating the spine, and examine the spine when evaluating the feet.
- Scoliosis may or may not have associated back pain. It is helpful to classify scoliosis into four different types: idiopathic, congenital, syndromic, and neuromuscular. This helps with determining associated workup needed, natural history, treatment, and appropriate referral.

Ten History Red Flags
- Children under age 10 years
- Loss of function related to the pain
- Recurring or worsening pain
- Early morning stiffness
- Night pain
- Localized pain
- A child that stops walking or playing
- Fever or weight loss
- Postural change
- Limp or altered gait

Physical Examination

William Osler taught the four key components of the physical examination: inspection, palpation, auscultation, and contemplation. Inspection starts when you first meet the child and family. Inspect the child's appearance and behavior. Palpation can start with a handshake, if appropriate, and later during the actual hands on physical examination. In a patient with back pain, auscultation occurs with careful listening to the child's story. General recommendations are as follows: The child needs to have shorts on and shoes and socks off. Pay attention to overall features such as height, weight, BMI, and rate of growth since previous visits. Look at the child's appearance and comfort. Does she look ill? Check nutrition. Check developmental stages, Tanner stage, and other measures of maturity. Menses typically occurs after the growth spurt. Growth spurt is typically during Tanner stage 2 or 3. Inspect with your mind wide open. Look for syndromic or associated conditions. Check posture, balance, motion, strength, and reflexes including the abdominal reflex (Video 7.1). Evaluate trunk core muscle strength by asking the patient to do things such as get off the floor (Gower sign), squat, perform push-ups and sit-ups, and walk and run down the hall. Examine the child supine and prone. Always examine the bare feet. A screening spine examination can be completed in under 2 minutes (Video 7.2). Finally, the most important phase of the examination is contemplation. Pause and reflect about the findings and what might be the underlying cause.

Ten Red Flags of Physical Examination
- Child impossible to examine due to pain
- Poor nutrition
- Fever and tachycardia
- Deformity of the spine—scoliosis, kyphosis, and lordosis
- Lymphadenopathy or other masses
- Back tenderness
- Stiffness
- Limp, reluctance to walk, or altered gait
- Any neurological deficit
- Bowel or bladder dysfunction

Pitfalls to Avoid
- An overly aggressive workup of nonspecific back pain. A laboratory and radiographic workup may not reveal the underlying cause, sometimes because there is no underlying disease.
- Going straight to MRI or CT scan.
- Although rare, be aware of the disasters to avoid such as tumor or infection.
- Examining the patient only one time—If unsure, see the patient again.
- Referral to the orthopedic surgeon for back pain without doing a workup.
- If still unsure after a workup, obtain a consult, or discuss the case over the phone with your orthopedic colleague.
- Think outside the spine box.

Referring Patients

What to Keep
- Nonspecific back pain or no specific diagnosis in a child >10 years old with a normal exam and worku
- Postural kyphosis
- Spondylolysis or grade 1 spondylolisthesis responsive to rest and therapy (Fig. 7.1)
- Mild adolescent scoliosis (AIS) measuring <20 degrees on x-ray
- Apical trunk rotation (ATR) on the scoliometer <7 degrees

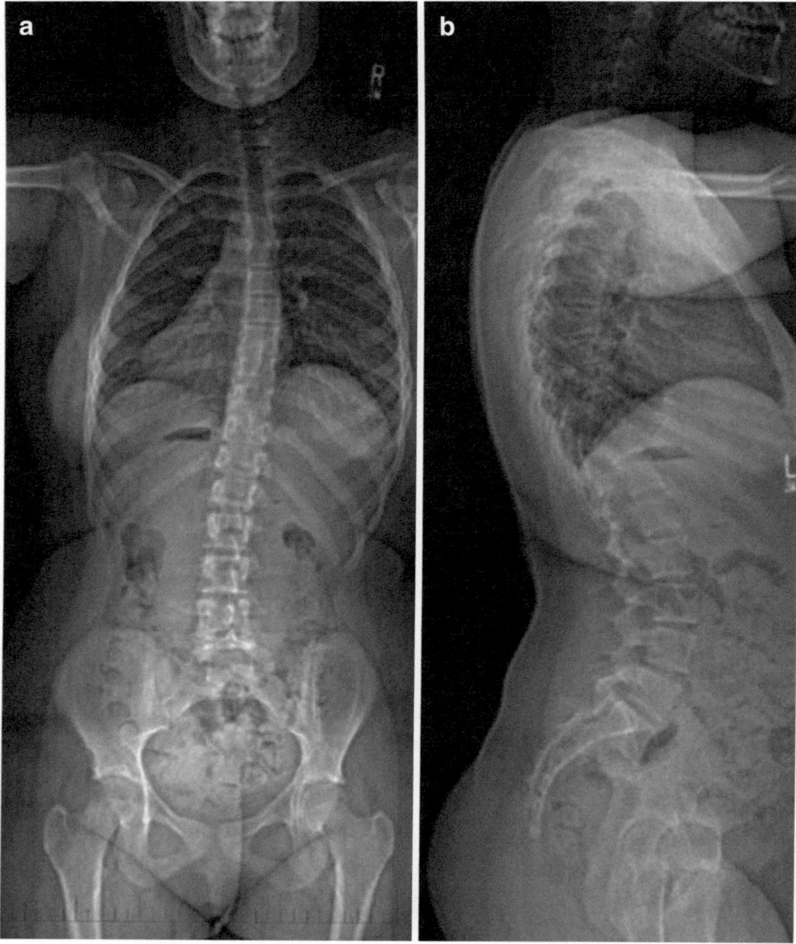

Fig. 7.1 A 12-year-old girl had a 3-month history of low back pain after starting volleyball. Pain was worse by end of the day and after practice or games. It was relieved by a 2-week period of rest. There was no radiation of the pain to the lower extremities or weakness. She had not started menses. Examination showed that she was overweight with a BMI of 26. She stood with mild trunk shift to the right, had a flexible spine, but noticed low back pain with hyperextension. Her core muscles were weak. Screening 2 minute spine exam was otherwise normal. (**a**) Posteroanterior (PA) radiograph shows mild trunk shift to the right with minimal scoliosis. (**b**) Lateral radiograph was normal. (**c**) Lateral radiograph focused at L5 S1 showed no evidence of spondylolysis or spondylolisthesis. The posterior elements of L5 appear normal. Clinically, she was felt to have spondylolisthesis. Core strengthening, nutrition counselling, and taking a break from volleyball were recommended by her pediatrician which helped initially. (**d**) Six weeks later, she was back competing in volleyball and the pain recurred. CT scan was performed, which showed a unilateral pars defect (open black arrow) on the axial image. The spondylolysis defect had minimal gap and appeared to be attempting to heal. Her symptoms eventually resolved by waiting out the volleyball season. She never needed a brace or surgery. This case is an example of a child with spondylolysis who was successfully treated without referral to the orthopedic service

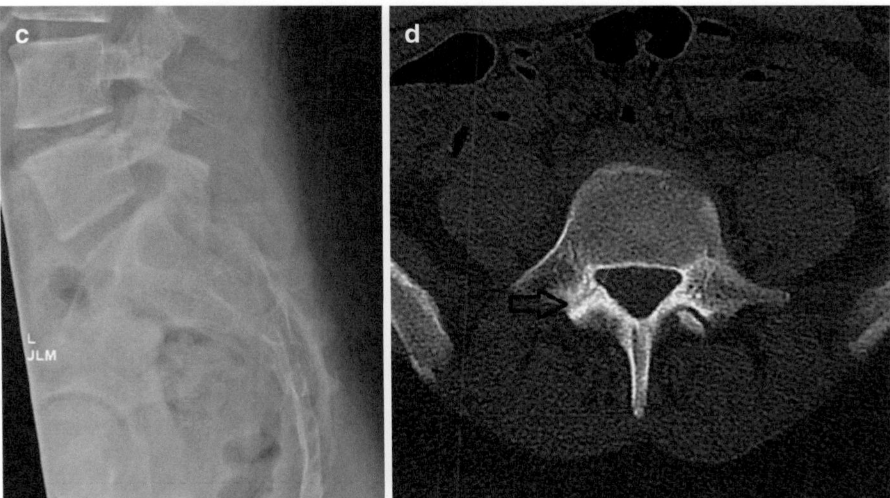

Fig. 7.1 (continued)

What to Refer
- In general, it is best to have a presumptive diagnosis for the back pain to better understand the condition and natural history and to whom the referral should go.
- Unexplained back pain in a young child <10 years old, especially if <5 years old.
- Scheuermann kyphosis in a growing child.
- Spondylolisthesis grade 0/1 not responsive to conservative treatment (Fig. 7.1).
- Grade 2 or greater spondylolisthesis (Fig. 7.2).
- AIS >20 degrees in a growing child.
- Apical trunk rotation (ATR) on the scoliometer >7 degrees.
- Underlying diagnosis of syndromic, congenital, or neuromuscular scoliosis or structural kyphosis.
- Neurological findings such as weakness, numbness, bowel or bladder involvement, clonus, and spasticity.
- Red flags of history or physical examination.
- If you are not sure if a patient should be referred, call your orthopedic colleague on the phone directly.

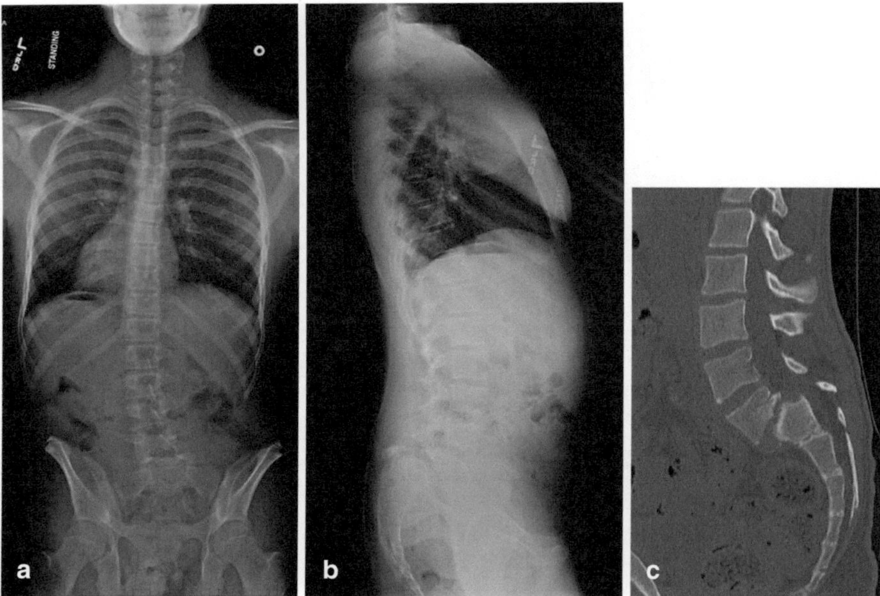

Fig. 7.2 A 14-year-old boy had a 3-year history of mild back pain. Over the past several months, the pain has increased in intensity and began to radiate down his right lower extremity to the foot. He also began walking with legs that were "stiff" and he had difficulty running fast. Parents noticed that his posture looked "odd." He was not an athlete. Physical examination showed him to have scoliosis, a posterior pelvic tilt, stiffness on forward bend, hamstring tightness, mild weakness of right ankle dorsiflexion, and short stride when walking. (**a**) Standing PA radiograph showed a long left apex scoliosis. This has an atypical appearance, which is frequently seen in painful spondylolisthesis. (**b**) Standing lateral radiograph shows a vertical sacrum, rounding of the dome of the sacrum, trapezoidal-shaped L5, and greater than 50% forward slip of L5 on S1 (grade 3). These features are typical for high-grade (>50% slip) dysplastic (abnormal-shaped bones) spondylolisthesis. (**c**) CT scan confirmed the high-grade forward slip of L5 on S1 as well as the dysplastic bony features of the L5 S1 articulation. Red flags include the back stiffness, gait abnormality, radiation of pain to the foot, weakness of dorsiflexion on examination, and the high-grade and dysplastic nature of the slip. Once a spondylolisthesis has slipped more than 50%, it frequently needs surgical treatment. Referral to orthopedic spine surgeon is indicated

Treatment

Treatment depends on the underlying diagnosis and anticipated natural history. Fortunately, most children with back pain have a self-limited condition related to sports activity, overuse, or deconditioning. The pain requires either no treatment or modification of risk factors such as weight management, rest, core strengthening, proper backpack wear, and modifying work schedules. Having the symptom of back pain is an opportunity for the physician to review lifestyle habits with the adolescent including sleep hygiene, nutrition, physical activity, stress, work, screen time, and posture. When a specific diagnosis is made, treatment can be prescribed or a referral to the appropriate specialist performed.

Summary

Back pain is very common in children and even more common in adults. Back pain is a symptom, not a diagnosis, so seek a deeper understanding of the condition. Always evaluate the child's development and growth. Be very concerned about a young child with a stiff spine, night pain, or abnormal neurological findings. Seek the underlying diagnosis in evaluating back pain or scoliosis. For the child under age 10 years, consider inflammation and the common pitfalls to avoid—especially tumors and infections. Stiffness can be a sign of inflammation. This inflammation can show up as night pain, limp, or refusal to walk. For the child older than age 10 years, think of mechanical origins, spondylolysis, spondylolisthesis, or Scheuermann kyphosis, but don't forget the possible pitfalls. After a thorough evaluation, there may be no specific diagnosis, and you then need to reassure the family and provide comfort.

References

1. Murphy RF, LaPorte DM, Wadey VM, American Academy of Orthopaedic Surgeons Orthopaedic Education Study Group. Musculoskeletal education in medical school: deficits in knowledge and strategies for improvement. J Bone Joint Surg Am. 2014;96(23):2009–14.
2. Peter Fabricant. The epidemiology of Back pain in children and adolescents: a cross-sectional study of 3,669 American youth. Paper presented at: American Academy of Orthopaedic Surgeons. 2019 March 13;Las Vegas.
3. Schwend RM, Geiger J. Outpatient pediatric orthopedics: common and important conditions. Pediatr Clin N Am. 1998;45(4):943–71.
4. Hensinger RN. Acute back pin in children. Instr Course Lect. 1995;44:111–26.
5. Brooks TM, Friedman LM, Silvis RM. Back pain in a pediatric emergency department: etiology and evaluation. Pediatr Emerg Care. 2018;34(1):e1–6.
6. Selbst SM, Lavelle JM, Soyupack SK, Markowitz RI. Back pain in children who present to the emergency department. Clin Pediatr. 1999;38(7):401–6.
7. Feldman DS, Hedden DM, Wright JG. The use of bone scan to investigate back pain in children and adolescents. J Pediatr Orthop. 2000;20(6):790–5.
8. Miller R, Beck NA, Sampson NR, Zhu X, Flynne JM, Drummond D. Imaging modalities for low back pain in children: a review of spondylolysis and undiagnosed mechanical back pain. J Pediatr Orthop. 2013;33(3):282–8.
9. Korovessis P, Koureas G, Papazisis Z. Correlation between backpack weight and way of carrying. J Spinal Disord Tech. 2004;17(1):33–40.
10. Talbott NR, Bhattacharya A, Davis KG, Shukla R, Levin L. School backpacks: it's more than just a weight problem. Work. 2009;34(4):481–94.
11. Ladenhauf HN, Fabricant PD, Grossman E, Widmann R, Green DW. Athletic participation in children with symptomatic spondylolysis in the New York area. Med Sci Sports Exerc. 2013;45(10) 1971–4.
12. Jones GT, MacFarlane GJ. Epidemiology of low back pain in children and adolescents. Arch Dis Child. 2005;90(3):321–6.
13. Hestbaek L, Leboeuf-Yde C, Kyvik KO, Manniche C. The course of low back pain from adolescence to adulthood: eight-year follow-up of 9600 twins. Spine. 2006;31(4):468–72.
14. Junge T, Wedderkopp N, Boyle E, Kjaer P. The natural course of low back pain from childhood to young adulthood- a systematic review. Chiropr Man Therap. 2019;27:10.

15. Coenen P, Smith A, Paananen M, O'Sullivan P, Beales D, Straker L. Trajectories of low back pain from adolescence to young adulthood. Arthritis Care Res (Hoboken). 2017;69(3):403–12.
16. Wedderkopp N, Leboeuf-Yde C, Anderson LB, Froberg K, Hansen HS. Back pain reporting pattern in a Danish population-based sample of children and adolescents. Spine. 2001;26(17):1879–83.

Resources

Good site for 5 simple steps to a pain free back. https://www.health.harvard.edu/pain/5-steps-to-a-pain-free-back . Accessed May 7, 2019.

Part II
Case Studies

Chapter 8
Case of an Adolescent Male with Back Pain and Poor Posture: Scheuermann's Kyphosis

Stephanie B. Ihnow and Peter F. Sturm

Brief Case Presentation

Chief Complaint

Two-year history of worsening upper back pain and poor posture.

History

This is a 16-year-old male with no significant past medical history who presents with 2 years of worsening upper back pain and "poor posture." Per the parents, their son hunches over constantly. His back pain started 2 years ago when he was playing baseball. There is no history of trauma or injury. The back pain has progressed to the point that it now limits his ability to participate in sports and other activities. Additionally, the parents have noticed that he has been leaning forward more, and he agrees that he hunches over more than other kids his age. Sitting or standing for prolonged periods of time makes the pain worse, while laying down makes it better. The pain does not wake him up at night. He has been taking anti-inflammatory medications for the pain without much relief. He has also tried physical therapy and activity modification but has had little relief of his pain or improvement in his

S. B. Ihnow
Division of Pediatric Orthopaedic Surgery, Cincinnati Children's Hospital Medical Center, Cincinnati, OH, USA

P. F. Sturm (✉)
Spine Surgery, Crawford Spine Center, Division of Pediatric Orthopaedic Surgery, Cincinnati Children's Hospital Medical Center, Cincinnati, OH, USA
e-mail: Peter.Sturm@cchmc.org

© Springer Nature Switzerland AG 2021
R. M. Schwend, W. L. Hennrikus (eds.), *Back Pain in the Young Child and Adolescent*, https://doi.org/10.1007/978-3-030-50758-9_8

posture. He has no numbness, tingling, radicular pain, and bowel or bladder incontinence or retention. There is no family history of spine problems, and he has normal physical development for his age.

Physical Examination

Weight 85 kg, height 174.6 cm, and BMI 27.9. He is a well-developed, mildly overweight adolescent male. He stands with a rounded thoracic spine and lumbar hyperlordosis. There was hyperkyphosis in the thoracic region with forward bend but no scoliosis noted. He had tenderness to midline palpation and over the paraspinal muscles in the thoracic spine. There was no tenderness to palpation in the cervical and lumbar spine. The neurologic examination, including lower extremity sensory, motor, and reflexes, Babinski test, and gait were normal. He was able to touch his mid-shins on forward bend. Popliteal angle was 30 degrees bilaterally when supine.

Imaging and Radiographic Studies *(Figs. 8.1 and 8.2)*

Questions About the Case the Reader Should Consider
1. What could be the cause of the patient's "poor posture"?
2. Why does the patient have back pain?
3. What is the appropriate referral?
4. What is the next diagnostic test that should be considered?
5. What are the possible treatment options?
6. What operative treatment could be recommended?

Discussion

Kyphosis, or an outward curvature of the spine, is normal in the thoracic spine, to an extent. On the other hand, lordosis, or an inward curvature of the spine, is normal in the cervical and lumbar spines. When a patient has excessive kyphosis, it can be considered abnormal. The excessive kyphosis can have several underlying causes (see below), including postural kyphosis, fixed kyphosis due to Scheuermann's disease, kyphosis due to compression fractures, or kyphosis due to other spinal abnormalities. Postural kyphosis is common in children and adolescents and is correctable with postural training [1]. With postural kyphosis, radiographs are typically normal, and the kyphosis is flexible. In Scheuermann's kyphosis, on the other hand, radiographs show increased (>45 degrees) thoracic kyphosis which does not correct very much with back extension. Other radiographic findings, as identified by Sørensen [2], include wedging of at least three consecutive vertebral bodies by 5°, Schmorl's

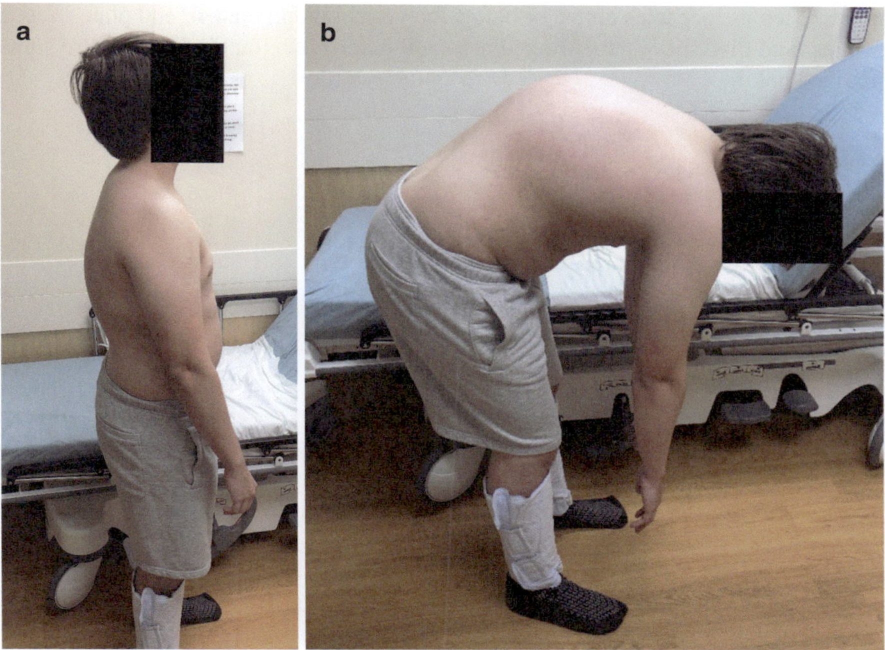

Fig. 8.1 (**a**) Standing lateral spine. Noticeable hyperkyphosis in the thoracic region and hyperlordosis in the lumbar region. (**b**) Forward bend lateral spine. Notice the area of increased focal kyphosis

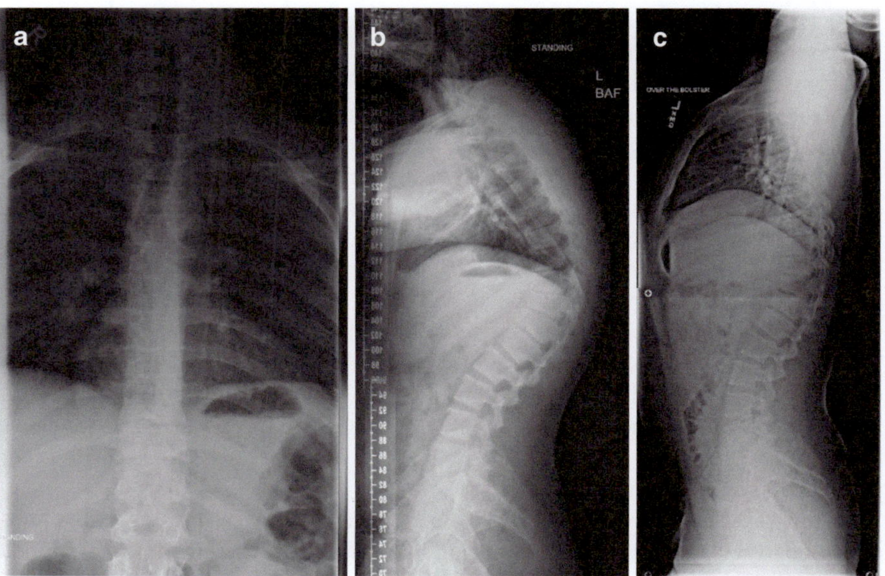

Fig. 8.2 (**a**) Posteroanterior (PA) and (**b**) lateral standing radiographs. There is thoracic kyphosis of 87 degrees with an apex at T7. The pelvis is Risser stage 5. There is no associated scoliosis. (**c**) Lateral radiograph over a bolster. The thoracic kyphosis corrects to 50 degrees when the patient lays on a bolster

nodes (seen as lucencies above or below the vertebral end plates), end plate irregularities, and disc space narrowing. These and other radiographic findings are summarized below.

Differential Diagnosis of Kyphosis
- Postural kyphosis
- Scheuermann's kyphosis
- Compression fracture
- Congenital kyphosis
- Neuromuscular kyphosis

Radiographic Features of Scheuermann's Kyphosis
- Thoracic kyphosis >45 degrees
- Anterior wedging of 5 or more degrees in three adjacent vertebral bodies
- Disc space narrowing
- End plate irregularities
- Presence of Schmorl's nodes (due to herniation of disc into vertebral end plates)
- Limited correction of kyphosis on an extension radiograph
- Hyperlordosis of the lumbar spine (compensatory in thoracic Scheuermann's kyphosis)

Scheuermann's kyphosis is the number one cause of thoracic-level back pain in children and adolescents [2], with as many as 60% of patients with Scheuermann's kyphosis having associated back pain [3, 4]. As many as 50% of patients present with back pain as their initial symptom [2]. Associated lumbar back pain is not uncommon and can be from spondylosis or spondylolisthesis, which is found in approximately 11% of these patients [5]. This high prevalence of concomitant lumbar spine pathology is thought to be from the added stress on the pars interarticularis from the compensatory hyperlordosis of the lumbar spine [5]. Additionally, many patients with Scheuermann's kyphosis have tight hamstrings, which contribute to the lumbar hyperlordosis and resulting back pain [6].

Patients with mild Scheuermann's kyphosis (less than 60 thoracic kyphosis degrees) and associated back pain can be referred to physical therapy and followed with radiographs of the spine to check for progression [7]. Once the kyphosis reaches 60 degrees, the patient should be referred to a pediatric spine specialist for further evaluation and management.

In this case, the only further imaging to consider is focused imaging of the lumbar spine to rule out spondylolysis or spondylolisthesis if that cannot be determined from the full-spine radiographs. If neurologic changes had been present, advanced

Table 8.1 Treatment Options in Scheuermann's Kyphosis

Classification	Treatment
Mild (kyphosis of 45 to 60 degrees). Mild Scheuermann kyphosis often resembles postural kyphosis and may require a radiograph to distinguish the two	Observation if asymptomatic Anti-inflammatories, physical therapy, and/or activity modification if symptomatic
Moderate (kyphosis 60 to 75–80 degrees)	Bracing if growth remaining Observation if asymptomatic and reached skeletal maturity Anti-inflammatories, physical therapy, and/or activity modification if reached skeletal maturity and symptomatic
Severe (kyphosis >75 degrees)	Observation if no significant discomfort or symptoms Operative treatment: posterior spinal instrumentation and fusion ± osteotomies (depends on severity and stiffness of curve)

imaging, specifically an MRI of the spine, would be recommended. However, for this case, with a kyphosis of 87 degrees, he will be referred to a pediatric spine surgeon, and any further specialized imaging should be obtained by the specialist.

Treatment options for Scheuermann's kyphosis include conservative measures (medications, stretching, physical therapy), bracing, or surgery. Table 8.1 lists the treatment options according to severity of the kyphosis. For mild kyphosis and back pain, the patient should be referred to physical therapy for core strengthening and stretching exercises, including the back and hamstrings. Over-the-counter anti-inflammatory medications can be used as well. Bracing is indicated when the curve is over 60 degrees and the patient has growth remaining. Bracing is difficult because of the type of brace needed to control the kyphosis (Milwaukee brace). Patient acceptance of the Milwaukee brace is usually poor; however, when the patient is compliant with brace wear, the outcomes are good, with skeletally immature patients having curves between 55 and 80 degrees achieving 27% and 40% improvement of the kyphosis [8]. There is some evidence that a thoracolumbar sacral orthosis (TLSO) can be effective in the treatment of Scheuermann's [9, 10]. Additionally, new lower-profile braces are in development and have shown promising results in kyphosis treatment [8].

Operative intervention is considered when the kyphosis approaches 75–80°, especially when having pain or functional problems. Surgery consists of a posterior spinal fusion with or without osteotomies depending on the flexibility of the kyphosis. Screws are placed at the top (usually upper thoracic) and bottom (usually lumbar spine) of the construct along with the apex of the kyphosis. Rods are then attached to the screws, and a cantilever technique is used to straighten the spine. The lamina is decorticated, and allograft bone graft is added to help the spine fuse along the instrumentation. The rods and screws work to hold the spine in place until the vertebra fuse together.

How to Approach the Case

Poor posture is common in adolescents; however, progressive hunching over and uncontrolled back pain are not typical. Progressive kyphosis of the spine should be investigated as this is not typical of postural kyphosis. When the kyphosis is progressive or is associated with back pain, imaging (i.e., a radiograph) should be obtained to rule out causes other than postural kyphosis. A careful history from both the patient and the parent/caregiver is important. This patient did not have neurologic deficits, but a careful history should be elicited, and physical examination should be performed to ensure the patient is neurologically intact, as this is a reason for an urgent referral to a specialist. For this patient, his degree of kyphosis and lack of neurologic involvement should prompt a nonurgent referral to a specialist before initiating treatment, including physical therapy.

Final Diagnosis

Scheuermann's kyphosis.

Natural History and Treatment Considerations

Scheuermann's kyphosis can be progressive, especially in skeletally immature patients. For this reason, these patients need to be followed for worsening of the kyphosis and treated with bracing or surgery, when indicated. Patients with mild Scheuermann's kyphosis often do not have any long-term complications from their deformity; however, those with moderate to severe kyphosis tend to have higher rates of back pain in adulthood. In one study by Murray et al. [11], 67 patients with Scheuermann's kyphosis were followed for an average of 32 years. Their mean kyphosis was 71 degrees. Compared to age-matched controls, patients with Scheuermann's kyphosis had more intense thoracic back pain, less thoracic extension, and less demanding jobs but were similar in terms of missed days from work, social limitations, pain medication use, and activity level. Overall, the long-term consequences of mild to moderate kyphosis are low. However, in those patients with kyphosis greater than 100 degrees, there is a higher incidence of restrictive lung disease along with increased pain [11]. Lastly, the effect on self-image secondary to the deformity should not be underestimated and is another factor to take into consideration when discussing treatment options with patients. In this case, the above factors were discussed in detail with the patient and parents, and it was decided to proceed with surgery in the form of posterior spinal fusion (Fig. 8.3).

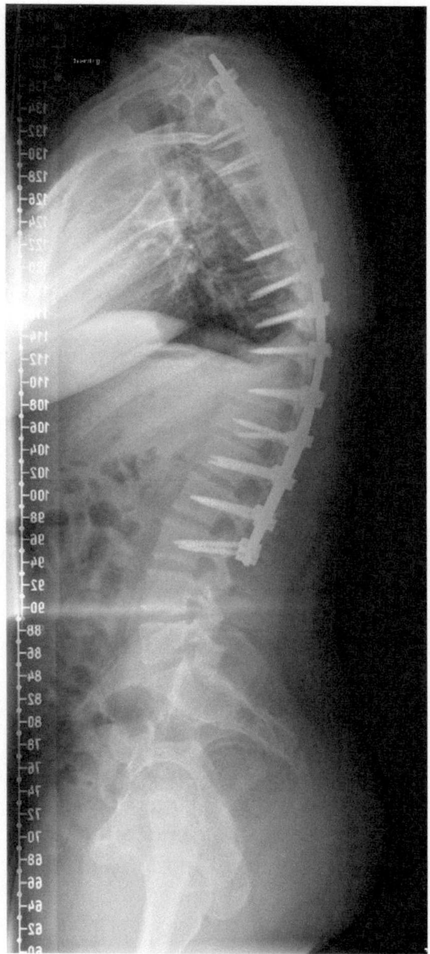

Fig. 8.3 Postoperative lateral radiograph showing improvement in kyphosis

Referral: Emergency, Urgent, or Routine—And to Whom?

Fixed kyphosis with radiographic features of Scheuermann's disease should be referred to a spine specialist (i.e., orthopedic surgery) for further evaluation, management, and follow-up. Mild disease (up to 60 degrees) can be a routine referral. More severe kyphosis (above 60 degrees) that would qualify for brace and/or surgical treatment should be referred on a more urgent basis, within about a month. If neurologic changes are present, the patient should be seen urgently, within a day, by a pediatric spine specialist to rule out more dangerous, acute causes.

Key Features and Pearls

- Thoracic kyphosis can have multiple underlying causes, both postural and structural. Mild kyphosis associated with back pain can initially be treated with anti-inflammatories, physical therapy (hyperextension exercises and core strengthening), and activity modification.
- Fixed kyphosis of the thoracic spine (does not correct with extension) is concerning for Scheuermann's kyphosis. Patients with fixed kyphosis should be referred to a specialist for further evaluation and treatment.
- Scheuermann's kyphosis in the thoracic spine is often associated with back pain that can persist into adulthood. Severe Scheuermann's kyphosis can be treated with surgery during adolescence to minimize complications later in life.

Brief Summary

Postural abnormalities, especially kyphosis, are common in children and adolescents. This is often due to postural kyphosis and can be corrected with reinforcement or physical therapy. Fixed, progressive kyphosis is more worrisome and can be caused by structural changes in the spine, such as from fractures or Scheuermann's kyphosis. The back pain associated with kyphosis is treated based on the underlying cause and the severity. When not accompanied by neurologic changes, physical therapy is a reasonable initial treatment. This can improve postural kyphosis and/or the back pain associated with Scheuermann's kyphosis. When the deformity becomes severe and the back pain is chronic, a specialist should be involved, and treatment may include bracing or operative intervention. With severe Scheuermann's kyphosis, surgery in the form of posterior spinal instrumentation and fusion may improve the back pain associated with the kyphosis and can improve patient self-image.

Editor Discussion

Scheuermann's kyphosis is an osteochondrosis—a growth disturbance producing vertebral wedging, shortening of the anterior column of the spine, and kyphosis. The deformity is named after Danish surgeon Holger Scheuermann. Boys are affected more often. Scheuermann's is partly a cosmetic problem. Milan Lucic, NHL hockey star, and Hunter Pence, major league baseball star, both had Scheuermann's—treated conservatively. Some children can hide their deformity when standing up, only to be revealed when bending forward. Many children with Scheuermann's kyphosis also have spondylolysis. In cases of severe, painful and stiff Scheuermann's deformity, some surgeons perform an anterior release and fusion followed by a posterior fusion and instrumentation.

W.L. Hennrikus

Besides presenting as a significant thoracic deformity, Scheuermann kyphosis can also present as severe pain, but with little in the way of a deformity. We see this frequently in teenage boys who are overtraining for a sport that they are required to be very strong, such as before summer football tryouts. The teen, who is still growing, may do weight training with excessive loads or poor technique but certainly more weight than the body can handle. During growth, the cartilaginous vertebral end plates are sensitive to excessive anterior pressure. Repetitive injury can create disc, end plate, and even vertebral body changes that are quite severe, often resembling cystic bone lesions or even a tumor. These changes are typically seen more in the lumbar or thoracolumbar spine. The pain can be disabling, yet it can still take a lot of discussion to convince athletes to stop this overtraining, since they are so motivated to succeed. With a change in activity, the pain can resolve, but the radiographic abnormality may persist permanently.

R.M. Schwend

References

1. Feng Q, Wang M, Zhang Y, Zhou Y. The effect of a corrective functional exercise program on postural thoracic kyphosis in teenagers: a randomized controlled trial. Clin Rehabil. 2018;32(1):48–56.
2. Sørensen K. Scheuermann's Juvenile kyphosis: clinical appearances, radiography, aetiology, and prognosis. Copenhagen: Munksgaard; 1964.
3. Bradford D. Juvenile kyphosis. In: Bradford D, Lonstein J, Moe J, Ogilvie J, Winter R, editors. Moe's textbook of scoliosis and other spinal deformities. 2nd ed. Philadelphia: WB Saunders; 1987. p. 347–68.
4. Tribus CB. Scheuermann's kyphosis in adolescents and adults: diagnosis and management. Am Acad Orthop Surg. 1998;6(1):36–43.
5. Tomé-Bermejo F, Tsirikos AIF. Current concepts on Scheuermann kyphosis: clinical presentation, diagnosis and controversies around treatment. Rev Esp Cir Ortop Traumatol. 2012;56(6):491–505.
6. Patel DR, Kinsella E. Evaluation and management of lower back pain in young athletes. Transl Pediatr. 2017;6(3):225–35.
7. Lowe TG. Scheuermann's disease. Orthop Clin North Am. 1999;30(3):475–87, ix
8. Weiss HR, Turnbull D, Bohr S. Brace treatment for patients with Scheuermann's disease – a review of the literature and first experiences with a new brace design. Scoliosis. 2009;4:22.
9. Gutowski WT, Renshaw TS. Orthotic results in adolescent kyphosis. Spine (Phila Pa 1976). 1988;13(5):485–9.
10. Riddle EC, Bowen JR, Shah SA, Moran EF, Lawall H Jr. The duPont kyphosis brace for the treatment of adolescent Scheuermann kyphosis. J South Orthop Assoc. 2003;12(3):135–40.
11. Murray PM, Weinstein SL, Spratt KF. The natural history and long-term follow-up of Scheuermann kyphosis. J Bone Joint Surg Am. 1993;75(2):236–48.

Chapter 9
The Gymnast's Gripe: A Case of a Teenager with Back Pain and Spondylolysis of L5

Andrew J. M. Gregory

Brief Case Presentation

Chief Complaint

Two-month history of low back pain.

History

This 14-year-old female gymnast has been having low back pain for about 2 months. She reports that the pain is in the midline of her lower back and is worse with activity, particularly back bends (hyperextension). Over time, the pain has slowly gotten worse and is affecting her ability to perform. She has experienced no radiating pain, burning, numbness or tingling in either leg, nor bowel or bladder incontinence. She has been treating this with ice, heat, ibuprofen, and chiropractic manipulation without improvement. Her past medical history includes seasonal allergies and ADHD. She has had no previous low back problems. She has not reached menarche. She eats a normal diet and is not trying to lose weight.

A. J. M. Gregory (✉)
Department of Orthopedics, Vanderbilt University Medical Center, Nashville, TN, USA
e-mail: Andrew.Gregory@vumc.org

© Springer Nature Switzerland AG 2021
R. M. Schwend, W. L. Hennrikus (eds.), *Back Pain in the Young Child and Adolescent*, https://doi.org/10.1007/978-3-030-50758-9_9

Physical Examination

Weight: 50 kg, height: 152 cm, and BMI: 19.5. She is healthy and athletic appearing and developmentally normal. There is no scoliosis, excessive kyphosis, or lordosis. She has tenderness to palpation of the L5 spinous process but not in the adjacent muscles. She has full range of motion but pain with stork testing (single-leg hyperextension) bilaterally. She has normal hamstring flexibility and a negative straight leg raise bilaterally. There are no midline skin changes. Screening neurologic examination and gait are normal.

Physical Exam Tests (Fig. 9.1)

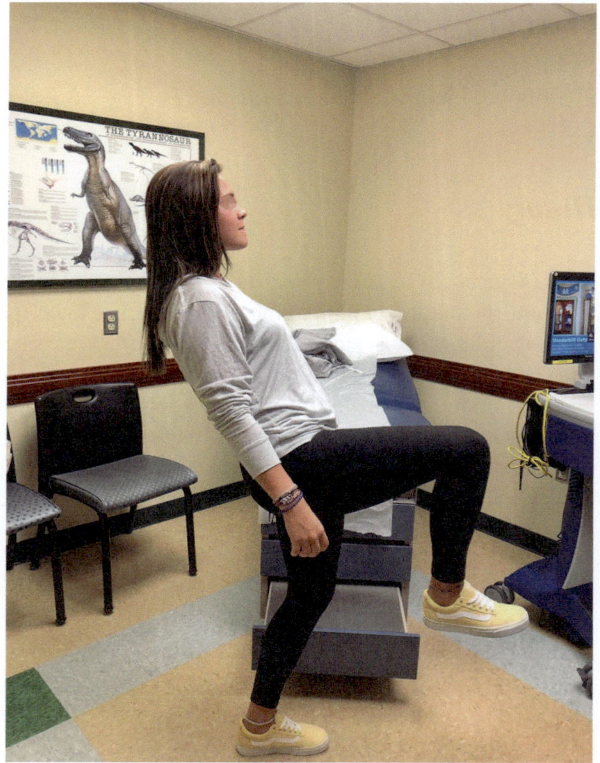

Fig. 9.1 Stork Test. Single-leg hyperextension exacerbates pain with spondylolysis. It is mildly to moderately sensitive but not specific to the condition. Palpation of the spinous processes may be the best examination test available

Imaging and Radiographic Studies (Fig. 9.2)

Questions About the Case the Reader Should Consider
1. How common is spondylolysis in adolescent athletes?
2. Is the stork test specific to spondylolysis?
3. Are plain radiographs helpful in making the diagnosis?
4. What is the best advanced imaging modality?
5. What is appropriate treatment in this case?

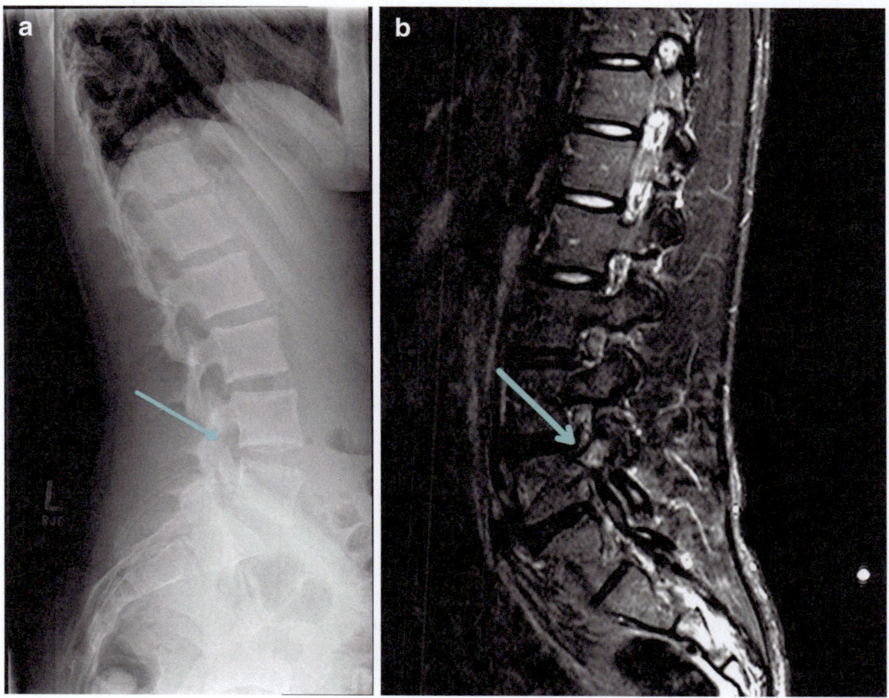

Fig. 9.2 (**a**) Lateral standing radiograph. This demonstrates pars fractures particularly if chronic and present bilaterally but may often be subtle. They can also show spina bifida occulta which is a risk factor for the development of spondylolysis. Spondylolisthesis is clearly visible on lateral radiographs and does not require advanced imaging. Oblique radiographs are not recommended as they add additional and excessive radiation and add expense, and it is difficult to distinguish pars fractures from overlying bowel gas or stool. (**b**) Sagittal (STIR looks at water content, think stirrring water) MRI of the lumbar spine. Specific STIR sequences that best demonstrate the lesion are often not included on standard protocols and have to be ordered separately. If you are not familiar with evaluating MRI imaging, then refer to a specialist for review

Discussion

Spondylolysis is one of the most common causes of low back pain in adolescent athletes. The incidence varies depending on the population. In the classic study on this topic, Micheli studied 100 adolescents (12–18 yo) vs. 100 adults (21–77 yo) with low back pain. Sixty-two percent of adolescents had derangements of the posterior elements compared to 5% in adults. Of those, 47% were stress fractures of the pars. Only 11% of adolescents had discogenic back pain compared to 48% of adults, and similarly, only 6% had muscle strains compared to 27% of adults [1]. More recent studies have not demonstrated as high a prevalence of pars fractures. In a prospective study with 153 pediatric patients with low back pain of at least 2 weeks, Nitta showed the prevalence of lumbar spondylolysis was 40%, but all patients with spondylolysis were athletes [2]. Kaneko performed a retrospective evaluation of 312 patients (under 18 years of age) with sports-related low back pain lasting for ≥ 7 days who underwent MRI, with 33% having lumbar stress injuries. Lumbar stress injuries were more common in males, and 50% of the patients who participated in soccer or track and field had lumbar stress injuries [3]. Selhorst looked at 1025 athletes with low back pain, and spondylolysis was identified in 308 (30%). The risk of spondylolysis differed by sex, with baseball (54%), soccer (48%), and hockey (44%) having the highest prevalence in males and gymnastics (34%), marching band (31%), and softball (30%) for females [4].

The Stork test (single-leg hyperextension) is a physical exam maneuver that has long been used to make the diagnosis of spondylolysis. As extension places stress on the posterior elements of the spine, other conditions such as facet joint irritation will also produce pain. Fortunately, tenderness to palpation of the spinous processes may be the best test to make the diagnosis. In a systematic review, Alqarni et al. showed the single-leg hyperextension test demonstrated low to moderate sensitivity (50–73%) and low specificity (17–32%) to diagnose lumbar spondylolysis, while lumbar spinous process palpation had high specificity (87–100%) and moderate to high sensitivity (60–88) values [5].

When looking at a radiograph, it is important to have a systematic method to examine all important aspects of the image. These include the areas outside the spine such as overall spine balance, evaluation of the soft tissues of the chest and abdomen, and other bones beyond the spine such as the pelvis, ribs, and long bones. It is very possible, even for an experienced radiologist reading many films during a typical day, to miss one seemingly small detail, such as the appearance of a pedicle. Pedicles on the anteroposterior (AP) film can be either missing or sclerotic. Unless one is actively looking at each pedicle, it is possible even for the most experienced of observers to miss such details. Once a radiology report describes "normal anatomy," further questioning by the clinician may not happen. Instead, we encourage the primary care doctor to review the image in person with the radiologist if any questions arise.

When spondylolysis is suspected, based on history and physical exam, plain radiographs with two views (AP and lateral) should be ordered. After a systematic review, Tofte recommends two-view radiographs as the best initial study due to efficacy, low cost, and low radiation exposure [6]. However, with an unusual presentations or a refractory course, advanced imaging should be pursued with MRI in early diagnosis and CT in more persistent courses. MRI is currently the gold standard for imaging for spondylolysis. In a systematic review, Dhouib showed the pooled sensitivity and specificity of the MRI for the diagnosis of a pars defect were 81% (95% CI 54–94%) and 99% (95% CI 98–100%), respectively [7]. If plain radiographs are not diagnostic and advanced imaging is needed, referral to a specialist is recommended as specific MRI sequences (STIR) are required to best detect the lesion and familiarity with reading MRI or CT is necessary.

Certain treatment aspects of spondylolysis are controversial, but conservative management seems to work for most. Sousa identified and contacted 295 patients who were at least 2 years out from diagnosis of spondylolysis and who were treated conservatively. Sixty subjects completed the follow-up survey, with 35/60 (58%) reporting no pain, 47/60 (78%) rating their pain at three or less, and 22% (13/60) rating their pain as four or higher. Of the 60 patients, 50 (82%) returned to sports, 8 (13%) did not return, and 5 (8%) returned to most but not all of their sports. No correlation was observed between radiographic healing and return to sports [8]. Klein et al. performed a meta-analysis of 665 young athletes with spondylolysis treated nonoperatively for at least 1 year and found a pooled success rate of 84% [9]. The clinical outcome of patients treated with a brace to patients treated without a brace was not significantly different. Radiographic healing of the defects had a pooled success rate of 28% ($n = 847$). Unilateral defects healed at a pooled and weighted rate of 71% ($n = 92$), significantly more than bilateral defects at 18% ($n = 446$). Acute defects healed at a rate of 68% ($n = 236$).

Conservative management may consist of activity modification, physical therapy, bracing, and ultrasound bone stimulation. There is evidence to support early physical therapy treatment. Selhorst studied 196 young athletes with acute spondylolysis and found a median of 115 days to a full return to activity for the group that had PT within 10 weeks and 140 days for those that had PT after 10 weeks [10]. There is also some evidence to support the use of a bone stimulator for treatment. Tsukada found the median time to return to previous sports activities was 61 days in the 35 young athletes treated with low-intensity pulsed ultrasound, which was significantly shorter than that of the 47 treated without (167 days) [11].

How to Approach the Case

Always be suspicious of activity-related pain in a young athlete, which may indicate spondylolysis. Midline pain to palpation and pain with stork test on examination are findings that should warrant plain radiographic imaging. Careful history, physical examination, and review of plain radiographs are the essential three aspects of making an accurate diagnosis. Advanced imaging studies such as MRI should be used to more accurately define and *confirm* the underlying diagnosis, rather than to *search* for a diagnosis.

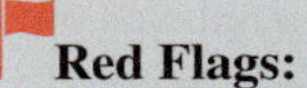

Red Flags: Key Common Risks and Findings with Spondylolysis
- Adolescent athlete.
- Midline low back pain.
- Pain with activity (particularly back extension).
- Pain with stork test.
- Pain on palpation of the spinous process.
- Plain radiographs may be normal.
- MRI is the definitive diagnostic study although CT can show long-standing lesions.

Short Differential Diagnosis
- Disc disease – usually associated with flexion-based pain. May or may not have associated radiation and paresthesias. Pain with forward flexion and radiating pain with straight leg raise test. Normal plain films. MRI is diagnostic.
- Muscle strain – bilateral low back with no radiation or paresthesias. Pain with all motions. Tender to palpation in the paraspinous muscles. Negative straight leg raise test. Normal imaging.
- Spondylolisthesis – more significant form of spondylolysis. Same history and examination. Plain films are diagnostic.

Final Diagnosis

Spondylolysis of L5.

Referral: When and to Whom?

If an adolescent athlete has a suspected spondylolysis with negative radiographs, a trial of rest and physical therapy is appropriate. If he/she does not respond within 1–2 months, then he/she should be referred to an orthopedic specialist who has training, expertise, and experience in pediatric sports medicine. If there is a specific diagnosis of spondylolisthesis of the spine, especially if there is significant slipping of one vertebrae on another, referral to an orthopedic surgeon with expertise in spine surgery is appropriate.

> **Key Features and Pearls**
> - Activity-related pain in a young athlete should prompt suspicion.
> - Normal exam except for pain with stork test and palpation of the spinous processes.
> - Plain films may be normal particularly early in the process.
> - MRI is the study of choice.
> - Limiting painful activities and physical therapy are the mainstays of treatment. Bracing does not seem to be very effective.

Editor Discussion

Dr. Lyle Micheli of Boston Children's Hospital, many years ago, taught us that back pain in an athlete is very commonly caused by spondylolysis. Pain during or after physical activity is the hallmark. Pain with palpation of the spinous processes or specific bone lesions seen on plain radiographs are also of concern.

W.L. Hennrikus

As discussed by Dr. Gregory, it is very possible for a radiologist or a clinician to miss noticing a lesion on a plain radiograph. It is especially possible if the radiologist has given the image a "normal read" that the clinician will be influenced by the radiologist's report and either not directly examine the images or accept the normal report as accurate. When the clinical findings do not seem straightforward, or there are sufficient atypical findings, go back over the history, physical and plain imaging studies, preferably with a wise colleague, and re-examine the evidence.

R.M. Schwend

References

1. Micheli L. Back pain in young athletesSignificant differences from adults in causes and patterns. Arch Pediatr Adolesc Med. 1995;149(1):15–8.
2. Nitta et al. Spondylolysis in pediatric patients. Orthopedics. 2016;39(3):e434–7.
3. Kaneko, et al. Prevalence of sports-related lumbosacral stress injuries in the young. Arch Orthop Trauma Surg. 2017;137(5):685–91.
4. Selhorst M, et al. Prevalence of spondylolysis in symptomatic adolescent athletes. CJSM. 2017;29:421–5.
5. Alqarni AM, Schneiders AG, Cook CE, Hendrick PA. Clinical tests to diagnose lumbar spondylolysis and spondylolisthesis: a systematic review. Phys Ther Sport. 2015;16(3):268–75.
6. Tofte, et al. Imaging pediatric spondylolysis: systematic review. Spine. 2017;42(10):777–82.
7. Dhouib, et al. Diagnostic accuracy of MRI for direct visualization of lumbar pars defect in children and young adults: a systematic review and meta-analysis. Eur Spine J. 2018;27(5):1058–66.
8. Sousa T, Skaggs DL, Chan P, Yamaguchi KT Jr, Borgella J, Lee C, Sawyer J, Moisan A, Flynn JM, Gunderson M, Hresko MT, D'Hemecourt P, Andras LM. Benign natural history of spondylolysis in adolescence with midterm follow-up. Spine Deform. 2017;5(2):134–8.

9. Klein G, Mehlman CT, McCarty M. Nonoperative treatment of spondylolysis and grade I spondylolisthesis in children and young adults: a meta-analysis of observational studies. J Pediatr Orthop. 2009;29(2):146–56.
10. Selhorst M, Fischer A, Graft K, Ravindran R, Peters E, Rodenberg R, Welder E, MacDonald J. Timing of physical therapy referral in adolescent athletes with acute spondylolysis: a retrospective chart review. Clin J Sport Med. 2017;27(3):296–301.
11. Tsukada M, Takiuchi T, Watanabe K. Low-intensity pulsed ultrasound for early-stage lumbar spondylolysis in young athletes. Clin J Sport Med. 2017;29:262.

Chapter 10
Teenage Weightlifter with Back Pain and a Fractured Vertebral End Plate

Ashley Startzman and William A. Phillips

Brief Case Presentation

Chief Complaint

Acute onset of low back pain and radicular symptoms.

History

A 15-year-6-month-old football player was lifting weights when he felt a snap in his lumbar spine. He was doing squats at the time. He had immediate back pain. Over the next few days, he had increasing pain down both legs, with left leg pain worse than the right. He notes some subjective weakness but no numbness. He has not had any changes in bowel or bladder function.

Physical Exam

General – Muscular teenage boy in some distress.

Back examination – Severe pain with flexion of his lumbar spine; not much pain with extension. Markedly positive straight leg raise (pain in left lower limb) on the left side (at 15 degrees of elevation) as well as a cross straight leg raise on the right side at 30 degrees.

A. Startzman · W. A. Phillips (✉)
Department of Orthopaedic Surgery, Texas Children's Hospital, Baylor College of Medicine, Houston, TX, USA
e-mail: Waphilli@Texaschildrens.org

© Springer Nature Switzerland AG 2021
R. M. Schwend, W. L. Hennrikus (eds.), *Back Pain in the Young Child and Adolescent*, https://doi.org/10.1007/978-3-030-50758-9_10

Motor examination reveals five out of five strength in bilateral lower extremities. Sensation is intact throughout lower extremities to light touch and sharp pain. Reflexes trace at both the knees and ankles. No clonus. He walks with a tentative and protective slow gait.

Imaging and Radiographic Studies

Posteroanterior (PA) and lateral views of the lumbar spine are unremarkable – no scoliosis and no spondylolysis (Fig. 10.1). An MRI shows a ring apophyseal fracture at L2–3 that is compressing the spinal canal on the left side (Fig. 10.2). A CT scan shows ossification in the spinal canal at the L2–3 level (Fig. 10.3).

Questions About the Case the Reader Should Consider
1. Acute onset of low back pain can be common in weightlifters. What are the most common cases of low back pain in weightlifters? What makes this case different?
2. Muscular back pain is not typically associated with radicular symptoms of leg numbness and tingling. What is the cause of the radicular symptoms?

Fig. 10.1 Lateral radiograph of lumbar spine. No abnormality is appreciated

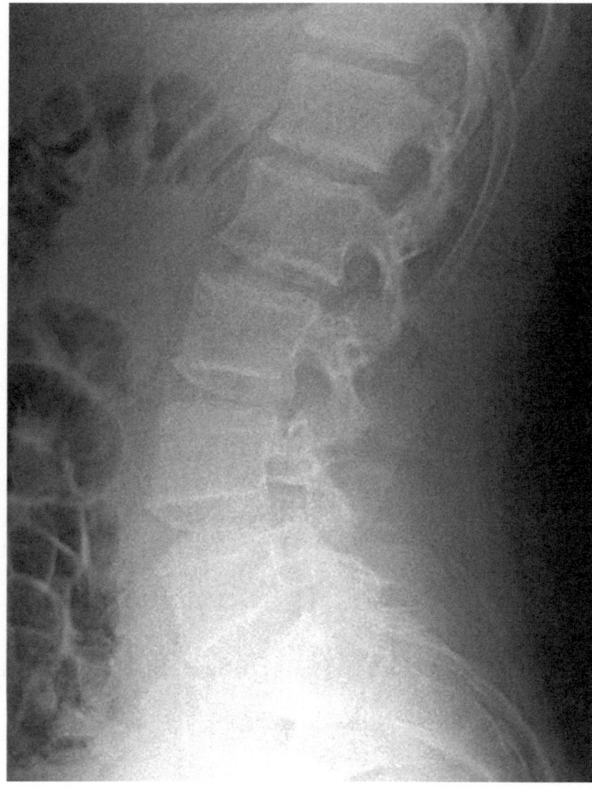

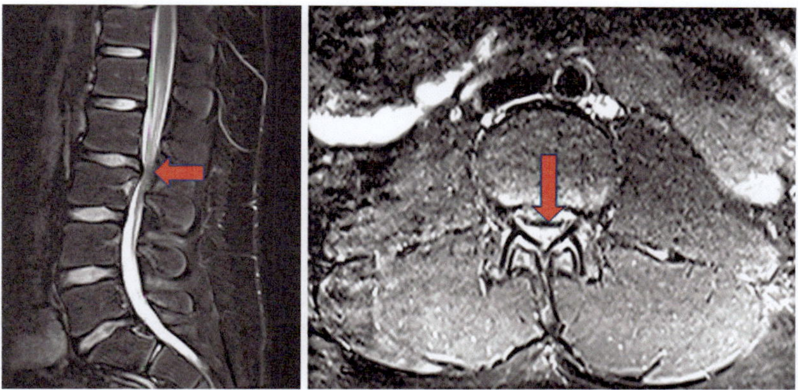

Fig. 10.2 Sagittal and axial T2 sections of lumbar spine showing compression of cauda equine at L2–3 level (*arrows*)

Fig. 10.3 Sagittal CT reconstruction showing L3 ossified superior end plate fragment in canal (*arrow*)

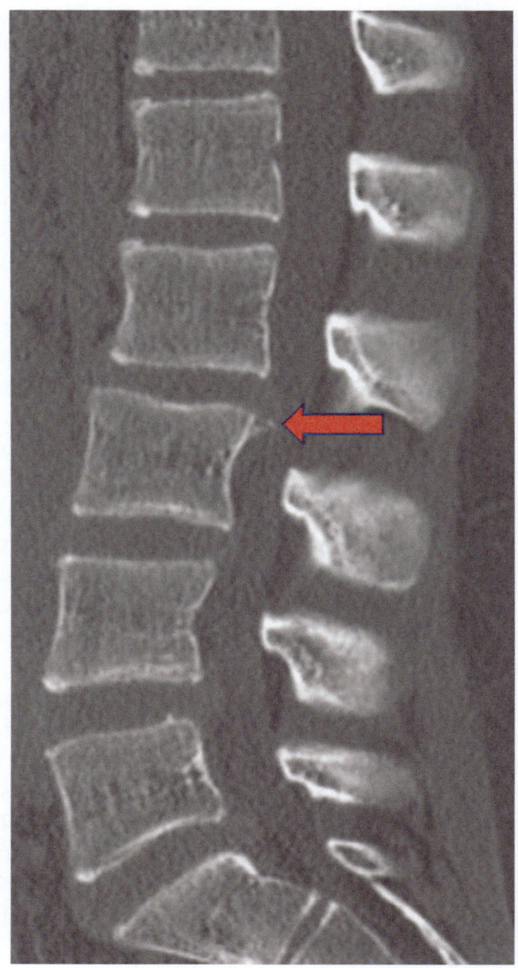

3. What is the appropriate referral?
4. What is the next diagnostic test that should be considered?
5. What are the possible treatment options?

Discussion

Teenagers often have benign low back pain with no identifiable etiology. Back pain may be related to improper lifting technique, overtraining, injury, spasms, and weak abdominal musculature [1, 2]. Back pain that causes radicular symptoms and pain below the knee is less common and is a red flag. Weightlifters may be at a higher risk for acute onset of back pain, especially if poor form is utilized [3–5]. During weightlifting, the spine can twist, hyperextend, or hyperflex to cause injury [2–6]. The mechanics utilized in some weightlifting maneuvers may lead to a higher risk of spondylolysis, disc herniation, or, unique in teenagers and young adults, ring apophysis avulsion fractures [2, 4]. All of the above may lead to radicular symptoms and should be high on a list of differential diagnoses in a teenage weightlifter with low back and radicular pain [2, 3].

Back pain with leg pain has several different etiologies. It is important to decipher where and if the leg pain travels. Pain in the back and leg that stops above the knee is less cause for concern and may be due to piriformis syndrome, sciatica, or other peripheral neuropathic diseases. Sciatica and piriformis syndrome will be clinically defined by tenderness or elucidation of symptoms with palpation of the piriformis (posterior hip) and reproduction of symptoms with flexion, adduction, and internal rotation of the hip [7, 8]. Back pain with leg pain that radiates down the leg to below the knee is more likely a result of nerve root irritation from an intraspinal etiology such as a disc herniation, ring apophyseal avulsion fracture, tumor, or infection. These patients will have pain with leg extension (straight leg raise), forward flexion, and maneuvers that cause tension on the spinal nerve roots. Sometimes these two diagnoses can overlap, but leg pain that is isolated to the thigh is typically unrelated to intraspinal pathology. In the teenager, always consider a slipped capital femoral epiphysis when there is unexplained hip, thigh, or knee pain.

Once a patient is identified to have back pain with leg pain traveling below the knee, a referral to a pediatric spine surgeon should be made. Based on the history and clinical exam, the spine surgeon will initially order a radiograph. In the case of an end plate fracture, a section of the posterior aspect of the superior or inferior end plate may be found to be avulsed in the canal on the lateral view plain radiograph. This fracture segment may contain the disc, ring apophysis, and a portion of metaphyseal bone [3, 9]. Avulsion fractures can be difficult to identify radiographically, so it is possible that no abnormality of the end plate will be seen on a plain radiograph, especially if the fractured portion is still cartilaginous and not completely ossified [6, 9].

Next, the specialist may order an MRI or CT of the lumbar spine without contrast. An MRI is ideal for evaluating intraspinal pathology, which is important when considering causes for radicular symptoms [6]. Key images are the sagittal and axial sections, which show osseous or cartilaginous material within the central portion of the spinal canal at the involved level. A CT scan can better identify osseous material within the spinal canal and is sometimes more effective at making the diagnosis of a ring apophyseal fracture than MRI [3, 6, 10, 11].

This boy's MRI showed a large central extruded disc at L2/L3 with associated fracture of the L3 ring apophysis causing moderate narrowing of the bilateral lateral recesses.

End plate fractures with displacement into the spinal canal will not resorb on their own. Nonsurgical management is rarely successful [3, 6, 11]. The avulsion fracture may unite with the posterior elements of the spine and lead to spinal stenosis [9]. Persistent back pain with or without radicular symptoms is expected. Weakness and sensory deficits are not common early on, but may present later if spinal stenosis occurs once the fragment heals [6, 9]. Surgical intervention with laminectomy, spinal decompression, and removal of the extruded fragment is indicated [3, 6, 10, 11]. If there is associated instability of the vertebral segment, fusion may be required at the time of surgery [6, 11]. Open excision and decompression have higher success rates than minimally invasive procedures such as microdiscectomy [10]. No long-term sequela are expected following adequate decompression of the spinal canal, but occasionally, late segmental instability or recurrence of disc herniation can occur [6].

How to Approach the Case

Teenagers with low back pain are commonly seen in the pediatric office. The difference here is the presence of acute onset of low back pain with associated radicular symptoms traveling below the knee. Numbness, tingling, leg pain, and leg weakness are findings of concern in the face of back pain. Leg pain (defined as pain going below the knees as opposed to thigh pain) or leg symptoms in the presence of low back pain suggest nerve root irritation. Obtaining a clear history and physical exam is the key to this case [3]. Advanced imaging with an MRI or CT should be used to delineate the specific etiology of leg pain in the face of back pain and is better ordered by the sub-specialist who can order the correct levels and sequences and justify the indication to the patient's insurer. The treatment of a disc herniation and end plate fracture is different in that the disc herniation being soft tissue can resorb over time [6].

Red Flags for Back Pain in Weightlifters
- Back pain under age 17 years
- A "pop" during injury
- Radicular symptoms including leg pain and leg tingling
- Numbness in the foot
- Weakness in the foot or leg

> **Short Differential Diagnosis**
> - Muscular back pain
> - Ring apophyseal avulsion fracture
> - Spondylolysis
> - Compression fracture
> - Disc herniation
> - Intraspinal tumor

Final Diagnosis

End plate (ring apophysis) fracture at L3.

Natural History and Treatment Considerations

Symptomatic herniated discs are uncommon in teens [10, 11]. In children with a disc herniation, a ring avulsion fracture will be present in 15–32% of these cases [10]. The ring apophysis inserts at the site of the posterior ligamentous structures [3, 4, 10]. Ring apophyseal fusion is expected to occur around age 17–25 years old [3, 4, 10]. During a disc herniation, there is increased tension on the posterior ligamentous structures of the spine. The tension placed on the apophysis during the disc herniation can lead to a shearing force and subsequent fracture with extrusion into the spinal canal [4, 10].

An end plate fracture of the apophysis may displace within the spinal canal and mimic a disc herniation [6, 9, 11]. The difference between a disc herniation and a ring apophysis fracture is the material that is extruded within the spinal canal. In a disc herniation, the material is gelatinous and consists of proteoglycans, water, and collagen. In teenagers and young adults, the end plates of the vertebrae are not yet completely ossified. If a ring apophysis avulses into the spinal canal, the material will consist of disc, bone, and cartilage [9, 11]. Disc herniations often resorb overtime, and symptoms may dissipate with nonsurgical management. In a ring apophysis avulsion, the osseous material within the spinal canal will not resorb [6]. The intraspinal fragment may ossify in place and lead to spinal stenosis [9]. Since the bone fragment will not resorb, the radicular symptoms in a patient with a ring apophysis or end plate avulsion fracture are not expected to improve and may actually worsen over time. An urgent referral to an orthopedic spine surgeon or neurosurgeon should be made in the setting of a teenage weightlifter with back pain and radicular symptoms.

In this patient, surgical laminectomy with decompression and removal of the entrapped fragment was performed. The patient had immediate relief of radicular symptoms and back pain.

Referral: Emergency, Urgent, or Routine – And to Whom?

End plate fractures with displacement within the spinal canal and radicular symptoms that travel below the knee should be referred urgently to a pediatric orthopedic spine surgeon or neurosurgeon. Unlike a disc herniation, the ossified fracture fragment will not resorb. Radicular symptoms are not expected to improve over time if a large fracture fragment is found within the spinal canal. The treatment of an end plate fracture involves surgical excision of the fragment and discectomy, with or without spinal fusion (based on associated spinal instability and the surgical approach performed at the time of surgery).

Brief Summary

Back pain in teenagers is very common, but back pain in teenagers associated with radicular symptoms is much less common. Lifting, twisting, and falls may place abnormal stress on the spine. In children and adolescents, the ring apophysis along the posterior elements of the spine is not yet completely ossified. Weightlifting and its associated mechanics may lead to the development of a disc herniation with a ring apophysis fracture. Plain radiographic imaging is challenging and is not always possible to identify an apophyseal ring avulsion fracture. Back pain with a radiculopathy that radiates below the knee merits urgent referral to a pediatric spine surgeon. Once seen by the specialist, CT or MRI will be ordered. In a ring apophysis avulsion fracture, the extruded fragment within the spinal canal will not likely resorb independently and often requires surgical decompression and fragment removal.

Key Features and Pearls
- The ring apophysis is located on the posterior elements of the spine, inserts onto the ligaments, and ossifies around age 17 years.
- In a ring apophysis fracture, the avulsed material may include disc material, cartilage, and/or metaphyseal bone.
- Radicular symptoms and leg pain are common.
- Nonsurgical treatment is rarely successful, and decompression with removal of the fragment often relieves symptoms with no long-term sequelae.

Editor Discussion

The vertebral end plate, vertebra, and disc have an important structural and nutritional relationship. Nutrients must traverse the vertebral end plate to supply nutrition to the disc. The end plate must be porous but still strong enough to resist fracture, while giving three-dimensional growth to the vertebral body. Porcine studies have shown that younger spines can have end plate fractures from rapid over-pressurization of the normal disc nucleus [12]. The disc annulus is also believed to be susceptible to injury when the end plate fractures [13]. There are probably no pure disc herniations in young patients who are still growing, since the end plate often becomes injured as well, just not as obvious and large as seen in this case.

R.M. Schwend

Classic radicular pain as seen in this case is felt in the leg and foot, below the knee. However, teenagers more commonly present with isolated back pain from pathology such as spondylolysis, Scheuermann kyphosis, or nonspecific back pain that does not radiate. Teenagers, especially overweight teenagers, with pain that is located in the hip area, thigh, or knee can have an underlying slipped capital femoral epiphysis (SCFE). In a study of 107 children undergoing surgery for a SCFE, 52 hips (43%) had atypical pain – with the three most common locations for this pain in the thigh, knee, or groin [14]. Always consider the diagnosis of SCFE! A frog lateral pelvis radiograph should be obtained when there is suspicion of SCFE. If the diagnosis is confirmed, urgent referral to a pediatric orthopedic surgeon is then recommended.

W.L. Hennrikus

Acknowledgment   The authors would like to thank Dr. Darrell Hanson for allowing us to use his patient's history and imaging as the basis for this case.

References

1. Yang S, Werner B, Singala A, et al. Low back pain in adolescents: a 1-year analysis of eventual diagnoses. J Pediatr Orthop. 2017;37:344–7.
2. Bono C. Current concepts review: low-back pain in athletes. JBJS. 2004;86-A(2):382–96.
3. Wu X, Ma W, Du H. A review of current treatment of lumbar posterior ring apophysis fracture with lumbar disc herniation. Eur Spine J. 2013;22:475–88.
4. Sward L, Hellstrom M, Jacobsson B, et al. Vertebral ring apophysis injury in athletes is the etiology different in the thoracic and lumbar spine? Am J Sports Med. 1993;26(6):841–5.
5. Shimozaki K, Nakase J, Yoshioka K, et al. Incidence rates and characteristics of abnormal lumbar findings and low back pain in child and adolescent weightlifter: a prospective three-year cohort study. PLoS One. 2018;13(10):e0206125.
6. Sink E, Flynn J. Thoracolumbar spine and lower extremity fractures. Lovell and Winters' Pediatric Orthopaedics (7th Edition) Lippincott, Williams & Wilkins, Philadelphia; 2014. p. 1774–6.
7. Benson E, Schutzer S. Posttraumatic piriformis syndrome: diagnosis and results of operative treatment. JBJS. 1999;81(7):941–9.
8. Toda T, Koda M. Rokkaku et al. sciatica caused by pyomyositis of the piriformis muscle in a pediatric patient. Orthopedics. 2013;36(2):e257–9.
9. Ogden JA. Skeletal injury in the child (3rd Edition) Springer, New York; 2000. p 760–3.
10. Singhal A, Mitra A, Cochran D, et al. Ring apophysis fracture in pediatric lumbar disc herniation: a common entity. Pediatr Neurosurg. 2013;49:16–20.

11. Frino J, McCarthy R, Sparks C, et al. Trends in adolescent lumbar disk herniation. J Pediatri Orthop. 2006;26:579–81.
12. Brown SH, Gregory DE, McGill SM. Vertebral end-plate fractures as a result of high rate pressure loading in the nucleus of the young adult porcine spine. J Biomech. 2008;41(1):122–7.
13. Snow CR, Harvey-Burgess M, Laird B, Brown SHM, Gregory DE. Pressure-induced end-plate fracture in the porcine spine: is the annulus fibrosus susceptible to damage? Eur Spine J. 2018;27(8):1767–74.
14. Uvodich M, Schwend R, Stevanovic O, Wurster W, Leamon J, Hermanson A. Patterns of pain in adolescents with slipped capital femoral epiphysis. J Pediatr. 2019;206:184–189.e1.

Chapter 11
A Girl with Low Back Pain due to Spondylolisthesis

John F. Sarwark, Kristine Santos Martin, and Ayesha Maqsood

Brief Case Presentation

Chief Complaint

Four-year history of chronic low back pain

History

This 18-year-old female has had chronic low back pain for the last 4 years. There was no trauma or an inciting incident. She has the pain when she wakes up, if she stands or sits for long periods of time and when she runs. She works at a cable factory for 40 hours a week, mostly sitting. She notices the mid to low back pain towards the end of her day, but with some relief with changing positions and stretching. She also occasionally has shooting pain on the lateral aspect of her right thigh and right foot plantar paresthesia when the back pain occurs. She has been managing her pain with physical therapy (PT), a lumbosacral orthosis (LSO) and nonsteroidal anti-inflammatory drugs (NSAIDs). She was taking the NSAID daily, until a few months ago when she started to have gastrointestinal (GI) symptoms. Her primary care physician (PCP) then prescribed acetaminophen 325 mg, which she

J. F. Sarwark (✉)
Division of Orthopaedic Surgery & Sports Medicine, Department of Surgery,
Ann & Robert H. Lurie Children's Hospital of Chicago, Chicago, IL, USA
e-mail: jsarwark@luriechildrens.org

K. Santos Martin · A. Maqsood
Department of Surgery, Ann & Robert H. Lurie Children's Hospital of Chicago,
Chicago, IL, USA

© Springer Nature Switzerland AG 2021
R. M. Schwend, W. L. Hennrikus (eds.), *Back Pain in the Young Child and Adolescent*, https://doi.org/10.1007/978-3-030-50758-9_11

can tolerate daily, with some pain relief. She now also takes diazepam at night, to ease the pain enough to sleep.

Physical Examination

Weight 103.8 kg, height 171.3 cm, BMI 35. She is healthy and well-nourished. Her stance and gait are normal. She has no pain with right left or forward bending. Her single leg hyperextension (stork) test was positive with the left foot raised and negative with the right foot raised. Neurologic, motor, sensory and reflex exams are normal. Bowel and bladder functions are normal as well. She had difficulty doing more than one push up and more than five sit ups.

Imaging and Radiographic Studies (Figs. 11.1 and 11.2)

Questions About the Case the Reader Should Consider
1. Was there increased physical activity or repetitive motions by the patient?
2. What is the appropriate referral?
3. What is the next diagnostic test that should be considered?
4. Why is a combination of PT, LSO and NSAIDs not alleviating her symptoms?
5. What are possible treatments in this case?

Discussion

In the paediatric population, the clinical manifestations of spondylolisthesis can vary greatly. Most cases are asymptomatic but symptoms, most commonly low back pain, can arise during pubertal growth. The pain can occasionally radiate in a sciatic distribution to the buttock or posterior thigh [1]. Patients who are athletes and compete in high-risk sports, such as gymnastics and football, can have injuries as their inciting incident or trauma. Other causes include minor overuse trauma, in particular repetitive hyperextension movements of the lumbar spine [2]. In adolescence and adulthood, the increased physical activity in addition to the wear-and-tear of daily life can result in spondylolisthesis, making it very common in this age range. In this case the young woman did not remember an inciting incident or trauma, but indicated that her job led to sitting 40 hours a week. The erect posture produces a constant downward and forward loading force on the lumbar vertebrae. This daily stress and repeated force being applied to the spine can wear out or degenerate it. Her obesity and weak core muscles may have contributed to the pain she had been experiencing.

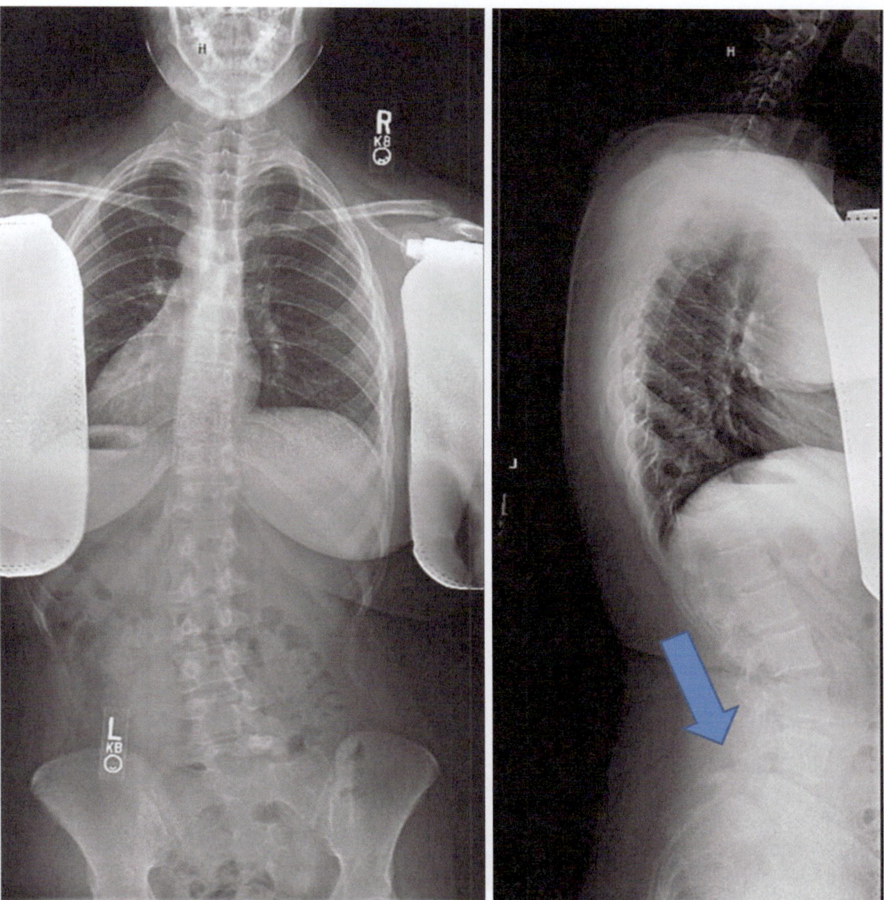

Fig. 11.1 PA and lateral radiograph; bilateral pars interarticularis defects at L5 with mild forward slip of L5 on S1. Note the secondary mild with apex left scoliosis which is frequently seen associated with painful spondylolisthesis. Apex of the secondary scoliosis may be to the left or to the right and is often a long neuromuscular appearing curvature

A spinal and lumbosacral AP and lateral radiographs are used to make a diagnosis of spondylolisthesis. If suspected, referral to an orthopaedic spine surgeon or sports medicine specialist if the patient is an athlete is appropriate. Neurologic findings such as weakness or decreased sensation especially need a referral to a spine surgeon. Advanced imaging such as MRI or CT are best ordered by the specialist. These radiological assessments give a better visualization of the bone morphology, making it check for the alignment of the facet joint and the degenerative changes that have occurred [3]. The need for advanced imaging arises when the patient is exhibiting significant and progressing neurologic claudication, bladder or bowel complaints, radiculopathies and the clinical suspicion that another condition such as space-occupying lesion such as disc, tumour or infection [4]. This patient had an

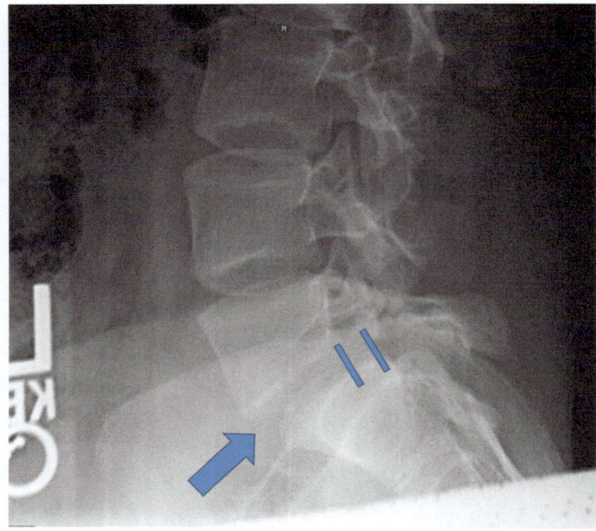

Fig. 11.2 Lateral lumbar radiograph; there is a loss of height observed between the vertebral bodies (*arrow*) and also a vertebral displacement observed at L5-S1 (*lines*); diagnosis is isthmic spondylolisthesis grade 1

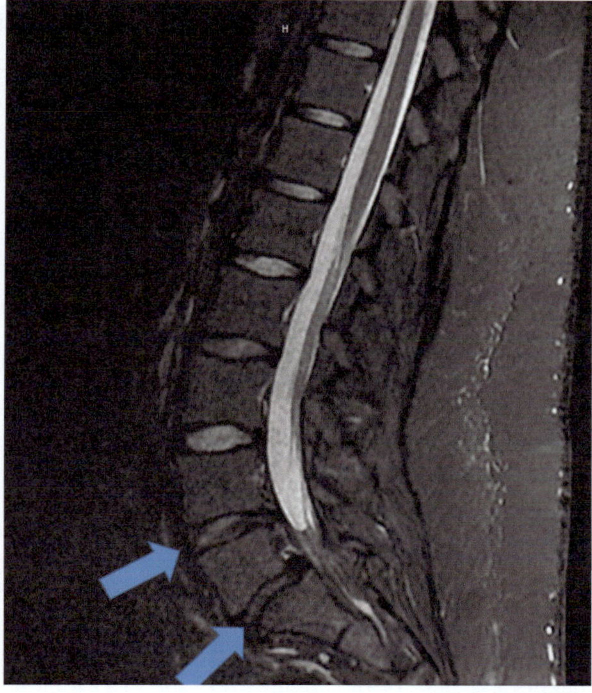

Fig. 11.3 Lateral lumbar MRI; degenerative disc findings associated with L4-L5 and L5-S1 discs (*arrows*). No spinal canal or foraminal narrowing associated with this level. Notice the mild forward slip of L5 on S1, which on a supine film or supine MRI is often less noticable than seen on the standing radiograph

MRI of the lumbar spine ordered by the referred orthopaedic surgeon. It showed a progression of the grade 1 anterolisthesis of L5 upon S1, sclerosis in the bilateral L5 pars interarticularis with persistent bony change on the right L5-S1 facet and progressive degenerative disc findings at the L4-L5 level (Fig. 11.3).

Normally in cases of low-grade spondylolisthesis, patients will respond to conservative, nonsurgical treatment. This includes activity restriction and physical therapy to strengthen the core muscles. If they get little relieve with these measures, nerve blocks, intralesional injection of Marcaine or steroid injection can be used [5]. In this case she was able to achieve some pain relief with physical therapy, a brace and NSAIDs (later switching to acetaminophen due to GI issues she encountered). However, her pain has not fully resolved, and she now needed to take diazepam nightly to achieve some pain relief.

Although the majority of patients will improve with conservative treatments, surgical options are warranted after 6 months of failed conservative treatments for patients who have radiculopathy. Patients with neurogenic claudication, progressive neurological deficits, high-grade slips or bladder and bowel symptoms may require more immediate surgery [6]. A posterolateral fusion with instrumentation is the typical operative treatment for low-grade isthmic spondylolisthesis. It involves a single-level L5-S1 fusion of the transverse processes; this can extend upward to L4 for more severe slippages [7]. In this case the patient has persistent pain with degenerative disc changes of two discs at L4-S1, and for this reason stabilization surgery was recommended. She received posterior spinal fusion with instrumentation from L4 to the sacrum with allograft bone graft, removal of the two degenerated discs and replacement with anterior structural bone graft. Often children have a degree of dysplastic spondylolisthesis with deficient posterior bony anatomy, requiring the addition of disc surgery to provide anterior structural support in addition to posterior rods and bone graft. The posterior operation has a fusion rate of up to 90% and good long-term clinical outcomes [7], although more recently anterior structural support between the vertebral bodies is being used.

How to Approach the Case

Start with a detailed history. Ask the patient specific questions about their pain, including trauma or inciting event, location, severity, duration, quality, exacerbating and alleviating factors and how it is in the morning compared to the night. Next perform a physical examination focusing on the spinal alignment and range of motion of the lumbosacral spine as well as a neurologic examination assessing the distal strength, sensation and reflexes [1]. A radiographic evaluation can provide diagnostic information and determine the grade of slippage. Start with a standing lumbosacral AP and lateral radiograph. If these views are not diagnostic and you still suspect a spondylolysis, oblique views can be obtained, but these may not be diagnostic [6]. Advanced imaging techniques, such as CT and MRI, can be used obtained by the spine specialist on a case-by-case basis, especially when neurological symptoms are present.

**Red Flags for Back Pain due to Spondylolisthesis**
- Late childhood, early adolescence
- Lumbosacral region of spine
- Repetitive hyperextension
- Numbness or tingling in the feet
- Pain radiates to thighs or legs

Short Differential Diagnosis
- Lumbosacral Spondylolysis – typically occurs in young people (teens), low back pain aggravated by activity, particularly hyperextension.
- Lumbosacral Discogenic Pain Syndrome – found in athletes and non-athletes; typically pain increases with sitting and other activities that increase intradiscal pressure.
- Lumbosacral Radiculopathy – onset of symptoms is sudden, sitting can exacerbate the pain, and it can refer to the anterior aspect of the thigh.

Final Diagnosis

Grade 1 L5/S1 spondylolisthesis; stable

Natural History and Treatment Considerations

The increased growth rate during the adolescent period is associated with the greatest slip progression in those patients who had spondylolisthesis [8]. If a slip angle (angle between the top of L5 and the top of the sacrum) is greater than 25°–30° [9], there is severe spinal instability or chronic disabling pain, and then surgical intervention may be required. In this young woman, the pain started in her adolescent years and progressed to chronic pain, which eventually underwent correction via spinal fusion and instrumentation.

Referral – Emergency, Urgent, or Routine: And to Whom?

If the inciting incident was a new sports-related injury, urgent referral to a sports medicine specialist would be warranted. If there is a high-grade vertebral slippage or symptoms are refractory to conservative treatment and surgical intervention is being considered, referral to an orthopaedic surgeon, spine surgeon or neurosurgeon would be appropriate.

Brief Summary

Most low-grade cases of spondylolisthesis tend to be asymptomatic or can be resolved with conservative treatment. However, in some cases, the condition may cause chronic low back pain, neurologic symptoms and pain resistant to conservative treatment and require surgical intervention. In order to assess a child with low back pain, form a diagnosis and treatment plan, a detailed history, physical examination and review of radiographs is important. A referral to an orthopaedic surgeon or a neurosurgeon is recommended if spondylolisthesis does not respond to conservative care.

Key Features and Pearls
- Repetitive hyperextension causes stress on the pars interarticularis, which can eventually lead to a stress fracture. A bilateral pars defect allows for forward slippage of the vertebra (usually L5, S1), resulting in spondylolisthesis.
- Associated pain radiating from the low back to the thigh, buttocks and leg may present in the L5 or S1 distribution as a result of nerve root compression.

  An erect posture produces a constant downward and forward loading force on the lumbar vertebrae. The daily stresses that are put on a spine or the repeated forces being applied to the spine can wear out or degenerate it.

Editor Discussion

Spondylolysis usually refers to a stress or fatigue fracture of the pars interarticularis caused by hyperextension of the lumbar spine. Certain sports such as gymnastics or weight lifting stress the spine and have a higher incidence of this lesion. Unilateral spondylolysis is stable and is more likely to heal with conservative treatment. Bilateral spondylolysis disengages the neural arch from the body and allows the body to slip relative to the adjacent neural arch resulting in spondylolisthesis. Hyperlordosis and a horizontal sacrum increase the likelihood of slippage. Hamstring tightness is a common secondary finding. The majority of patients can be treated conservatively. Fusion and instrumentation is indicated for unstable lesions. Decompression is indicated for neural signs and symptoms. Reduction of deformity is controversial but is occasionally indicated to achieve better spine and pelvic balance. Sagittal balance of the spine is the most sensitive measure related to quality of life.

W.L. Hennrikus

Spondylolisthesis in children with normal posterior spine anatomy can occur from repetitive stress. This is what typically happens to a girl in gymnastics who repeatedly does back bends or back flips. The normal L5 pars interarticularis gets overstressed until it fractures (termed isthmic spondylolisthesis since the pars is the narrowest part of this anatomy). With loss of the posterior "tether", the L5 vertebra can slip forward. Typically, the L5 disc is healthy and so the slippage is only slight (typically called grade 1). However, some children are born with deficient bony anatomy in both the posterior pars interarticularis and surrounding tissues. Early in life there can be slippage of L5 on S1, even without the stress of athletics. These children have "dysplastic" spondylolisthesis and can present early in childhood with more severe grades of spondylolisthesis that involves changes in the disc. Low-grade dysplastic spondylolisthesis is less than 50% slippage of L5 on S1. These require continued follow-up to make sure progression of deformity is not happening. High-grade spondylolisthesis is greater than 50% forward slippage, is usually dysplastic in nature, has a high risk of deformity progression and generally requires preventive spine fusion and at least partial reduction, to prevent further slippage.

R.M. Schwend

References

1. Attiah MA, Macyszyn L, Cahill PJ. Management of spondylolysis and spondylolisthesis in the pediatric population: a review. Semin Spine Surg. 2014;26(4):230–7.
2. Mac-Thiong JM, Duong L, Parent S, Hresko MT, Dimar JR, Weidenbaum M, et al. Reliability of the spinal deformity study groups classification of lumbosacral spondylolisthesis. Spine. 2012;37(2):95–102.
3. Tsirikos AI, Garrido EG. Spondylolysis and spondylolisthesis in children and adolescents. J Bone Joint Surg Br. 2010;92(6):751–9.
4. Pizzutillo PD, Hummer CD. Nonoperative treatment for painful adolescent spondylolysis or spondylolisthesis. J Pediatr Orthop. 1989;9(5):538–40.
5. Kalichman L, Hunter DJ. Diagnosis and conservative management of degenerative lumbar spondylolisthesis. Eur Spine J. 2008;17:327–35.
6. Metzger R, Chaney S. Spondylolysis and spondylolisthesis: what the primary care provider should know. J Am Assoc Nurse Pract. 2014;26(1):5–12.
7. Frennered AK, Danielson BI, Nachemson AL, Nordwall AB. Midterm follow-up of young patients fused in situ for spondylolisthesis. Spine. 1991;16(4):409–16.
8. Fredrickson BE, Baker D, McHolick WJ, Yuan HA, Lubicky JP. The natural history of spondylolysis and spondylolisthesis. J Bone Joint Surg Am. 1984;66(5):699–707.
9. Lundine KM, Lewis SJ, Al-Aubaidi Z, Alman B, Howard AW. Patient outcomes in the operative and nonoperative management of high-grade spondylolisthesis in children. J Pediatr Orthop. 2014;34(5):483–9.

Chapter 12
A Girl with Low Back Pain due to Deconditioning

John F. Sarwark, Kristine Santos Martin, and Ayesha Maqsood

Brief Case Presentation

Chief Complaint

Many years history of low back pain

History

This 11-year-old girl had been having low back pain for the past few years. She describes that pain in her low, central back, with no radiation. She has pain with running and standing from a seated position. There was no history of trauma. She manages the pain with anti-inflammatory medication and heat packs applied to the area of pain. There is no pain, numbness, or weakness in other joints or systematic symptoms. Bowel and bladder functions are normal.

J. F. Sarwark (✉)
Division of Orthopaedic Surgery & Sports Medicine, Department of Surgery, Ann & Robert H. Lurie Children's Hospital of Chicago, Chicago, IL, USA
e-mail: jsarwark@luriechildrens.org

K. Santos Martin · A. Maqsood
Department of Surgery, Ann & Robert H. Lurie Children's Hospital of Chicago, Chicago, IL, USA

© Springer Nature Switzerland AG 2021
R. M. Schwend, W. L. Hennrikus (eds.), *Back Pain in the Young Child and Adolescent*, https://doi.org/10.1007/978-3-030-50758-9_12

Physical Examination

Weight 34.8 kg, height 147 cm, BMI 16. She is a healthy well-nourished child. There are no deformities of her trunk or lower extremities. Her stance and gait are normal. She has pain with forward spine flexion. When asked to do 5 pushups she has marked difficulty maintaining proper plank position and cannot complete them. Popliteal angle on the left is 45° and on the right is 40°.

Imaging and Radiographic Studies (Figs. 12.1 and 12.2)

Questions About the Case the Reader Should Consider
1. Did an event or trauma occur before the pain began?

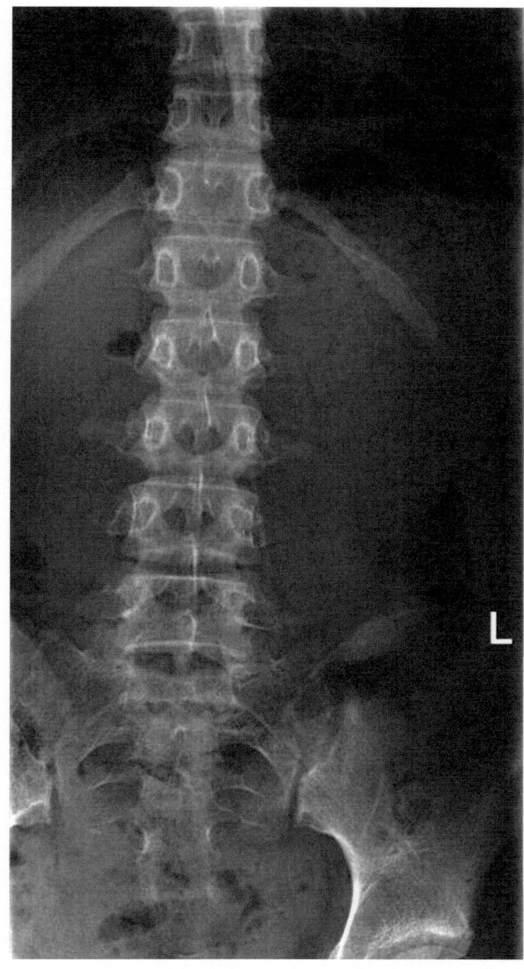

Fig. 12.1 PA standing lumbar sacral radiograph. No abnormalities are present

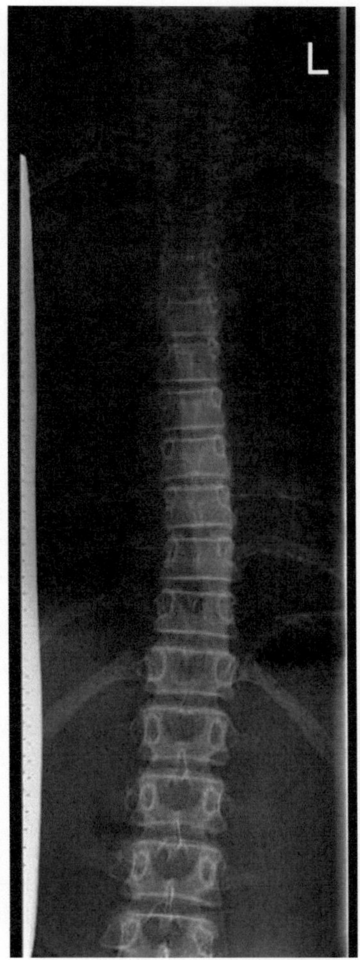

Fig. 12.2 PA standing thoracic lumbar radiograph. Mild asymmetry is noted. However, there is no rotation of the spinous process; therefore no significant scoliosis is present

2. Why does she experience pain when standing from a seated position?
3. What is the appropriate referral?
4. What is the next diagnostic test that should be considered?
5. What are possible treatments in this case?

Discussion

Nonspecific low back pain is the most common type of back pain among young children and especially adolescents [1]. Risk factors for low back pain in children include inactivity such as sitting and watching television or excessive time playing video games, obesity, sedentary lifestyle, sports participation, and a positive family history [2]. For children involved in sports, it is important to ask if there was an event or trauma that occurred before the onset of pain, as this could be a cause of spondylolysis and spondylolisthesis. For this patient there was no inciting incident. She may also have trouble standing from a seated position due to low back pain from underuse and deconditioning.

If her symptoms do not improve after 2–4 weeks, a referral may be made for physical therapy. A referral for specialty evaluation is made to a pediatric orthopedic surgeon and/or a neurosurgeon if the patient exhibits progressive neurologic deficit, conservative therapy fails, or the diagnosis is serious or uncertain. Serious conditions would include cauda equina syndrome, herniated disk, spinal stenosis, tumor, infection, or fracture [3].

If a patient with nonspecific low back pain does not improve after 6 weeks of conservative treatment including therapy, then laboratory tests and spine radiographs should be obtained. CBC, ESR, and CRP can help to evaluate the presence of inflammation, infection, or tumor. Excess imaging with limited benefit in the evaluation of low back pain in children has been reported [4]. For this reason, in nonspecific cases a radiograph is recommended if no improvement occurs after 6 weeks of follow-up, rather than sooner. On the other hand, if the history and physical examination suggest serious pathology, urgent referral to a pediatric spine specialist should be made. The specialist can then order advanced imaging, CT or MRI, as needed for diagnostic purposes and potential surgical planning. For this patient, routine referral was made to a pediatric orthopedic surgeon, but no advanced imaging was ordered because at her follow-up appointment, her pain had improved with physical therapy.

Low back pain is nonspecific when no definable cause can be identified. In such cases, the cause of the pain may be deconditioning combined with a strain of ligaments or muscles or other minor strains to the intervertebral disks or facet joints. Unfortunately, the exact cause of the pain is not always discernable—the diagnosis of nonspecific low back pain is a diagnosis of exclusion [2]. Treatment for nonspecific low back pain is conservative care with 4–6 weeks of physical therapy, observation, and reassurance. In addition, acetaminophen, NSAIDs, rest, application of cold/heat, or massage therapy can also be prescribed [2]. Parental involvement increases the child's compliance with treatment. In this case, she completed physical therapy, and at her last follow-up, her low back pain was markedly improved.

How to Approach the Case

Nonspecific low back pain is common. One goal of evaluation is to rule out potentially serious causes. A detailed history and physical is key to making an accurate diagnosis and guiding treatment. Specific questions to include are the onset of symptoms, description of the pain, location, duration, exacerbating and alleviating factors, presence or lack of pain radiation, family history, and if there is morning stiffness [2]. A complete neurological examination including deep tendon reflexes, strength, sensation, and gait should be performed. Core strength and stability should be examined to determine if the pain stems from weakness of the paraspinal and lateral abdominal muscles [2]. In cases of nonspecific back pain, radiographs are recommended if no improvement occurs after 6 weeks of conservative care. Advanced imaging such as bone scan, CT, or MRI can be ordered by the specialist on a case-by-case basis to rule out suspected serious conditions such as tumor, infection, or fracture [5].

> **▐ Red Flags for Back Pain due to Deconditioning**
> - Unexplained weight loss or loss of appetite
> - Fever and chills
> - Pain at rest
> - Pain that awakens the child from sleep at night
> - Recent onset of bladder dysfunction
> - Neurologic deficit

> **Short Differential Diagnosis**
> - Muscular strain—low back pain that can sometimes radiate to the buttocks, muscle spasms, back stiffness.
> - Spondylolysis—often occurs in teenage athletes, low back pain that is aggravated by hyperextension of the spine.
> - Spondylolisthesis—vertebral slippage can cause radiculopathy by irritation of the nerve roots.

Final Diagnosis

Chronic low back pain without sciatica due to muscular deconditioning

Natural History and Treatment Considerations

Nonspecific low back pain is self-limited in most patients. The natural history is gradual improvement over a few weeks. Persistent low back pain lasting more than 6 weeks needs a workup including standing AP and lateral radiographs of the painful area. If a patient demonstrates a neurologic deficit, leg pain worse than their back pain, no response to conservative treatment after 6 weeks, or radiographs that demonstrate a lesion, then referral to a pediatric spine specialist is indicated. In this case of nonspecific back pain, her back pain improved with physical therapy, and no additional workup was indicated.

Referral—Emergency, Urgent, or Routine: And to Whom?

A patient with nonspecific low back pain can be routinely referred to a physical therapist. If the back pain is not improving after 6 weeks with conservative care, then routine referral to a pediatric non-operative musculoskeletal physician, sports medicine physician if the child is an athlete, a pediatric orthopedic surgeon, and/or a neurosurgeon is appropriate. On the other hand, urgent referral to a pediatric spine specialist should be done in cases of back pain due to a specific cause such as a tumor, infection, or fracture.

Brief Summary

Low back pain is a common complaint in children and adolescents. In most cases the pain is nonspecific and self-limiting. Conservative treatment with physical therapy, NSAIDs, and rest is appropriate. However, if after 6 weeks of conservative care the pain does not improve, then standing PA and lateral radiographs of the painful area of the back and a referral to a pediatric orthopedic surgeon or neurosurgeon are indicated.

Key Features and Pearls
- Nonspecific back pain is self-limited and will resolve by 6 weeks.
- For patients with nonspecific low back pain, the primary treatment is conservative care, time, reassurance, and education.
- Possible risk factors for nonspecific low back pain in children include obesity, sedentary lifestyle, and psychosocial difficulties.
- Nonspecific back pain that does not resolve by 6 weeks needs radiographs and possible referral.

Editor Discussion

Nonspecific mechanical back pain in children and adolescents is common. A careful history and exam should be done on every patient who complains of back pain. Know the red flags of pediatric back pain. Remember that not all back pain in children stems from the spine—don't forget to consider pulmonary, renal, abdominal, and gynecological causes. In addition, obesity and depression can contribute to pediatric back pain. If nonspecific back pain does not resolve with 6 weeks of therapy, NSAIDs, and rest, standing AP and lateral radiographs of the painful area should be obtained and referral to a pediatric spine specialist considered.

W.L. Hennrikus

When a child complains of back pain and the worrisome causes have been excluded, this is an opportunity to evaluate their lifestyle and habits. Ask about nutrition, sleep (best to have a consistent wakeup time and minimum of 8 hours sleep), exercise, posture, screen time, carrying a heavy backpack, and other habits. If they are overweight and especially if they are obese (BMI >30). this is an opportunity to evaluate their and the family's nutrition. During the physical examination, evaluate core muscle strength. I ask the child to demonstrate ability to do 10 pushups with quality plank position. Also the child should demonstrate ability to hold a "V" position (with both lower extremities extended up in the air 30 degrees with their shoulders and chest also lifted off the table) for minimum of 10 seconds (see Chapt. 5). Know how to efficiently do a screening neurological examination, which can be done in less than 2 minutes (see Chap. 5). When we order spine radiographs, we typically obtain a standing PA and lateral film of the entire spine (cervical, thoracic, lumbar, and sacral) since this also gives us useful information of posture and balance.

R.M. Schwend

References

1. Jones GT, Macfarlane GJ. Epidemiology of low back pain in children and adolescents. Arch Dis Child. 2005;90(3):312–6.
2. Kordi R, Rostami M. Low back pain in children and adolescents: an algorithmic clinical approach. Iran J Pediatr. 2011;21(3):259–70.
3. Atlas SJ, Deyo RA. Evaluating and managing acute low back pain in the primary care setting. J Gen Intern Med 2001;16(2):120–31.
4. Auerbach J, Ahn J, Zgonis M, Reddy SC, Ecker ML, Flynn JM. Streamlining the evaluation of low back pain in children. Clin Orthop Relat Res. 2008;466(6):1971–7.
5. Taxter AJ, Chauvin NA, Weiss PF. Diagnosis and treatment of low back pain in the pediatric population. Phys Sportsmed. 2014;42(1):94–104.

Chapter 13
A Case of a Child with "Idiopathic" Scoliosis

George J. Richard, Stephanie B. Ihnow, and Laurel C. Blakemore

Brief Case Presentation

Chief Complaint

Six months of back pain

History

This is a 12-year-old female who presents for a clinic visit with 6 months of mild back pain. There has been no trauma or injury. She describes her pain as having an insidious onset and aggravated by standing, but it has not worsened over the past 6 months. She initially thought the pain was from overexertion with sports, but it did not resolve with periods of rest, prompting this visit. The pain was not related to the time of day and did not awaken her at night. The pain was located in her mid-back in a nonspecific area and did not radiate. Upon further prompting, she noted that she would occasionally have episodes of paresthesias affecting bilateral upper extremities, back of her neck, and parts of her upper back, which were short lasting

G. J. Richard (✉)
Department of Orthopaedic Surgery, University of Florida, Gainesville, FL, USA
e-mail: richaGJ@ortho.ufl.edu

S. B. Ihnow
Division of Pediatric Orthopaedic Surgery, University of Florida, Gainesville, FL, USA

L. C. Blakemore
Division of Pediatric Orthopedics, University of Florida, Gainesville, FL, USA

© Springer Nature Switzerland AG 2021
R. M. Schwend, W. L. Hennrikus (eds.), *Back Pain in the Young Child and Adolescent*, https://doi.org/10.1007/978-3-030-50758-9_13

and associated with sneezing or coughing. She reported transient occipital headaches associated with sneezing or coughing, which never required treatment or over-the-counter medications. She has had no recent fevers, night sweats, chills, or weight loss.

She had not had bladder or bowel incontinence. She was the product of a full-term vaginal delivery with no perinatal issues. Menses first began 1 month ago. There is no family history of scoliosis.

Physical Examination

She was afebrile with normal vital signs. Her weight is 38.6 kg, height 146.4 cm, and BMI 18.03 kg/m^2. She appeared healthy, Tanner stage IV, and was developmentally normal. No ligamentous laxity was appreciated. While standing upright, the right shoulder was elevated, her pelvis was level, and she had a left trunk shift and waistline asymmetry. She had no focal tenderness to palpation along her entire spine. On Adam's forward bend test, there was a large left thoracic prominence measuring 21° apical trunk rotation measured by the scoliometer. The patient had normal and painless forward flexion and extension. Neurological examination demonstrated a normal gait, negative Hoffman's test, and downgoing Babinski reflexes bilaterally. Brachioradialis, patellar tendon, and Achilles reflexes were 2+ bilaterally. There were abnormal abdominal reflexes in all four quadrants. Motor strength was full and symmetric in bilateral upper and lower extremities. Sensation was intact in all dermatomes in upper and lower extremities. Clinical appearance and radiographs are shown as follows.

Imaging and Radiographic Studies (Figs. 13.1, 13.2, and 13.3)

Questions About the Case the Reader Should Consider
1. What is the typical presentation of adolescent idiopathic scoliosis?
2. What features make this an atypical presentation for scoliosis?
3. What are the necessary referrals, and what diagnostic testing is required?
4. What is the differential diagnosis for atypical scoliosis?
5. Why does this patient have back pain?

Discussion

Adolescent idiopathic scoliosis (AIS) is defined as lateral spinal curvature greater than 10° diagnosed in a patient 10 years of age or older. Patients with typical AIS curves tend to present with a painless subtle thoracic and/or lumbar prominence

Fig. 13.1 (**a**) Patient standing upright with notable right trunk crease (*red arrow*), right shoulder elevation (*black arrow*), and left thoracic curvature (*black line*). No cutaneous abnormalities are evident. (**b**) Patient during the Adam's forward bending examination demonstrating the large left thoracic prominence (*black arrow*)

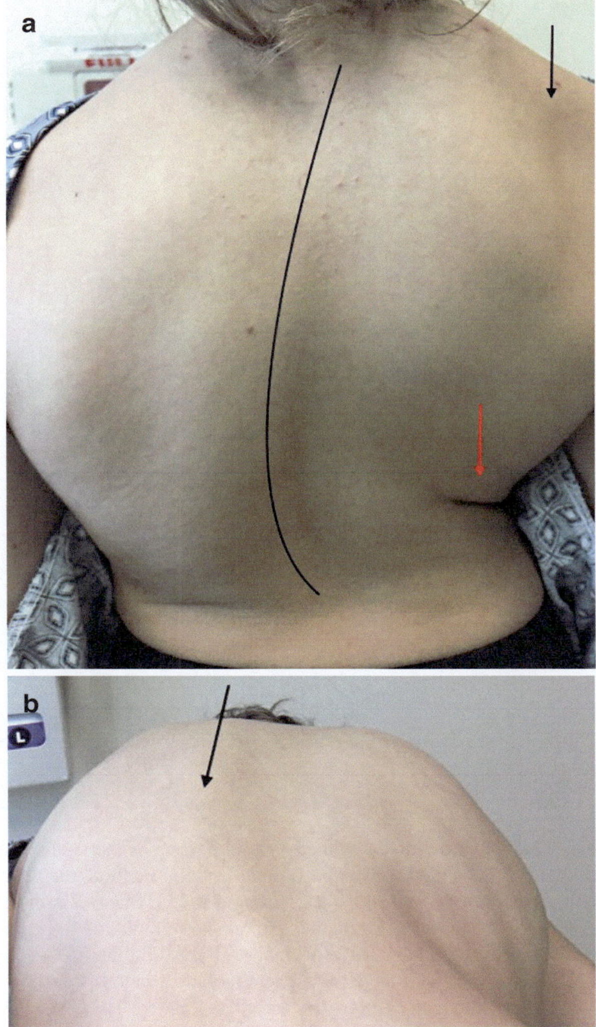

noted by the patient, parent, and pediatrician or on school screening [1]. Over 90% of patients with scoliosis will have curves with right-sided convexity [2]. AIS affects a reported 4 in 100 adolescents, having a female predominance, with studies reporting as high as a 3:1 ratio that increases with age [3]. Neurologic symptoms and signs such as headaches, hyperreflexia, and extremity numbness or weakness are not typically seen. Imaging will normally demonstrate a Cobb angle of <25° at initial presentation, as most patients present with curves below the threshold of treatment. By the end of skeletal maturity, only 10% of patients will progress to a curve beyond 45–50°, a degree deformity that may undergo spinal deformity surgery [4].

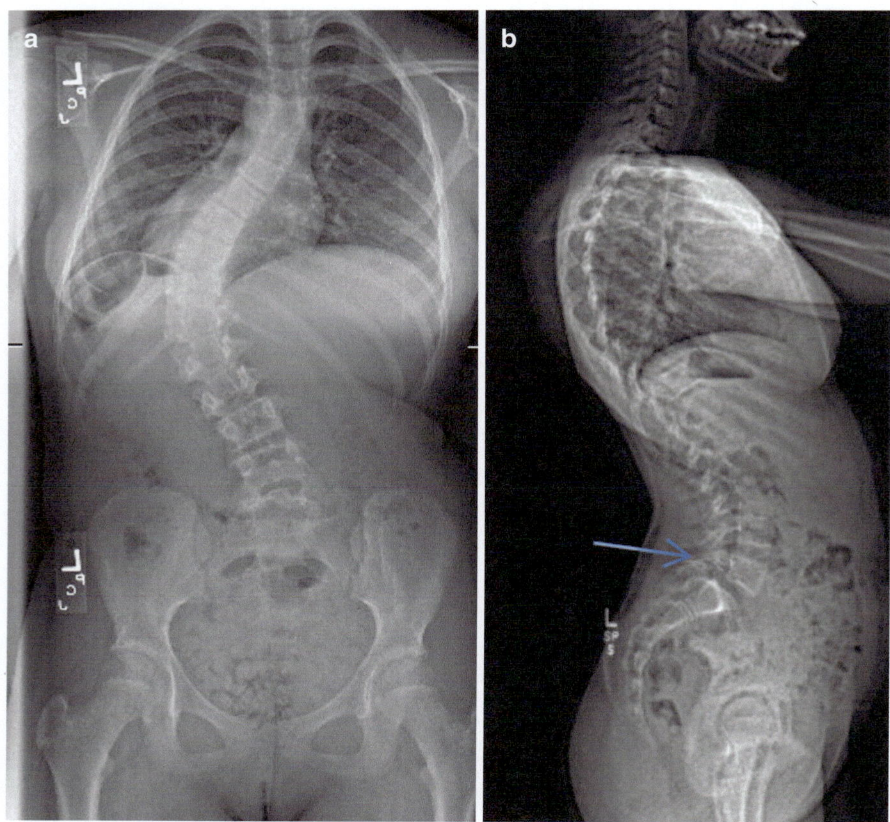

Fig. 13.2 (**a**) Low-dose biplanar PA radiograph of the spine. There is a large C-shaped thoracic curve with left-sided convexity. Using the Cobb method, the primary curve is 68° measured from end vertebrae T8 to L2 and apex vertebrae at T11. She is Risser Stage 1 and the triradiate cartilage is closed. (**b**) Low-dose biplanar lateral radiographs of the spine. Note thoracic hyperkyphosis measuring 58° from T2-T12 (normal <40°). Additionally, there is a grade 1 spondylolisthesis at L5-S1 (*blue arrow*). Pelvic parameters include a sacral slope of 55° (increased), pelvic tilt of 10°, and a pelvic incidence of 65° (increased)

In this case presentation, the patient had several red flag findings in the history, physical examination, and imaging that are not consistent with a diagnosis of AIS. These include as follows: (a) history of headaches occurring during times of Valsalva, (b) the presence of abnormal abdominal reflexes on physical exam, (c) reports of cape-like distribution paresthesias associated with Valsalva, and (d) left thoracic curve on imaging [5]. Findings that represent an atypical presentation of scoliosis are found in all portions of a patient encounter. Back pain is frequently reported in adolescents but is not directly linked to the presence of idiopathic scoliosis. Characteristics of atypical scoliosis include as follows: chronic back pain or headaches, abnormal neurological findings (i.e., absent or asymmetric reflexes,

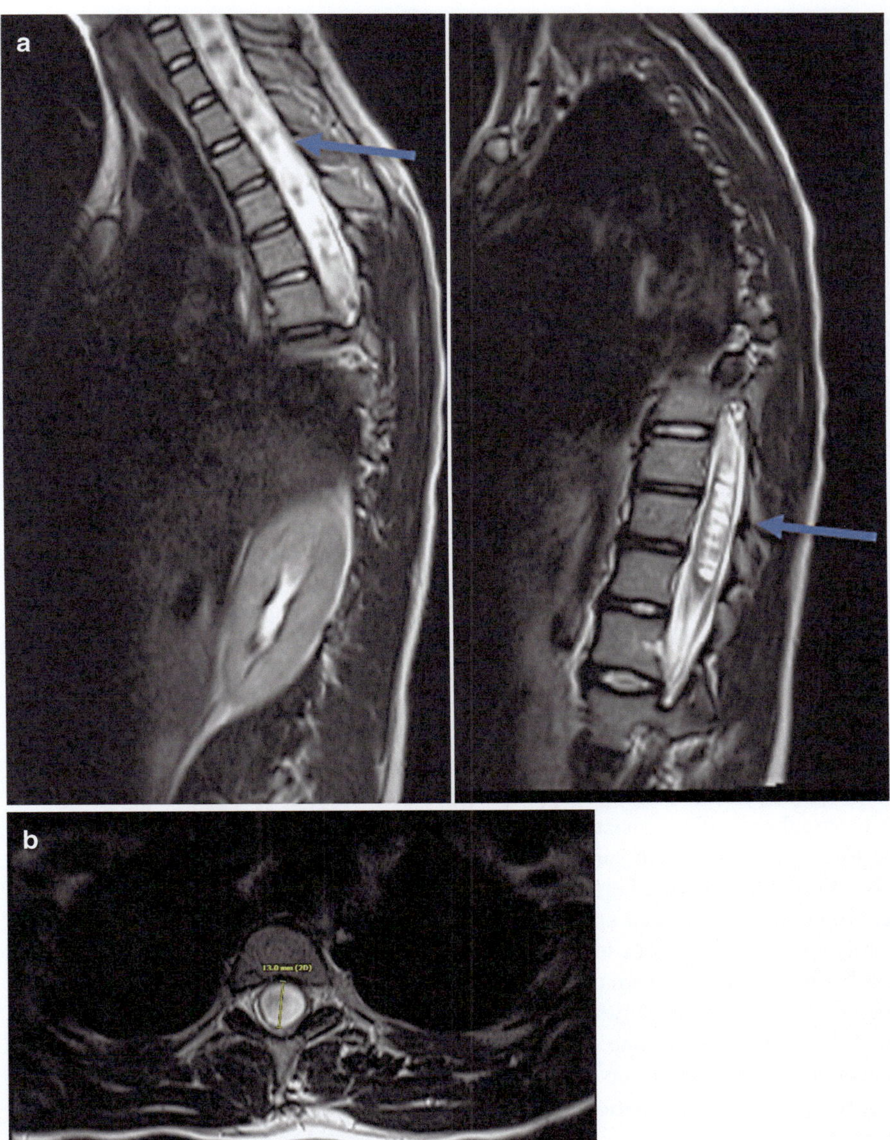

Fig. 13.3 (**a**) Sagittal T2-weighted MRI of the spine. This demonstrates large fluid-filled cyst within the spinal cord extending from the cervicomedullary junction to the conus medullaris consistent with a holocord syrinx (*blue arrows*). Not shown is 1 cm of cerebellar tonsillar herniation through the foramen magnum. (**b**) Axial T2-weighted MRI of the cervical spine demonstrating a 13-mm-diameter syrinx within the spinal cord

motor or sensory deficits), left thoracic curves, diagnosis at an early age (less than 10 years), severe curves (>45°) at a young age, and rapid progression of the curve (>1 degree progression per month).

> **Red Flags for Atypical Scoliosis**
> - Chronic back pain or headaches
> - Abnormal neurological findings (i.e., absent or asymmetric reflexes, motor or sensory deficits)
> - Left thoracic curve
> - Diagnosis at an early age (less than 10 years)
> - Severe curves (>45°) at a young age
> - Rapid progression of the curve (>1 degree progression per month)

The initial workup and diagnostic testing in cases of atypical scoliosis is similar to that of typical adolescent idiopathic scoliosis. This includes a complete birth history, past medical history, past surgical history, and family history. Complete examination must include examination of the spine for overlying cutaneous abnormalities (which can suggest an underlying neurologic abnormality), spinal and trunk alignment, Adam's forward bend test, and a complete neurologic examination including strength, sensation, reflexes, and abdominal reflexes.

If available, low-dose biplanar imaging can provide excellent image quality at a lower radiation dose than standard radiographs. If this is available through the pediatric spine specialist, then it is appropriate to defer radiographs until that visit. Initial radiographs should consist of standing posterior-anterior (PA) and lateral (Lat) radiograph of the entire spine. The PA view is preferred to the AP view to reduce radiation to the breasts. Performing multiple short cassette radiographs of the cervical, thoracic, and lumbar spine individually are rarely adequaete and can unnecessarily expose the patient to increased levels of radiation. If evidence of atypical scoliosis is found on exam and/or imaging, the child should be referred to an orthopedic specialist preferably within 1 month [1]. Further testing or in this case MRI imaging of the entire spine should be left to the pediatric spine specialist. If there is concern for an acute issue requiring immediate evaluation, such as a progressive neurologic deficit, the patient should be sent to the emergency room rather than a referral placed.

The imaging for this patient demonstrated a severe 68-degree *left-sided* thoracic curve on the PA view and thoracic hyperkyphosis of 58° on the lateral view. Additionally, a grade 1 spondylolisthesis and abnormal pelvic balance parameters were observed. Adolescent idiopathic scoliosis is more commonly associated with relative hypokyphosis on the lateral view, and hyperkyphosis suggests an atypical scoliosis. In this case, the spondylolisthesis did not correlate to the location of her back pain and was felt to be an asymptomatic incidental finding.

This child's large thoracic curvature and relative hyperkyphosis suggest an underlying etiology for this patient's scoliosis [6]. The differential diagnosis of occult etiologies in "idiopathic" adolescent scoliosis includes neurologic causes.

Congenital, neoplastic, and syndromic etiologies often present as cases of early-onset scoliosis, although they can sometimes be missed until early adolescence. The atypical findings discussed above were noted by a primary care physician and prompted an urgent orthopedic surgery evaluation. Once the patient was evaluated by an orthopedic surgeon and imaging was reviewed, an MRI was ordered, which demonstrated cerebellar tonsillar herniation and a large holocord syrinx (Fig. 13.3). These findings are consistent with the diagnosis of Chiari malformation and syrinx-associated scoliosis.

> **Underlying Causes of Atypical Scoliosis**
> - Back pain is not the most common presenting chief complaint in patients with syrinx-associated scoliosis, as syringomyelia is more often associated with headache and neck pain.
> - Less frequently patients present with a neurologic sensory deficit or complaints of pain in a cape-like distribution.

How to Approach the Case

Primary care physicians are the front line for the screening of many treatable conditions. In the setting of adolescent scoliosis, it is important to know the typical presentation in order to differentiate an idiopathic spinal curvature from an atypical curves or underlying etiologies. This allows for appropriate referral and timely evaluation and treatment. Important atypical symptoms include neurologic symptoms or signs, headaches, night pain, fevers, a left-sided curve, large curve magnitude at presentation, and rapid curve progression. Any of these findings in an adolescent patient should especially raise red flags. Back pain may or may not be a complaint. In our case, the differential diagnosis included tethered cord, syrinx, and Chiari malformation, with other causes (neoplastic, neurologic conditions, congenital) less likely. When presentation and plain radiographs suggest that a curve is atypical, referral to a pediatric spine specialist is indicated. The pediatric spine specialist will order MRI imaging of the entire spine.

Final Diagnosis

Chiari malformation and syrinx-associated scoliosis

Natural History and Treatment Considerations

A syrinx is a fluid filled cavity within the spinal cord and, when combined with neurologic symptoms, is referred to as syringomyelia. There is an approximate 25–85% association between syrinx and Chiari malformation [7]. The pathophysiology for this association has been hypothesized to be due to fourth ventricular outflow obstruction and subsequent forces (i.e., Valsalva maneuvers, intracranial arterial pulsation, etc.) acting to push CSF into a created spinal space [8]. The pathophysiology of the resulting scoliosis is much less clear. The most accepted etiology is anterior horn cell dysfunction causing paraspinal muscle imbalance and resultant scoliosis [9, 10]. However, others have posited that it is the Chiari malformation, tonsillar herniation, and subsequent cervicomedullary compression that propagate the spinal deformity [11].

Syrinx-associated scoliosis, as demonstrated in the above patient case, presents with uncommon manifestations. The most typical presenting symptoms are Valsalva-associated headache and neck pain [12]. Complaints of sensorimotor deficits and hyperreflexia are much less common findings at presentation, and their absence does not rule out a syrinx in the setting of scoliosis. Patients with syrinx-associated scoliosis are seen in an equal male to female ratio and first present with larger, more severe spinal curvatures. Also important is the increased frequency of left-sided curvatures, which occur in much higher frequency (reported up to 50%) in syrinx-associated cases. This is compared to 10% in the AIS literature [2]. Other common findings are large "C-shaped" curves, thoracic hyperkyphosis, and abnormal pelvic indices, which are all demonstrated in the patient case [13, 14].

Once the diagnosis of Chiari malformation was established, the patient was referred by the pediatric orthopedic surgeon to neurosurgery and underwent posterior fossa decompression with duraplasty (PFDD). Some evidence suggests that PFDD may halt curve progression in syrinx-associated scoliosis [15, 16]. However, due to this patient's curve magnitude at presentation, she will require a posterior spinal instrumentation and fusion. This will occur after follow-up MRI (hopefully) demonstrates successful syrinx resolution and she is cleared by the treating neurosurgeon to proceed.

Referral: Urgent to Orthopedic Surgery

Scoliosis with atypical features such as neurologic symptoms (headaches, paresthesias, weakness, hyperreflexia, primitive reflexes, etc.), left-sided curvature, and large curve magnitude should be urgently referred to an orthopedic surgeon who has training and expertise in treating pediatric spinal deformities. The diagnosis of Chiari I malformation and syrinx requires neurosurgical evaluation.

Brief Summary

Back pain is a frequent chief complaint in a pediatric primary care physician office. While back pain is not uncommon in children and adolescents, it is not typical of adolescent idiopathic scoliosis. A child presenting with back pain and scoliosis must undergo a thorough history and physical examination to rule out features of atypical scoliosis including headaches, night pain or fevers, or abnormal neurologic findings. If those findings are identified, or if radiographs suggest an atypical scoliosis, urgent referral to an orthopedic surgeon trained in pediatric spinal deformity is indicated. Radiographic findings on PA and lateral views of the entire spine can include large curves, left thoracic curves, and curves associated with hyperkyphosis. In this case, MRI of the entire spine demonstrated a Chiari malformation and a large thoracic syrinx. She was referred to a pediatric neurosurgeon who treated her surgically prior to orthopedic intervention.

> **Key Features and Pearls**
> - Features of atypical scoliosis include chronic back pain or headaches, abnormal neurological findings on exam, left thoracic curve, diagnosis of scoliosis at an early age, large curves >45°, and curves with rapid progression.
> - The presence of features of atypical scoliosis should prompt urgent referral to an orthopedic surgeon who has training and expertise in treating pediatric spinal deformities.
> - Patients with Chiari malformation and syrinx often require neurosurgical intervention prior to treatment of their scoliosis.

Editor Discussion

Atypical scoliosis is uncommon but always concerning. As illustrated in this classic chapter, a case of left thoracic scoliosis and back pain can stem from a Chiari malformation type I (CM-I) with syrinx. In addition, headaches, neck pain with extension, ataxia, weakness, and a cavus foot are additional red flags to urgently refer the patient to a pediatric spine specialist and obtain an MRI of the entire spine [17].

W.L. Hennrikus

The asymmetric abdominal reflex is a useful clinical finding that should be noted on each new patient evaluation for scoliosis (Video 7.1 in Chap. 7). You can use the back of your pen or other rough but not sharp or painful instrument. Scratch each of the four quadrants overlying the rectus femoris muscle on either side of the navel. Normally, there should be a contraction of the ipsilateral rectus femoris muscle. With a large syrinx, the reflex may be asymmetric, contracting on one side and no motion on the other, or there may be absence of the reflex altogether.

R.M. Schwend

References

1. Janicki JA, Alman B. Scoliosis: Review of diagnosis and treatment. Paediatr Child Health [Internet]. 2007;12(9):771–6.
2. Choudhry MN, Ahmad Z, Verma R. Adolescent idiopathic scoliosis. Open Orthop J. 2016;10:143–54.
3. Konieczny MR, Senyurt H, Krauspe R. Epidemiology of adolescent idiopathic scoliosis. J Child Orthop. 2013;7(1):3–9.
4. Asher MA, Burton DC. Adolescent idiopathic scoliosis: natural history and long term treatment effects. Scoliosis. 2006;1(1):2.
5. Qin X, Sun W, Xu L, Qiu Y, Zhu Z. Effectiveness of selective thoracic fusion in the surgical treatment of syringomyelia-associated scoliosis. Spine (Phila Pa 1976). 2016;41(14):E887–92.
6. Sha S, Qiu Y, Sun W, Han X, Zhu W, Zhu Z. Does surgical correction of right thoracic scoliosis in syringomyelia produce outcomes similar to those in adolescent idiopathic scoliosis? J Bone Jt Surg. 2016;98(4):295–302.
7. Kennedy BC, Kelly KM, Anderson RCE, Feldstein NA. Isolated thoracic syrinx in children with Chiari I malformation. Childs Nerv Syst. 2016;32(3):531–4.
8. Sharma M, Coppa N, Sandhu FA. Syringomyelia: a review. Semin Spine Surg. 2006;18:180–4.
9. Huebert HT, MacKinnon WB. Syringomyelia and scoliosis. J Bone Joint Surg Br. 1969;51(2):338–43.
10. Isu T, Iwasaki Y, Akino M, Abe H. Hydrosyringomyelia associated with a Chiari I malformation in children and adolescents. Neurosurgery. 1990;26(4):591–6; discussion 596–7.
11. Hankinson TC, Klimo P, Feldstein NA, Anderson RCE, Brockmeyer D. Chiari malformations, syringohydromyelia and scoliosis. Neurosurg Clin N Am. 2007;18(3):549–68.
12. Goel A, Vutha R, Shah A, Dharurkar P, Jadhav N, Jadhav D. Spinal kyphoscoliosis associated with Chiari formation and syringomyelia 'recovery' following atlantoaxial fixation: a preliminary report and early results based on experience with 11 surgically treated cases. World Neurosurg. 2019;125:e937–46.
13. Ferguson RL, DeVine J, Stasikelis P, Caskey P, Allen BL. Outcomes in surgical treatment of idiopathic-like scoliosis associated with syringomyelia. J Spinal Disord Tech. 2002;15(4):301–6.
14. Farley FA, Song KM, Birch JG, Browne R. Syringomyelia and scoliosis in children. J Pediatr Orthop. 1995;15(2):187–92.
15. Brockmeyer D, Gollogly S, Smith JT. Scoliosis associated with Chiari I malformations: the effect of suboccipital decompression on scoliosis curve progression. Spine (Phila Pa 1976). 2003;28(22):2505–9.
16. Sha S, Zhu Z, Qiu Y, Sun X, Qian B, Liu Z, et al. Natural history of scoliosis after posterior fossa decompression in patients with Chiari malformation/syringomyelia. Zhonghua Yi Xue Za Zhi. 2014;94(1):22–6.
17. Schwend RM, Hennrikus W, Hall JE, Emans JB. Childhood scoliosis: clinical indications for magnetic resonance imaging. J Bone Joint Surg Am. 1995;77(1):46–533.

Chapter 14
Low Back Pain in an Adolescent with Core Weakness, Hamstring Tightness, and Increased Body Mass Index

Mary E. Dubon, Dana H. Kotler, and Cynthia R. LaBella

Brief Case Presentation

Chief Complaint

A 13-year-old boy presents to you with a 2-week history of insidious onset, low back pain.

History

The pain is dull and ranges from a pain intensity of 5/10 to 9/10. He has no numbness, tingling, weakness, radicular symptoms, bowel/bladder incontinence, or night pain. His back pain is worse when sitting or walking for long periods of time but is unchanged with running in physical education class. It is improved with heat,

M. E. Dubon (✉)
Pediatric Sports Medicine, Boston Children's Hospital, Boston, MA, USA

Pediatric Rehabilitation Medicine, Spaulding Rehabilitation Hospital Boston, Charlestown, MA, USA

Physical Medicine and Rehabilitation, Harvard Medical School, Boston, MA, USA
e-mail: Mary.Dubon@childrens.harvard.edu

D. H. Kotler
Physical Medicine and Rehabilitation, Harvard Medical School, Boston, MA, USA

C. R. LaBella
Department of Pediatrics, Northwestern University's Feinberg School of Medicine, Chicago, IL, USA

Institute for Sports Medicine at Ann & Robert H. Lurie Children's Hospital of Chicago, Chicago, IL, USA

© Springer Nature Switzerland AG 2021
R. M. Schwend, W. L. Hennrikus (eds.), *Back Pain in the Young Child and Adolescent*, https://doi.org/10.1007/978-3-030-50758-9_14

massage, or change of position. He does not recall any trauma or changes in activity when the pain first began. He is otherwise healthy without other medical conditions. He has never had any surgeries or previous back pain. He does not play sports and does not exercise regularly. He reports that he is overweight and is motivated to lose weight. There is no family history of back pain or orthopedic conditions.

Physical Examination

His body mass index (BMI) is 28 Kg/M^2. His general examination is otherwise unremarkable. His lumbar spine examination reveals no asymmetry, deformity, or curvature, but there is a postural increased lumbar lordosis. He has generalized tenderness to palpation of his L2-L5 spinous processes and throughout his lumbar paraspinal musculature bilaterally. He has no tenderness to palpation of his sacroiliac joints or sacral spine. He has pain with return to spine neutral position from lumbar flexion and is noted to perform thigh climbing (with his hands) from a lumbar flexed position to return to an upright position. He otherwise has no pain with lumbar range of motion. He has no pain with single leg/one-legged hyperextension testing (stork test, a test for spondylolysis that involves the patient standing on one leg with the other hip flexed and then performing active lumbar hyperextension) bilaterally. He has a negative bilateral slump test (a test performed with the patient in a seated position with flexion of the cervical, thoracic, and lumbar spine; the examiner then assists the patient in stretching each knee individually into extension and ankle into dorsiflexion, asking if it prompts leg symptoms. If it does, the patient is asked to release the cervical flexion to see if it resolves the symptoms. If there is leg pain that is resolved with cervical release, the test is positive). He also has a negative bilateral straight leg raise (a test for radicular leg pain in which the patient is supine and the examiner passively stretches a straight/knee-extended leg toward the head, evaluating for radicular symptoms). When in a prone position, he has tenderness to palpation along the same points of the lumbar spine as he did in a standing position. You then ask the patient to extend his arms and legs into a "superman" position and if palpation of these same locations produces no tenderness. He has popliteal angle complements of 80° bilaterally, indicating hamstring muscle tightness. Popliteal angle compliment is a measure of hamstring flexibility tested with the patient supine, hip flexed to 90°, and the knee then passively extended (see Fig. 14.3). He has normal strength, sensation, and deep tendon reflexes to the bilateral lower extremities.

Questions About the Case the Reader Should Consider
1. What are some of the reasons for his pain?
2. How does the "core" provide stability for the spine and trunk?
3. How can you measure core stability?
4. How do core stabilization exercise programs work?
5. What is the importance of the hamstring muscles in back pain?

Discussion

This patient's history and physical examination reveal some key factors that are associated with mechanical low back pain including increased body mass index (BMI), sedentary lifestyle, core instability, and hamstring tightness. In this chapter, we highlight these associations and review the evaluation and treatment options.

Increased BMI, Sedentary Lifestyle, and Low Back Pain

Childhood obesity is associated with low back pain [1]. The increased body weight results in an increased mechanical load on the spine and supporting soft tissues [2]. Additionally, in obese patients, adipose tissue functions as an endocrine organ and produces pro-inflammatory cytokines leading to chronic low-level inflammation [3]. Low-level inflammation is associated with musculoskeletal pain [4].

Sedentary lifestyle has also been associated with low back pain [5]. There are mixed results regarding the effect of exercise on chronic low-grade inflammation; however, there is some evidence suggesting decreased low back pain after adherence to an exercise regimen [3, 6].

Core Stability and Low Back Pain

The "core" refers to a box including the abdominal musculature anteriorly, the spinal and gluteal musculature posteriorly, the pelvic floor and hip girdle musculature inferiorly, and the diaphragm musculature superiorly [7]. The relationship of the core musculature to spine mechanics has been studied extensively. There are several points of view regarding the optimal core activity to maintain spine stability during functional activity [8, 9]. Spinal stability is dependent on the interaction of three interdependent systems: the osseoligamentous system, the musculature, and the neural control system [10].

Measuring Core Stability

A gold standard validated test to determine core stability in the clinic setting does not exist. However, there are some examination maneuvers that are helpful including the prone instability test [7, 11]. In children and adolescents, a simpler modified version of this examination maneuver can be utilized. This modification involves the patient lying prone on the examination table. The examiner then does a standard palpation examination of the lumbar spine. If tenderness is elicited with palpation, the examiner then asks the patient to extend his/her arms and legs into the

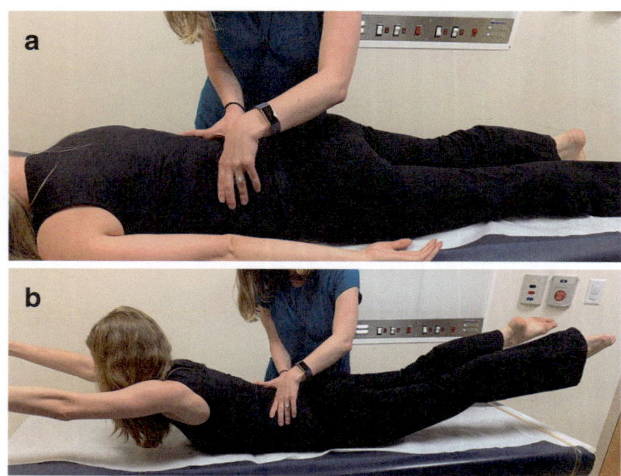

Fig. 14.1 Modified prone instability test. The patient lying prone on the examination table. The examiner then does a standard palpation examination of the lumbar spine (**a**). If tenderness is elicited with palpation, the examiner then asks the patient to extend his/her arms and legs into the "superman" position, and the examiner palpates the area of tenderness again (**b**). If tenderness is elicited with initial palpation but is not elicited with palpation of the same location while in the superman position, this is considered a positive test, suggestive of core instability and suggestive of the potential benefit of core stabilization exercises for the patient

"superman" position, and the examiner palpates the area of tenderness again. If tenderness is elicited with initial palpation but is not elicited with palpation of the same location while in the superman position, this is considered a positive test, suggestive of core instability and suggestive of the potential benefit of core stabilization exercises for the patient (Fig. 14.1). This test was performed and positive in this chapter's case presentation. In adults other examination findings that demonstrate core instability include a painful arc with lumbar flexion or with return to neutral from lumbar flexion as well as thigh climbing from a lumbar flexed position [12]. Some of these signs were seen in this chapter's case presentation.

Core Stability Exercise Programs

Exercise approaches to low back pain involve learning (or relearning) to recruit stabilizing muscles, progressively strengthening these muscles, and then translating this action to functional activity [13]. A core stability program is part of the standard of care for low back pain. Most clinical practice guidelines recommend exercise therapy. However, there is no evidence to support one specific type of exercise or the mode of administration [14].

A core stability exercise program begins with achieving the neutral spine position [7]. This may be accomplished through exercises such as pelvic tilts, pelvic

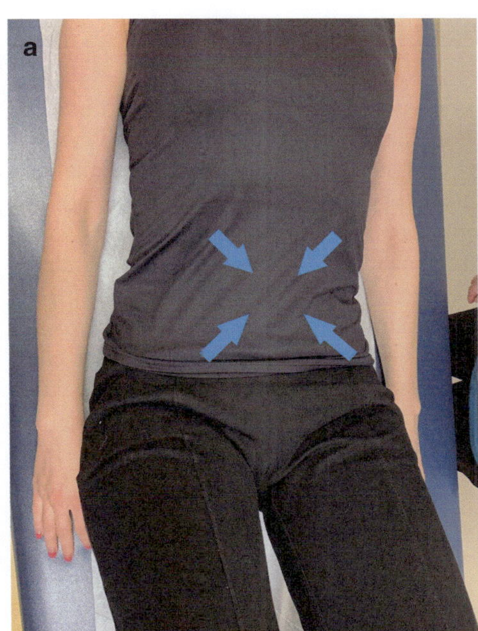
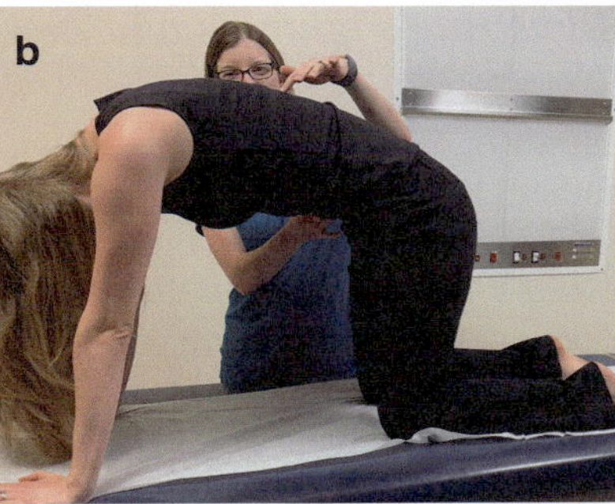
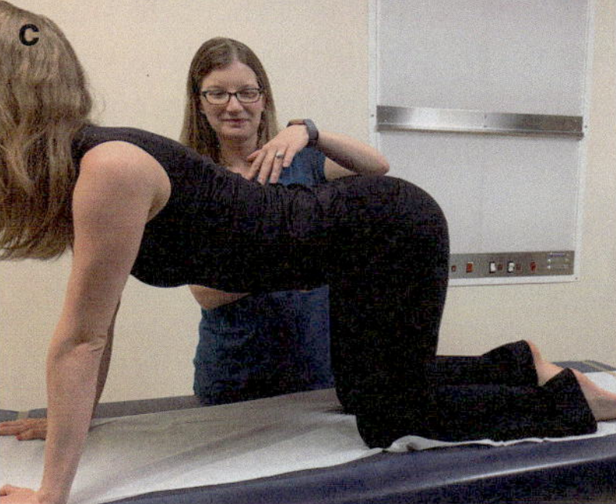

Fig. 14.2 Core stabilization exercises. Some examples of core stabilization exercises include as follows: (**a**) hollowing, navel to spine transverse abdominis activation and popular with yoga, the (**b**) cat pose, and (**c**) cow pose, which are performed one after another, starting in a neutral posture of the spine in a quadruped position. Core stabilization exercises are best learned under the guidance of a skilled physical therapist who can ensure that the exercises are performed properly

clocks (tipping the pelvis between 12 o'clock and 6 o'clock in an alternating fashion), or quadruped exercises such as "cat/camel" stretches. The patient must learn to activate the abdominal musculature in different fashions, including hollowing ("navel to spine"), which activates the transversus abdominis and internal obliques selectively and abdominal bracing, which activates the external obliques and lumbar extensors [15, 16] (Fig. 14.2). Once the patient is able to activate these abdominal muscles, there are a variety of potential exercises to build strength, address impairments, and improve movement quality.

Exercises can be progressed in multiple planes, including supine, side-lying, seated, kneeling, and standing. Typically the patient starts supine, learning how to activate and stabilize the core with the support of the examination table. The child then proceeds to more challenging exercises such as planks in a gradual and safe fashion over the course of weeks to months. Lastly, strategies such as unstable surfaces (balance boards, Bosu balls, etc.) can be utilized.

Hamstring Tightness and Low Back Pain

Hamstring tightness has been shown to be associated with low back pain in some studies [17]. Hamstring tightness/hamstring length can be measured using the popliteal angle complement (Fig. 14.3) [18]. Although some authors will use the term popliteal angle to refer to the popliteal angle complement, for the purposes of this paper, we will use the term popliteal angle complement to describe the angle in red pictured in Fig. 14.3. Popliteal angle complements of 50° or greater are considered to indicate tight hamstrings [19].

Research on the relationship between hamstring flexibility and low back pain is also limited as it is difficult to study these variables in isolation, as back pain etiology is often multifactorial, as seen in this case. Nonetheless, hamstring stretching exercises are frequently recommended for patients with low back pain and

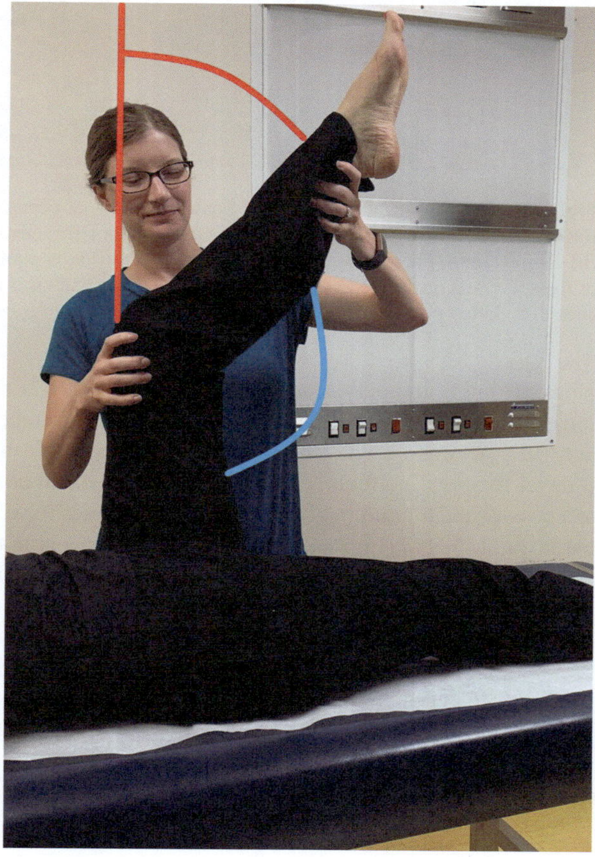

Fig. 14.3 Popliteal angle complement and popliteal angle. Popliteal angle complement, indicated by the curved red line, is often used to measure hamstring tightness. This is called the "popliteal angle" by many authors; however, the true popliteal angle is indicated by the blue curved line and is less commonly used when describing hamstring length. It is important to indicate which angle you are using clinically to properly communicate this with other providers. If the popliteal angle complement is greater than 30°, the hamstring muscles are considered tight

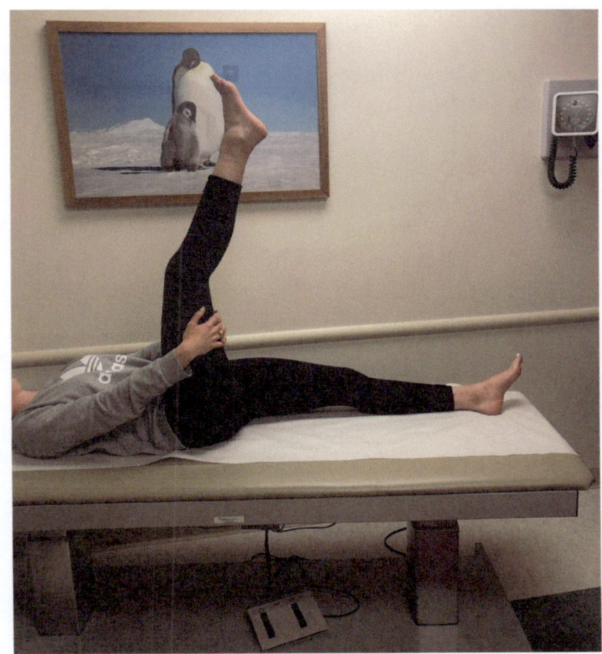

Fig. 14.4 Hamstring stretching in the supine spine neutral position

hamstring tightness. Hamstring stretches should be performed in a spine neutral position to avoid overstretching the ligaments of the spine instead of the hamstrings (Fig. 14.4).

How to Approach the Case

When evaluating an adolescent with mechanical low back pain, some factors that should be considered include the patient's activity level, core stability, hamstring flexibility, and body mass index. Examination maneuvers and treatment strategies discussed above can be helpful. Treatment requires an individualized approach based on underlying risk factors and may include weight loss, regular exercise, core stabilization exercises, and hamstring stretches.

Given the pattern of this patient's pain and examination findings, you diagnose him with mechanical low back pain and prescribe physical therapy for core strengthening and hamstring strengthening. You emphasize the importance of good core strength to support posture and reduce loading of the spine. You also explain that maintaining a healthy weight reduces load on the spine and therefore results in less back pain. You discuss some strategies toward weight loss.

> **🚩 Red Flags (Suggest Diagnosis Other Than Mechanical Back Pain and Warrant Imaging)**
> - Radicular signs/symptoms (radiating pain, positive straight leg raise test or seated slump test, paresthesias, numbness)
> - History of acute trauma
> - History of repetitive overuse (e.g., intensive training in a sport associated with risk for spondylolysis)
> - Pain with stork test (see chapter on spondylolysis)
> - Systemic symptoms

> **Short Differential Diagnosis**
> - Spondylolysis/spondylolisthesis
> - Herniated lumbar disc
> - Sacroiliitis or sacroiliac dysfunction
> - Facet joint arthropathy
> - Osteoid osteoma
> - Urinary tract infection/pyelonephritis

Final Diagnosis

Mechanical low back pain in the setting of core muscle weakness, elevated BMI, and tight hamstring muscles

Referral: When and to Whom?

You refer the patient to physical therapy with a focus on weekly core stabilization and hamstring stretching and a home exercise program. You reassure him that his pain should improve with physical therapy and that he should work with his physical therapist on healthy aerobic exercises he can do in addition to his strengthening and stretching. You also refer him to the interdisciplinary weight management clinic that includes a comprehensive exercise and nutrition program in addition to counseling and medical comorbidity screening resources. Over the course of several months of physical therapy, his low back pain gradually improves and he loses 20 pounds. At the 4-month return visit, he reports resolution of his low back pain. If there had been no improvement in his pain after doing physical therapy as prescribed, radiographs (AP and lateral) of the lumbar spine and a referral to a pediatric sports medicine specialist or pediatric orthopedic surgeon for further evaluation and treatment should be considered.

> **Key Features and Pearls**
> - Common risk factors for mechanical low back pain in adolescents are physical inactivity, overweight/obesity, and tight hamstrings.
> - Imaging is recommended only if there are one or more red flags (Box 1).
> - Treatment for mechanical low back pain in adolescents includes (1) physical therapy to guide core strengthening, posture training, and hamstring stretching, (2) regular aerobic physical activity, and (3) referral to weight management program if patient is overweight or obese.

Editor Discussion

Nonspecific mechanical back pain in children and adolescents is common. A careful history and exam should be done on every patient who complains of back pain. Know the red flags of pediatric back pain. In addition, obesity and depression can contribute to pediatric back pain. Be familiar with position statements by the American Academy of Pediatrics on obesity prevention, gaming, internet, television, and healthy lifestyles. All can be related to back pain. If nonspecific back pain does not resolve with 6 weeks of treatment with physical therapy, weight loss, and NSAIA's, standing AP and lateral radiographs of the painful area should be obtained and referral to a pediatric spine specialist considered.

W.L. Hennrikus

Back pain in a child should be viewed as an opportunity to address details of the child's diet as well as their overall fitness and exercise. Parents will appreciate your attention to their child's and the family's food choices, lifestyle, and exercise, which can be lifesaving. Although many who are obese or overweight have metabolic syndrome, not all do, and metabolic syndrome can be found in people who are of normal or low body weight. Insulin resistance is the hallmark of metabolic syndrome. Metabolic syndrome is a major public health problem in the United States and is increasingly a cause of death in the developing world, more so than from infectious diseases. According to Robert H Lustig MD, Director of UCSF Weight Assessment for Teen and Child Health Program, an excessive amount of dietary sugar and especially fructose, "the toxin," is a major contributor to obesity and metabolic syndrome in children [20]. Breakfasts cereals marketed to children can be up to 50% sugar. So, once you confirm that there is not an underlying pathological condition causing the back pain, use this opportunity to provide needed lifestyle guidance.

R.M. Schwend

References

1. Paulis WD, Silva S, Koes BW, Van Middelkoop M. Overweight and obesity are associated with musculoskeletal complaints as early as childhood: a systematic review. Obes Rev. 2014;15(1):52–67.
2. Bout-Tabaku S, Klieger SB, Wrotniak BH, Sherry DD, Zemel BS, Stettler N. Adolescent obesity, joint pain, and hypermobility. Pediatr Rheumatol. 2014;12:11.
3. da Cruz Fernandes IM, Pinto RZ, Ferreira P, Lira FS. Low back pain, obesity, and inflammatory markers: exercise as potential treatment. J Exerc Rehabil. 2018;14:168–74.
4. Briggs MS, Givens DL, Schmitt LC, Taylor CA. Relations of C-reactive protein and obesity to the prevalence and the odds of reporting low back pain. Arch Phys Med Rehabil. 2013;94:745–52.
5. Scarabottolo CC, Pinto RZ, Oliveira CB, Zanuto EF, Cardoso JR, Christofaro DGD. Back and neck pain prevalence and their association with physical inactivity domains in adolescents. Eur Spine J. 2017;26:2274–80.
6. Wasser JG, Vasilopoulos T, Zdziarski LA, Vincent HK. Narrative review exercise benefits for chronic low back pain in overweight and obese individuals. PM R. 2017;9(2):181–92.
7. Akuthota V, Ferreiro A, Moore T, Fredericson M. Core stability exercise principles. Curr Sports Med Rep. 2008;7:39–44.
8. Pope MH, Panjabi M. Biomechanical definitions of spinal instability. Spine (Phila Pa 1976). 1985;10:255–6.
9. Izzo R, Guarnieri G, Guglielmi G, Muto M. Biomechanics of the spine. Part I: spinal stability. Eur J Radiol. 2013;82:118–26.
10. Panjabi MM. The stabilizing system of the spine. Part I. Function, dysfunction, adaptation, and enhancement. J Spinal Disord. 1992;5:383–9; discussion 397.
11. Hicks GE, Fritz JM, Delitto A, Mishock J. Interrater reliability of clinical examination measures for identification of lumbar segmental instability. Arch Phys Med Rehabil. 2003;84:1858–64.
12. Ferrari S, Manni T, Bonetti F, Villafañe JH, Vanti C. A literature review of clinical tests for lumbar instability in low back pain: validity and applicability in clinical practice. Chiropr Man Therap. 2015;23:14.
13. Akuthota V, Nadler S. Core strengthening. Arch Phys Med Rehabil. 2004;85:86–92.
14. Oliveira CB, Maher CG, Pinto RZ, Traeger AC, Lin C-WC, Chenot J-F, van Tulder M, Koes BW. Clinical practice guidelines for the management of non-specific low back pain in primary care: an updated overview. Eur Spine J. 2018;27:2791–803.
15. Grenier SG, McGill SM. Quantification of lumbar stability by using 2 different abdominal activation strategies. Arch Phys Med Rehabil. 2007;88:54–62.
16. Richardson C, Jull GA, Hodges PW, Hides JA. Therapeutic exercise for spinal segmental stabilization in low back pain: scientific basis and clinical approach. Edinburgh: Churchill Livingstone; 1999.
17. Fasuyi FO, Fabunmi AA, Adegoke BOA. Hamstring muscle length and pelvic tilt range among individuals with and without low back pain. J Bodyw Mov Ther. 2017;21:246–50.
18. Lovell WW, Winter RB, Weinstein SL, Flynn JM. Lovell and Winter's pediatric orthopaedics. Philadelphia: Wolters Kluwer Health/Lippincott Williams & Wilkins; 2014.
19. Katz K, Rosenthal A, Yosipovitch Z. Normal ranges of popliteal angle in children. J Pediatr Orthop. 1992;12:229–31.
20. Lustig RH. Fat chance: beating the odds against sugar, processed food, obesity, and disease. New York: Penguin; 2013.

Chapter 15
Case of a Young Child Who Refuses to Bear Weight and Has Back Pain due to Leukemia

David Gendelberg and Todd J. Blumberg

Brief Case Presentation

Chief Complaint

A 4-week history of progressive weakness, weight loss, back pain, and 4 days of refusal to bear weight after a fall at home.

History

A 4-year-old boy has had progressive lower extremity weakness over the last month, increasing back pain, and a 3 kg weight loss and now won't stand up or walk. He had been playing outside a few weeks ago when his parents report that he had an accidental fall. He seemed to recover, but was notably clumsier and unsteady on his feet and has fallen several times in the last week. Four days ago he really slowed down, stopped walking, and began scooting, and now he is refusing to walk at all. He complains of pain when his parents lift him under his arms or with attempts to make him stand. When he is resting or seated, he seems comfortable. There has been no change in his bowel or bladder function. He has had no fevers recently, but he did have an upper respiratory illness about 2 weeks ago. This has since resolved. Family

D. Gendelberg (✉)
Department of Orthopaedics and Sports Medicine, Harborview Medical Center,
University of Washington, Seattle, WA, USA

T. J. Blumberg
Department of Orthopaedics and Sports Medicine, Seattle Children's Hospital,
University of Washington, Seattle, WA, USA

© Springer Nature Switzerland AG 2021
R. M. Schwend, W. L. Hennrikus (eds.), *Back Pain in the Young Child and Adolescent*, https://doi.org/10.1007/978-3-030-50758-9_15

history is notable for multiple family members with autoimmune diseases on the maternal side. There has been no recent travel out of the country or sick contacts.

Physical Examination

His weight is 20.2 kg, height 114 cm, and temp 36.2. He is not ill-appearing. Development is normal. There is no lymphadenopathy, but has notable pallor. There are no petechiae or organomegaly. He has no pain at rest while supine; however, he is uncomfortable with strength testing of the extremities. Lumbar spine tenderness to palpation is noted. No scoliosis is noted. Neurological examination is challenging given the patient's age, but he was noted to be spontaneously moving his upper and lower extremities with spontaneous knee flexion and extension, plantar flexion, dorsiflexion, and movement of all the toes in flexion and extension. He responds appropriately to light touch and tickling of his feet. There is no clonus. Babinski is down going. Reflexes are symmetric and 2+. He is unable to ambulate for gait assessment.

Imaging and Radiographic Studies (Figs. 15.1 and 15.2)

Questions About the Case the Reader Should Consider
1. What are the red flags in this patient's history that raise your concern?
2. What may be the possible cause of this patient's vertebral compression fracture?

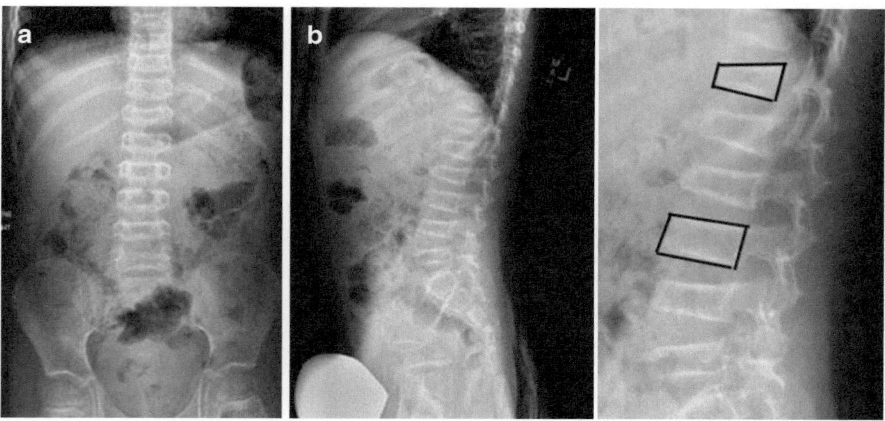

Fig. 15.1 (**a**) Full-length AP and lateral spine x-rays. (**b**). On closer inspection, there are multilevel compression fractures involving the thoracic and lumbar spine. The levels with most prominent height loss are T12, L4, and L5. Note the anterior wedging and height loss as compared to the adjacent normal vertebras. (Courtesy of Teresa Chapman, MD, Seattle Children's Hospital, Seattle, Washington)

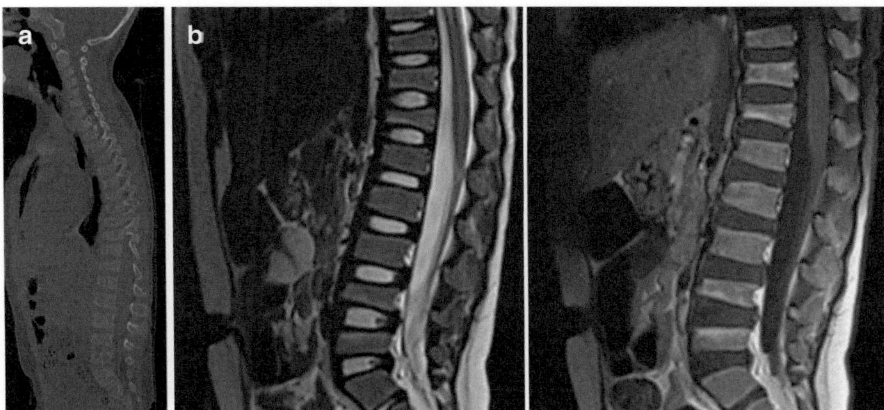

Fig. 15.2 (**a**) An CT ordered by the oncologist demonstrated diffuse osteopenia throughout the visualized axial skeleton with associated multilevel vertebral body height loss involving the thoracic and lumbar spine, in particular involving T12, L4, and L5 with at least 50% vertebral body height loss. These findings suggest a systemic underlying cause of demineralization and suspicion for pathologic vertebral body fractures. In this age group, leukemia is a primary consideration, although an underlying metabolic bone abnormality is also possible. (**b**) T2 sagittal and T1 contrast-enhanced sagittal images showing multilevel compression fractures and marrow enhancement of T12, L4, and L5. The oncologist or pediatric orthopedist will always obtain a contrast-enhanced MRI when evaluating for a tumor, inflammatory, or infectious process. (Courtesy of Teresa Chapman, MD, Seattle Children's Hospital, Seattle, Washington)

3. What tests should be ordered next?
4. What physical exam findings are often found with this diagnosis?
5. What is the appropriate referral?
6. What are the treatment options for this case?

Discussion

Leukemia can mimic several orthopedic pathologies in children at presentation. Therefore, it is important to obtain a thorough history and exam [1]. Many details in this patient's history should raise concern. Back pain in a 4-year-old is a red flag. Moreover, persistent back pain that wakes the child up at night and is debilitating to the point that the patient has difficulty ambulating requires an immediate and thorough evaluation [2–4]. As the child grows, gradual weight gain is expected. Therefore, unintended weight loss, especially over a short period of time, should raise concern. Increasing clumsiness or an unsteady gait is also very concerning. When encountering these symptoms, one should consider a differential diagnosis that includes tumor, infection, or systemic inflammatory arthritis [4].

The causes of bone demineralization during the course of leukemia are multifactorial, and it can be caused by the underlying infiltrative disease process, inactivity, chemotherapeutic agents, and abnormalities in bone mineral homeostasis. This in turn leads to decreased bone density, to weakening of the bony architecture of the vertebral body, and ultimately to the development of compression fractures, even without trauma. Following treatment, patients often experience some degree of remodeling and improvement of bone mineral density [5–9].

When approaching a pediatric patient with back pain, weight loss, and refusal to bear weight, it is important to establish a differential diagnosis to guide further diagnostic evaluation. Many conditions may present similar to the patient described above necessitating further testing. The most urgent diagnoses are malignancy and infection. Leukemia is a malignancy affecting the white blood cells, often leading to an infiltrative process of the bone marrow and ultimately changes in the patient's peripheral blood composition. Infection, especially when severe, may also present with abnormal findings in routine laboratory blood tests. Therefore, initial diagnostic tests for suspected malignancy or infection should consist of a complete blood count (CBC) with differential and a peripheral blood smear. In addition to a CBC, erythrocyte sedimentation rate (ESR) and C-reactive protein (CRP) should also be obtained, as inflammatory arthropathies and musculoskeletal infection may present similarly [10–13].

Leukemia can affect multiple organ systems throughout the body. Therefore, additional tests should be performed to evaluate the function of the additional viscera. This is achieved by ordering a basic metabolic panel (BMP), liver function tests, and coagulation studies.

Leukemia may present in multiple ways and mimics many self-limited diseases of childhood. Therefore, one needs to keep a certain index of suspicion and perform a thorough history and physical exam of the patient. A meta-analysis that included >3000 children from 33 studies found that more than half of the patients presented with at least one of the following exam findings: organomegaly, pallor, fever, or bruising. Organomegaly was found in over 60% of the cases and may manifest as weight loss, abdominal distension, or abdominal pain. Lymphadenopathy, which may be found in nearly half of the patients, typically presents as nontender, firm, and matted and does not respond to antibiotics. Lymphadenopathy in the posterior auricular, epitrochlear, or supraclavicular area should raise greater concern for malignancy. Fever is present in more than half of the patients with leukemia. Manifestation of hematologic abnormalities, such as bleeding (i.e., petechiae), pallor, and abnormal laboratory values are present in over 50% of patients. In addition, musculoskeletal pain has been found to be the presenting symptom in 43% of cases [14]. Less common findings include a mediastinal mass, headaches, or testicular enlargement. A mediastinal mass may cause swelling, dysphagia, or dyspnea secondary to compression of the superior vena cava or through direct compression [10].

Upon suspicion of leukemia, the patient should be referred to a pediatric oncologist for further workup and diagnosis. The first step taken will be to obtain a bone marrow biopsy. Once the tissue is obtained, the pathologist will perform further tests to confirm the diagnosis and detect the subtype of leukemia present. Workup of the bone marrow may include morphological assessment, cytochemical evaluation, or immunohistochemical analysis [10, 11]. When vertebral compression fractures or other fractures are present, the patient should be referred to a pediatric orthopedic surgeon for further evaluation and treatment. In these cases, CT or MRI may be ordered by the oncologist in collaboration with the pediatric orthopedist to better characterize the fractures and extent of disease.

Multidrug chemotherapy is the mainstay of treatment for leukemia. The exact regimen is dependent on the immunophenotype of the leukemia as well as the patient's risk category. Treatment is divided into multiple phases, and evaluation for central nervous system involvement with a lumbar puncture is necessary to determine if intrathecal chemotherapy is indicated (Fig. 15.3). Most treatment regimens take 2–3 years to complete. In addition, the patient should be treated whenever there is a suspected infection with broad-spectrum antibiotics, and any metabolic imbalances should be corrected. Back pain and joint pain will usually begin to improve a few weeks after the initiation of therapy. Typically, no active intervention is required. For multiple compression fractures, bracing may be helpful, but is sometimes not considered necessary unless there is the development of kyphosis on upright radiographs.

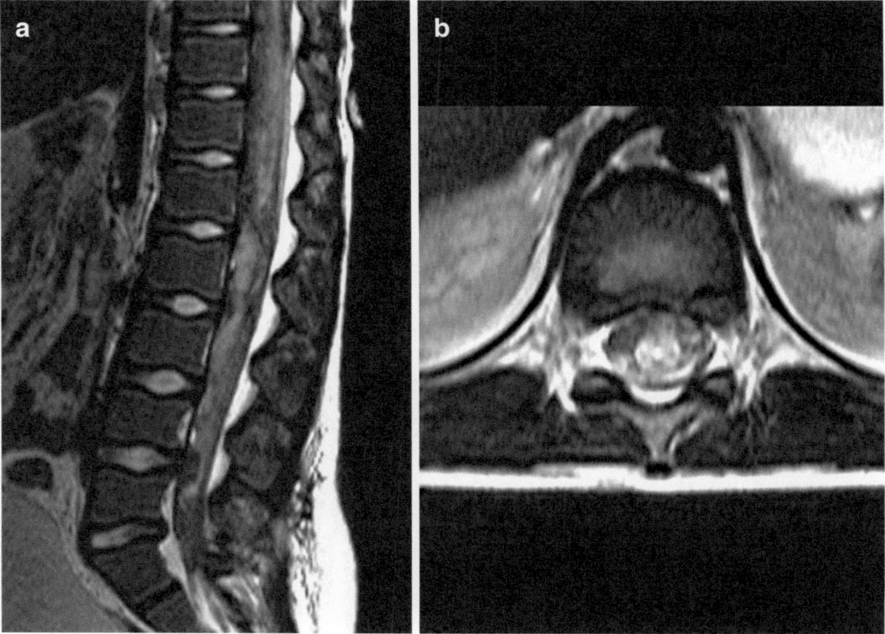

Fig. 15.3 T2-weighted sagittal and axial images displaying an example of central nervous system involvement with intradural enhancement in a patient with leukemia. (Courtesy of Teresa Chapman, MD, Seattle Children's Hospital, Seattle, Washington)

How to Approach the Case

Any young child who refuses to bear weight or is having unexplained weakness and clumsiness warrants further evaluation, with blood work and plain radiographs initially obtained to help narrow the differential diagnosis. Labs showed a normal white blood cell count of 6.1 K/mm^3, mild thrombocytopenia with a platelet count of 138 K/mm^3, and severe anemia, with a hematocrit 19.8%. CRP was mildly elevated at 1.8 mg/dL. ESR was markedly elevated at >140 mm/min.

In this case, there were no clear localizing symptoms, and the onset was fairly insidious over several weeks. Infection would also be possible given his clinical presentation; however, without fever and only mildly elevated CRP, this is less likely. A blood culture may be ordered. A decrease in the production of platelets and red blood cells with multilevel pathologic compression fractures is concerning for a systemic process, and additional imaging is indicated to better evaluate whether an oncologic, infectious, or inflammatory process is occurring.

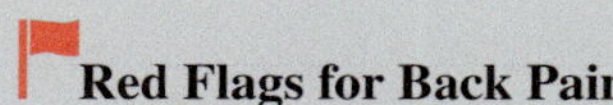

Red Flags for Back Pain
- Younger child
- Night pain
- Neurological findings
- Inability to bear weight
- Fevers
- Weight loss

Short Differential Diagnosis
- Infection – Always suspect infection when a tumor is suspected.
- Inflammatory arthritis – Juvenile idiopathic arthritis, reactive arthritis, inflammatory bowel disease-related arthritis.
- Other malignancies: Lymphoma, benign bone tumors, malignant bone tumors, tumors of the neural elements.
- Eating disorder or vitamin D deficiency.

Final Diagnosis

Leukemia in a 4-year-old boy.

Natural History and Treatment Considerations

Multilevel compression fractures in a young patient without kyphosis can be observed without bracing. Bracing, however, can be used to reduce pain in select cases. The compression fractures are pathologic fractures as the bone marrow has been replaced by rapidly dividing leukemic cells, in this case precursor B-cells. When this occurs, the energy needed to cause a compression fracture is markedly decreased, and even a simple fall in a young child may result in a fracture. Follow-up is needed with repeat upright radiographs to confirm that no kyphosis develops. Pain typically resolves with appropriate treatment of the underlying malignancy [6–9].

Referral – Emergency, Urgent, or Routine: And to Whom?

A young child presenting with back pain and refusal to bear weight should raise alarms and prompt immediate workup. Once there is suspicion for a malignant process, the patient should be *urgently* referred to a pediatric oncologist. In the event of a child with associated compression fractures, the patient should be referred to a pediatric orthopedic surgeon with expertise in spinal conditions for fracture management. In addition, the patient should be seen by a physician with experience in bone metabolism, such as an endocrinologist, for bone mineral density optimization. Many treatment regimens for leukemia include high-dose corticosteroids, which further weaken the bone density. Monitoring of bone mineral density should continue after remission as studies have found that bone metabolism and endocrine function continue to be affected into adulthood among pediatric cancer survivors [15].

Brief Summary

Refusal to bear weight in a young child is never normal and must be investigated until a cause is identified. While back pain is not uncommon in children, it is concerning if associated with refusal to bear weight, unintended weight loss, signs of motor weakness, and increased clumsiness or falls. In this case, the imaging helps to both explain the back pain and to identify a systemic cause for both the back pain and refusal to bear weight. Multiple compression fractures of the spine are not common in children without associated high-energy trauma. However, severe osteopenia and bone marrow infiltration predisposed this patient to them. The most common pediatric malignancy is leukemia, which accounts for nearly 30% of all pediatric cancers. Urgent referral to a pediatric oncologist and pediatric spine surgeon is indicated for appropriate staging and treatment for the malignancy and to assure no long-term sequelae from the compression fractures.

> **Key Features and Pearls**
> - Refusal to bear weight and persistent back pain in a young child should raise a red flag for a more involved process such as malignancy, infection, or inflammatory arthritis. These children should undergo a prompt workup and referral.
> - Patients with leukemia that have involvement of the spine may sustain compression fractures secondary to local osteopenia. These fractures usually do not need surgical intervention and need follow-up as well bone mineral density optimization.
> - Back pain will usually lessen a few weeks after treatment for the leukemia is initiated.

Editor Discussion

Leukemia is the most common cancer in childhood. Twenty percent of children with leukemia present with bone pain. Some children with leukemia will limp and some will stop walking. The most important aspect of this case is recognition! Keep leukemia high on your differential diagnosis in any child with back pain combined with fever, pallor, malaise, lymphadenopathy, hepatosplenomegaly, and easy bruising.

W.L. Hennrikus

Back pain in the child under 5 years of age is particularly concerning. Infection and tumor are both relatively rare in this age group, but a surprisingly common cause of back pain when an actual source is identified. So when you hear that a 3-year-old child has back pain, won't walk or walks very cautiously, and seems very stiff, think of inflammation in the spine. This could include discitis, a primary spinal cord tumor, or tumor affecting the spine such as leukemia. The hip joint in this age group is a more common reason a child might refuse to walk, either from transient synovitis or septic arthritis. So when the workup of the hip is negative, don't forget the spine!

R.M. Schwend

References

1. Sinigaglia R, Gigante C, Bisinella G, Varotto S, Zanesco L, Turra S. Musculoskeletal manifestations in pediatric acute leukemia. J Pediatr Orthop. 2008;28(1):20–8.
2. Hollingworth P. Back pain in children. Br J Rheumatol. 1996;35(10):1022–8.
3. Dissing KB, Hestbæk L, Hartvigsen J, et al. Spinal pain in Danish school children - how often and how long? The CHAMPS Study-DK. BMC Musculoskelet Disord. 2017;18(1):67.
4. Hasler CC. Back pain during growth. Swiss Med Wkly. 2013;143(0102):w13714.
5. te Winkel ML, Pieters R, Hop WCJ, et al. Bone mineral density at diagnosis determines fracture rate in children with acute lymphoblastic leukemia treated according to the DCOG-ALL9 protocol. Bone. 2014;59:223–8.
6. Newman AJ, Melhorn DK. Vertebral compression in childhood leukemia. Arch Pediatr Adolesc Med. 1973;125(6):863.

7. Hirji H, Saifuddin A. Paediatric acquired pathological vertebral collapse. Skelet Radiol. 2014;43(4):423–36.
8. Pandya NA, Meller ST, MacVicar D, Atra AA, Pinkerton CR. Vertebral compression fractures in acute lymphoblastic leukaemia and remodelling after treatment. Arch Dis Child. 2001;85(6):492–3.
9. Latha M, Thirugnanasambandam R, Venkatraman P, Scott J. Back pain: an unusual manifestation of acute lymphoblastic leukemia – a case report and review of literature. J Fam Med Prim Care. 2017;6(3):657.
10. Malogolowkin MH, et al. Clinical assessment and differential diagnosis of the child with suspected cancer. In: Pizzo P, Poplack D, editors. Principles and practice of pediatric oncology. 5th ed. Philadelphia: Lippincott Williams & Wilkins; 2006. p. 145.
11. Fletcher BD, Pratt CB. Evaluation of the child with a suspected malignant solid tumor. Pediatr Clin N Am. 1991;38(2):223–48.
12. Cabral DA, Tucker LB. Malignancies in children who initially present with rheumatic complaints. J Pediatr. 1999;134(1):53–7.
13. Murray MJ, Tang T, Ryder C, Mabin D, Nicholson JC. Childhood leukaemia masquerading as juvenile idiopathic arthritis. BMJ. 2004;329(7472):959–61.
14. Clarke RT, Van den Bruel A, Bankhead C, Mitchell CD, Phillips B, Thompson MJ. Clinical presentation of childhood leukaemia: a systematic review and meta-analysis. Arch Dis Child. 2016;101(10):894–901.
15. Brignardello E, Felicetti F, Castiglione A, et al. Endocrine health conditions in adult survivors of childhood cancer: the need for specialized adult-focused follow-up clinics. Eur J Endocrinol. 2013;168(3):465–72.

Chapter 16
Child with Back Pain due to Sickle Cell Crisis

Nattaly E. Greene, Natasha M. Archer, and Coleen S. Sabatini

Brief Case Presentation

Chief Complaint

A 16-year-old male with acute on chronic back pain.

History

A 16-year-old male with a known diagnosis of sickle cell disease (SCD) presents to the clinic with acute on chronic thoracic and lumbar back pain. He denies any acute traumatic event. He has been "working out" in recent days and admits that he has not been staying well-hydrated. In reviewing his history, he also has had recent subjective fevers and generally has not been feeling particularly well the last few days.

N. E. Greene
Harvard Combined Orthopaedic Residency Program, Boston, MA, USA

N. M. Archer
Department of Pediatrics, Dana Farber/Boston Children's Cancer and Blood Disorders Center, Harvard Medical School, Boston, MA, USA

C. S. Sabatini (✉)
Department of Orthopaedic Surgery, University of California San Francisco, UCSF Benioff Children's Hospital Oakland, Oakland, CA, USA
e-mail: Coleen.Sabatini@ucsf.edu

© Springer Nature Switzerland AG 2021
R. M. Schwend, W. L. Hennrikus (eds.), *Back Pain in the Young Child and Adolescent*, https://doi.org/10.1007/978-3-030-50758-9_16

Physical Examination

He is healthy, but tired-appearing. He is of normal height and weight. He is developmentally normal for age, Tanner 5. He has tenderness to palpation along the thoracic and lumbar spine both along the midline and in the paraspinal muscles. He moves slowly when changing positions but has a normal gait when walking in clinic. He is neurologically normal in the upper and lower extremities and has no bowel or bladder symptoms.

Imaging and Radiographic Studies (Figs. 16.1, 16.2, 16.3, and 16.4)

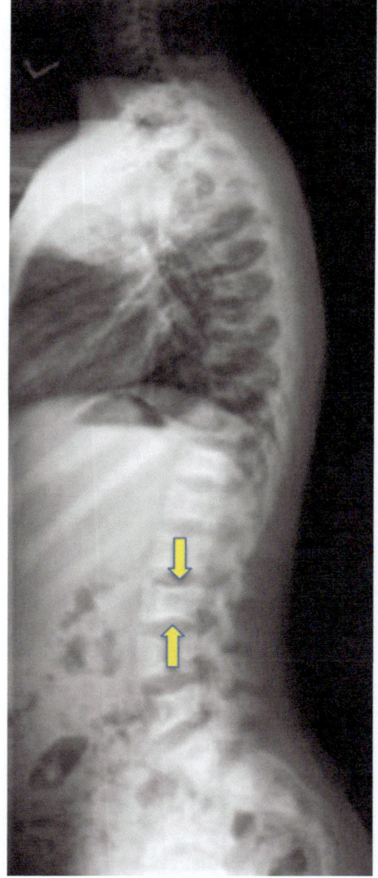

Fig. 16.1 A lateral radiograph of the spine which demonstrates marginated depression of the superior and inferior endplates of multiple adjacent vertebrae. These depressions are due to endplate necrosis from microvascular occlusions and are the typical "H-shaped" vertebrae seen in sickle cell disease. (Courtesy of Bamidele Kammen, MD. UCSF Benioff Children's Hospital Oakland)

Fig. 16.2 Close-up radiograph of spine demonstrating the typical "H-shaped" vertebrae seen in sickle cell disease. (Courtesy of Bamidele Kammen, MD. UCSF Benioff Children's Hospital Oakland)

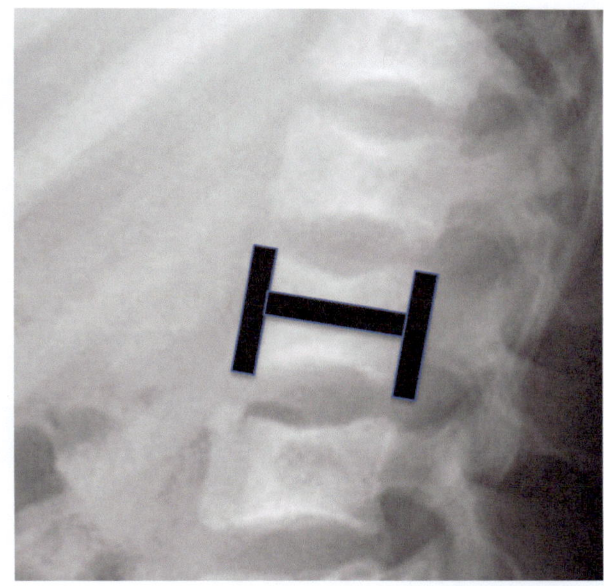

Fig. 16.3 Sagittal MR images of thoracic spine that demonstrates acute infarction with heterogeneous T2 prolongation of multiple vertebrae. (Courtesy of Bamidele Kammen, MD. UCSF Benioff Children's Hospital Oakland)

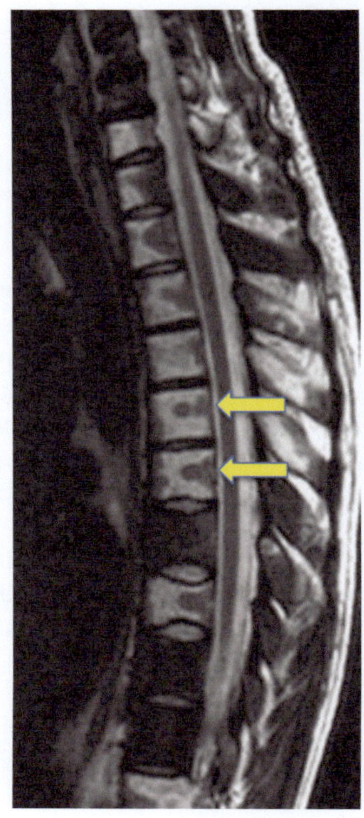

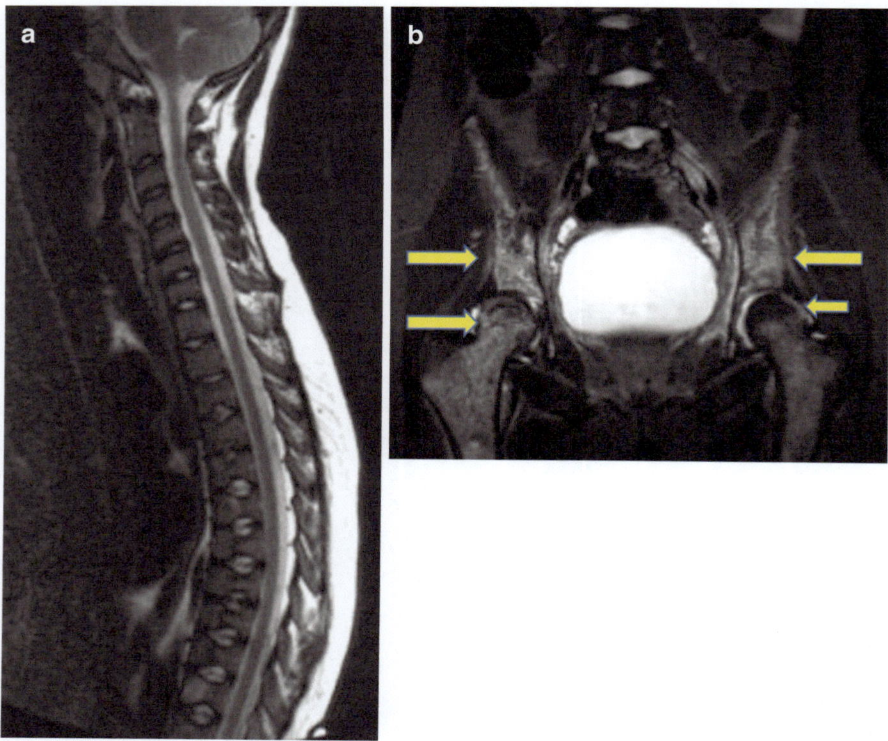

Fig. 16.4 (**a**, **b**) Whole-body coronal STIR-weighted MR images showing multiple irregular areas consistent with multiple infarcts. (Courtesy of Bamidele Kammen, MD. UCSF Benioff Children's Hospital Oakland)

Questions About the Case the Reader Should Consider

1. How does the sickle cell disease (SCD) diagnosis in this patient change the differential diagnosis of back pain in an adolescent?
2. How does SCD lead to back pain?
3. How does SCD often present as back pain in an adolescent? Which pieces of information in the health history point towards back pain due to SCD?
4. Could this be routine back pain like we would see in other adolescents without SCD?
5. Given the underlying diagnosis of SCD, what laboratory data and radiologic imaging studies would we do to make the appropriate diagnosis and make sure that we are not missing something in this patient?

Discussion

Given this patient's history of sickle cell disease, the differential diagnosis is broader than that of back pain in an adolescent without sickle cell disease (see below).

In understanding this patient's back pain, it is necessary to remember what sickle cell disease is and how the process of sickling in the body can lead to pain crisis events.

Sickle cell disease is a group of inherited blood disorders in which the RBCs change from their traditional flexible biconcave shape to a crescent or rigid, "sickled" shape [1]. This transformation is due to a point mutation in the β-globin gene resulting in a substitution of the amino acid valine for glutamic acid.

There is a long-standing association between people of African descent and SCD, although it also occurs in individuals from other ethnic backgrounds including Mediterranean, Indian, and the Middle Eastern [2]. This connection is thought to be due, in part, to the protective role the sickle cell mutation has provided against *Plasmodium falciparum* malaria in regions where malaria is endemic [3]. Although not exclusive to these ethnic backgrounds, this becomes an important portion of the health history and SCD is an important etiology to consider in patients presenting with back pain.

The process of sickling is due to conformational changes within the hemoglobin molecule between the deoxygenated and oxygenated states. This process leads to its change in shape into an elongated rigid form, a process known as "sickling," and it is the basis for the downstream effects of the disease [4]. Repetitive sickling and un-sickling leads to erythrocyte damage by rendering the membrane inflexible. The clinical complications caused by the anemia, repeated ischemia and reperfusion, and inflammation include vaso-occlusive bone pain, functional asplenia, acute chest syndrome (ACS), cerebrovascular events, pulmonary hypertension (PH), and multi-organ dysfunction syndrome [5].

Vaso-occlusive crises (VOC) result from end-tissue microinfarctions [6]. These episodes most often involve bone, lung, spleen, brain, and penis. When bone is involved, long bones are most commonly affected, but pain episodes can occur in any structure that contains bone marrow, including ribs, sternum, vertebral bodies, and the skull.

Vaso-occlusive crises are intense, and they vary in duration lasting from hours to days. They can present as early as 6 months of age with an average first time presentation at 6 years [7]. For young children, they frequently experience early vaso-occlusive pain in the bones of their hands and feet ("dactylitis") [8]. As a child gets older, the larger bones, spine, and joints tend to become involved, and he or she can have significant acute and chronic pain from vaso-occlusive events.

Differential Diagnosis for Back Pain in Patients with Sickle Cell Disease

Back pain as a chief complaint in patients with SCD can be attributed to various etiologies in addition to vaso-occlusive pain. It can also signal an impending pathology and be the preceding symptom to a syndrome.

Differential Diagnosis of Back Pain in Patient with Sickle Cell Disease
- Muscular back pain
- Vaso-occlusive episode
- Early phase of acute chest syndrome
- Delayed hemolytic transfusion reaction
- Fracture (in the setting of osteoporosis, avascular necrosis)
- Hematoma (due to cortical disruption and development of epidural hematoma)
- Infection – osteomyelitis

Vaso-occlusive Back Pain

Pain is the hallmark of vaso-occlusive crises. These episodes are attributed to vaso-occlusion involving the bone where bone infarctions occur due to intravascular sickling [9]. The clinical presentation of vaso-occlusive pain involving a bone is often acute, described as deep-rooted and severe, and can be accompanied by erythema, warmth, and fever [10]. In children, the spine is one of the most common sites of bony involvement, with the lumbosacral spine being the most common site within the spine [6]. A vaso-occlusive episode typically can last from 3 to 9 days.

Acute Chest Syndrome

Acute chest syndrome (ACS) is a form of acute lung injury caused by vaso-occlusion that is typically characterized by fever, respiratory symptoms, chest pain, and/or a new pulmonary infiltrate on chest radiograph. ACS is one of the most common reasons for hospitalizations, intensive care admissions, and blood transfusions in patients with SCD. It is associated with morbidity and mortality in children with SCD [11], and prevention of ACS is important because repetitive episodes can lead to worsening lung function and chronic lung disease [12].

A VOC involving the back can be a prodrome before an acute chest syndrome (ACS) episode in pediatric patients with SCD. About 50% of ACS episodes happen in children while they are hospitalized for another SCD-associated complication [13, 14]. The most common location of the VOC pain was the back (60%) followed by the chest (50%) with some of these patients reporting pain in both locations [15].

The presence of VOC of the chest or back may elucidate potential mechanisms of ACS including infarction and infection which could be progressing days before the ACS is diagnosed. Additionally, chest and back pain due to a VOE could add to the morbidity associated with ACS; this greatly limits a patient's mobility. Both the lack of activity due to pain and splinted breathing can result in decreased lung aeration.

Back pain may be a signal of an impending ACS episode in patients with SCD and should be considered a risk factor for ACS. Current ACS prevention strategies include pain management, bronchodilators, and the use of incentive spirometry [16, 17]. Thus, when a child with SCD develops back pain, it should be taken seriously.

Osteomyelitis

Patients with SCD have long been known to be at risk of infection, particularly osteomyelitis related to vaso-occlusion, hyposplenism, defective complement activity, and bone necrosis [10]. Areas of necrotic bone are a nidus for infection, and infection sets in via hematogenous spread [18, 19]. *Salmonella* and *Staphylococcus aureus* are common causes of osteomyelitis in this population [20, 21]. The most common sites for osteomyelitis include the femur, tibia, and humerus usually along the diaphysis [22]. Vertebral osteomyelitis is rare, but it should be considered within the differential for a patient with SCD presenting with back pain and a fever.

Patients with SCD have increased risk of infection over the course of their lives due to functional asplenia from splenic infarction. Therefore, in patients with SCD, it is important to always have infection on the differential when they present with pain and to do the necessary studies to distinguish between a vaso-occlusive event and osteomyelitis.

Differentiating between VOC and osteomyelitis can be challenging since there is overlap in both symptoms and findings on diagnostic studies. A patient with osteomyelitis often presents with pain, swelling, and fever, which can be seen in VOC as well. However, the symptoms in osteomyelitis often onset over a longer period of time than an acute VOC. Laboratory studies can be helpful – although both can show an elevation of CRP >2 mg/dL, in VOC it does not usually rise above 6 mg/dL, but in infection it often does. MRI and bone scans can be helpful in trying to differentiate these two diagnoses, as is discussed in imaging section below.

Delayed Hemolytic Transfusion Reaction

Transfusions continue to be one of the most important components of treatment for complications of SCD. Delayed hemolytic transfusion reactions (DHTRs), occurring more than 24 hours after a transfusion and up to 3 weeks following a transfusion, are very serious immune-mediated complications and could have lethal consequences when not recognized and treated appropriately [23].

The clinical presentation of a DHTR includes a sudden drop in hemoglobin, primarily hemoglobin A, following transfusions, or a lower than expected rise in hemoglobin after a transfusion. This is often accompanied by signs of extravascular hemolysis like fever, jaundice, and back pain among others [24]. The pain is frequently indistinguishable from pain caused by a VOE which leads to the underdiagnosis of DHTR. Moreover, in severe cases there can be destruction of the patient's own red blood cells in addition to the transfused red blood cells, a process called "hyperhemolysis" which can lead to multiorgan failure and death [25].

Back pain is closely associated with a DHTR and reported often as a symptom by patients experiencing a DHTR [26].

It is crucial to keep a high suspicion for DHTR in this patient population because treating the condition with further transfusion can only worsen the hemolysis and the patient's anemia. Patients with SCD are exposed to transfusions more often which makes them more vulnerable to a DHTR. Ultimately, it is important to be hypervigilant of this phenomenon when caring for patients with SCD who present with pain within days of a blood transfusion as further transfusions can worsen their condition.

Imaging of the Spine in Sickle Cell Disease

Acute vaso-occlusive events are not seen on imaging. This diagnosis is made based on history and physical examination. Repeated episodes of vaso-occlusion can lead to mottled appearance of the bones on radiographs. Infarction may be seen and appear as "high-density lesions" in the marrow cavity [27]. However, these findings are not specific and are time sensitive. A periosteal reaction is often the first and only change seen on radiographs [27]. Avascular necrosis (AVN) can occur in the femoral and humeral heads. Classically, AVN demonstrates cortex sparing; mixed sclerotic changes at the epiphyses, metaphyses, and medullary canals; and a "shell-like sclerosis" or border which looks similar to a "plume of smoke" [27]. AVN of the spine can also occur in late teen or adult patients [28].

Radiographs of the spine in SCD can have several characteristic features. Due to infarction of the endplates of the vertebral bodies that can occur with vaso-occlusion and attenuation of blood vessels, vertebrae often become flattened and develop a unique biconcave deformity, which is often referred to as "H-vertebrae" or "codfish vertebrae" [6, 29] (see Figs. 16.1 and 16.2). Additionally, "tower vertebrae" have also been described – these are vertebrae that are next to infarcted, short vertebrae, and they develop compensatory elongation.

Advanced imaging may be ordered by the orthopedic surgeon or sickle cell specialist caring for the child after referral. MRI can provide more detailed evaluation of bone and soft tissue and does not expose the child to radiation. MRI is helpful in identifying infarction and involvement of the spine, pelvis, and humeral and femoral heads (Figs. 16.3 and 16.4a/b). In trying to determine if pain is due to infarction versus infection, gadolinium can be helpful [30]. If MRI is not available or if MRI was not able to distinguish between infection and VOE/infarction, radionuclide bone scan or radionuclide bone marrow scan can be utilized. Osteomyelitis will show normal marrow uptake in an abnormal bone scan, and infarct shows decreased marrow uptake with an abnormal bone scan [31].

Management of Back Pain in Patients with Sickle Cell Disease

Management of pain crises and back pain in SCD includes hydration, analgesics, and supportive therapy. If at home, patients are encouraged to hydrate orally, use acetaminophen or NSAIDs like ibuprofen for pain, and apply warm packs to the affected area. Some patients have pain crises severe enough that admission to the hospital is necessary. In the hospital, the management of patients with back pain and SCD includes rehydration with IV fluids, oxygen, NSAIDs, opioids, patient-controlled analgesia, and warm packs to the back. The overall management of their SCD should be by a hematologist.

Editor Comment: For completeness, there are many standard as well as new therapies for the treatment of sickle cell disease. Each child should be followed closely by a Hematologist that is very involved in his or her care and will be up to date on the latest therapies.

How to Approach the Case

Always be wary of possible impending pain crises in patients with sickle cell disease and take their pain seriously. A thorough history is important that includes any recent pain crises, transfusion, sick contacts, traumatic injury, etc. Laboratory examinations can be considered to help sort through the differential – see Table 16.1 for details. Our patient's initial imaging studies showed H-vertebrae indicating that he has had endplate necrosis of the vertebral bodies due to past micro-occlusive events. His overall alignment of the spine however was within normal range with no evidence of acute compression fracture or kyphotic deformity.

Laboratory studies were ordered to try to differentiate between infection and VOE. CBC showed mild anemia. The reticulocyte count and LDH were elevated. The patient's CRP was high normal and the ESR was mildly elevated. Thus, these

Table 16.1 Laboratory studies to consider depending on differential for back pain in SCD

Diagnosis	Laboratory	Comments
Chronic back pain	Vitamin D* Consider if concern for non-SCD cause of chronic back pain: ANA HLA B27 RF	Greater risk of vitamin D* deficiency and osteoporosis in SCD due to chronic hemolytic anemia and compensatory erythropoiesis and resulting bone marrow increase [32]. Given the potential link between low vitamin D and both increased fracture risk and musculoskeletal pain, assessing the vitamin D level of sickle cell patients and supplementing as needed is important
Osteomyelitis	CBC with differential ESR CRP Blood cultures	Consider bone biopsy and culture if needed to guide treatment CRP usually >2 mg/dL and ESR >20 mm/hr
Acute back pain following a blood transfusion	Total Hgb HbA%* LDH Bilirubin (T and D) Direct Antiglobulin Test+ (DAT) CBC with differential Reticulocyte count	*HbA% is more specific given the hemolysis of transfused red blood cells. Hemoglobin drop of >25% should raise suspicion for a DHTR [25] +DAT does not always show alloantibodies
Acute back pain due to vaso-occlusive crisis	CBC with differential Reticulocyte count LDH	The reticulocyte count is a measure of immature red blood cells (RBC). During a VOE, with acute RBC destruction, the reticulocyte count is elevated. If the bone marrow fails to respond to the acute anemia due to RBC destruction, an aplastic crisis can occur. LDH may serve as a prognostic marker in acute disease but only when significantly elevated. LDH is elevated at baseline in SCA due to ongoing red cell death. During acute vaso-occlusive crises (VOC) however, LDH may increase due to added hemolysis and tissue infarction. With levels 4x the upper of limit of normal in an acute crisis, this can suggest impending severe disease

labs suggested a VOE episode rather than infection. At home, supportive treatment with oral hydration, NSAIDs, and Tylenol were recommended. Later, due to worsening pain not responsive to NSAIDs and Tylenol, he was admitted and treated with a PCA, NSAIDs, and warm packs. An MRI was obtained which showed infarctions at multiple levels (Fig. 16.3), but no evidence of an acute infection. His symptoms improved over the course of 3 days. He was discharged to home with outpatient physical therapy arranged.

Final Diagnosis

Vaso-occlusive crises in the setting of increased physical activity and limited hydration.

Natural History and Treatment Considerations

For this patient, he had been exercising recently and not hydrating well. His laboratory data was not concerning for infection, and his x-rays showed the typical "H-shaped" vertebrae that are due to endplate necrosis from microvascular occlusions seen in patients with SCD. Treatment for his vaso-occlusive episode entails the following: Nonsteroidal anti-inflammatory medications and acetaminophen are often first-line agents for pain control in patients with mild to moderate pain. For those in whom these medications are not enough, opioid pain medication is often added. Topical medication patches can be a helpful adjuvant option for children with back pain. Additionally, as with back pain in adolescents without sickle cell disease, patients with back pain in the setting of sickle cell who are not in an acute pain crisis can also benefit from physical therapy to improve core strength and posture to help prevent back pain. Physical therapy may include various modalities including heat, ultrasounds, and transcutaneous electrical nerve stimulation (TENS). Ensuring that the patient is well-connected to Hematology and that they are aware of the pain episode is crucial.

Referral: When and to Whom?

Patients with SCD should have a team approach to their care – including their pediatrician, hematologist, orthopedist (for AVN and osteomyelitis if those arise), social worker, perhaps a pain specialist, and others engaged in their health and well-being. In this patient's case, an orthopedic surgeon is not the person to manage his acute back pain – the pediatrician and hematologist are best for that. If there is pain that is related to fracture, spine deformity (e.g., kyphosis from fracture), infection, or AVN (particularly of the femoral heads or of the spine leading to deformity), an orthopedic surgeon should be involved in the assessment and plan development for the patient.

Key Features and Pearls
- Patients with sickle cell disease should be under the care of a hematologist for their baseline management of SCD.
- In the setting of acute-onset back pain, asking a history inclusive of recent transfusion is critical to make sure a delayed hemolytic transfusion reaction is not missed.

- Laboratory evaluation *may* be helpful to decide between a vaso-occlusive crises (low-grade fever, mildly elevated ESR and CRP) and infection (higher-grade fever, ESR and CRP elevated often above 40 mm/hr and 2 mg/dL – with VOC elevated usually only up to 6 mg/dL and infection can increase much higher) – but frequently not able to discern between the two with labs and temperature alone.
- Patients with SCD should be treated with a team approach to care for the medical, pain, and social challenges that patients face.

Editor Discussion

In patients with sickle cell disease and back pain, the most difficult decision is to differentiate a bone infarct from an infection. These two problems often have a similar presentation. ESR can be falsely low because of the abnormal red blood cells. If the presentation is suspicious for an infection, be sure to get blood cultures and consider an aspiration.
  W.L. Hennrikus

Patients with SCD have a variety of explanations for back pain, including vaso-occlusive episodes, osteomyelitis, hematomas after acute bone infarcts, a prodrome to ACS (acute chest syndrome), and DHTRs (delayed hemolytic transfusion reaction). The most common cause of back pain is micro-infarctions of the bone. DHTR can cause back pain following a blood transfusion and in the case of DHTR, back pain can be misinterpreted for a vaso-occlusive process and the subsequent delay in treatment can be fatal. Back pain accompanied by fever should warrant a workup for osteomyelitis.
  R.M. Schwend

References

1. Rees DC, Williams TN, Gladwin MT. Sickle-cell disease. Lancet. 2010;376:2018–31.
2. Herrick JB. Peculiar elongated and sickle-shaped red blood corpuscles in a case of severe anemia. JAMA. 2014;312:1063.
3. Allison AC. Protection afforded by sickle-cell trait against subtertian malarial infection. Br Med J. 1954;1:290.
4. Howard J, Telfer P. Overview of sickle cell disease. In: Sickle cell Disease in Clinical Practice. London: Springer; 2015. p. 3–28.
5. Ansari J, Moufarrej YE, Pawlinski R, Gavins FNE. Sickle cell disease: a malady beyond a hemoglobin defect in cerebrovascular disease. Expert Rev Hematol. 2018;11:45–55.
6. Roger E, Letts M. Sickle cell disease of the spine in children. Can J Surg. 1999;42:289–92.
7. Bainbridge R, Higgs DR, Maude GH, Serjeant GR. Clinical presentation of homozygous sickle cell disease. J Pediatr. 1985;106:881–5.
8. Quinn CT. Sickle cell disease in childhood: from newborn screening through transition to adult medical care. Pediatr Clin N Am. 2013;60:1363–81.
9. Barriteau CM, McNaull MA. Sickle cell disease in the emergency department: complications and management. Clin Pediatr Emerg Med. 2018;19:103–9.
10. Almeida A, Roberts I. Bone involvement in sickle cell disease. Br J Haematol. 2005;129:482–90.

11. Gladwin MT, Vichinsky E. Pulmonary complications of sickle cell disease. N Engl J Med. 2008;359:2254–65.
12. Sylvester KP, Patey RA, Milligan P, Rafferty GF, Broughton S, Rees D, Thein SL, Greenough A. Impact of acute chest syndrome on lung function of children with sickle cell disease. J Pediatr. 2006;149:17–22.
13. Vichinsky EP, Neumayr LD, Earles AN, Williams R, Lennette ET, Dean D, Nickerson B, Orringer E, McKie V, Bellevue R. Causes and outcomes of the acute chest syndrome in sickle cell disease. N Engl J Med. 2000;342:1855–65.
14. Platt OS, Brambilla DJ, Rosse WF, Milner PF, Castro O, Steinberg MH, Klug PP. Mortality in sickle cell disease – life expectancy and risk factors for early death. N Engl J Med. 1994;330:1639–44.
15. Creary SE, Krishnamurti L. Prodromal illness before acute chest syndrome in pediatric patients with sickle cell disease. J Pediatr Hematol Oncol. 2014;36:480–3.
16. Bellet PS, Kalinyak KA, Shukla R, Gelfand MJ, Rucknagel DL. Incentive spirometry to prevent acute pulmonary complications in sickle cell diseases. N Engl J Med. 1995;333:699–703.
17. Ahmad FA, Macias CG, Allen JY. The use of incentive spirometry in pediatric patients with sickle cell disease to reduce the incidence of acute chest syndrome. J Pediatr Hematol Oncol. 2011;33:415–20.
18. Booth C, Inusa B, Obaro SK. Infection in sickle cell disease: a review. Int J Infect Dis. 2010;14:e2–e12.
19. Neonato MG, Guilloud-Bataille M, Beauvais P, Bégué P, Belloy M, Benkerrou M, Ducrocq R, Maier-Redelsperger M, de Montalembert M, Quinet B, Elion J, Feingold J, Girot R. Acute clinical events in 299 homozygous sickle cell patients living in France. French Study Group on Sickle Cell Disease. Eur J Haematol. 2000;65:155–64.
20. Atkins BL, Price EH, Tillyer L, Novelli V, Evans J. Salmonella osteomyelitis in sickle cell disease children in the east end of London. J Infect. 1997;34:133–8.
21. Burnett MW, Bass JW, Cook BA. Etiology of osteomyelitis complicating sickle cell disease. Pediatrics. 1998;101:296–7.
22. Stark JE, Glasier CM, Blasier RD, Aronson J, Seibert JJ. Osteomyelitis in children with sickle cell disease: early diagnosis with contrast-enhanced CT. Radiology. 1991;179:731–3.
23. Vidler JB, Gardner K, Amenyah K, Mijovic A, Thein SL. Delayed haemolytic transfusion reaction in adults with sickle cell disease: a 5-year experience. Br J Haematol. 2015;169:746–53.
24. Josephson CD. Delayed hemolytic transfusion reactions. In: Transfusion medicine and hemostasis. Burlington, MA. Elsevier; 2009. p. 323–6.
25. Pirenne F, Yazdanbakhsh K. How I safely transfuse patients with sickle-cell disease and manage delayed hemolytic transfusion reactions. Blood. 2018;131:2773–81.
26. Aygun B, Padmanabhan S, Paley C, Chandrasekaran V. Clinical significance of RBC alloantibodies and autoantibodies in sickle cell patients who received transfusions. Transfusion. 2002;42:37–43.
27. Lafforgue P, Trijau S. Bone infarcts: unsuspected gray areas. Joint Bone Spine. 2016;83:495–9.
28. Balogun RA, Obalum DC, Giwa SO, Adekoya-Cole TO, Ogo CN, Enweluzo GO. Spectrum of musculo-skeletal disorders in sickle cell disease in Lagos, Nigeria. J Orthop Surg Res. 2010;5:2.
29. Westerman MP, Greenfield GB, Wong PWK. Fish vertebrae, homocystinuria, and sickle cell anemia. JAMA. 1974;230:261–2.
30. Umans H, Haramati N, Flusser G. The diagnostic role of gadolinium enhanced MRI in distinguishing between acute medullary bone infarct and osteomyelitis. Magn Reson Imaging. 2000;18:255–62.
31. Skaggs DL, Kim SK, Greene NW, Harris D, Miller JH. Differentiation between bone infarction and acute osteomyelitis in children with sickle-cell disease with use of sequential radionuclide bone-marrow and bone scans. J Bone Joint Surg Am. 2001;83-A:1810–3.
32. Lal A, Fung EB, Pakbaz Z, Hackney-Stephens E, Vichinsky EP. Bone mineral density in children with sickle cell anemia. Pediatr Blood Cancer. 2006;47:901–6.

Chapter 17
A Teenage Boy with Back Pain due to a Spontaneous Pneumothorax

Matthew M. Brown and M. Alison Brooks

Brief Case Presentation

Chief Complaint

Back pain and dyspnea.

History

This 17-year-old male noted an acute onset of upper back pain the evening before coming to the clinic. He initially attributed this to lifting some large items earlier in the day. He noted pain which initially felt like a muscle spasm in his upper back and progressed to include unilateral shoulder, neck, and chest pain associated with shortness of breath throughout the evening. He noted a positional nature to his pain, hurting more while lying on his right side or when lying flat on his back with his neck extended while in bed at night. He took NSAIDs, but this did not help his symptoms, and so he went to his primary care physician's office the next morning.

His past medical and surgical histories were otherwise unremarkable without back/neck or shoulder pain or chronic lung disease such as asthma. Other than NSAIDs, he was on no other medications. Family history was remarkable only for his mother with asthma. He lives with both of his parents. He does not smoke cigarettes; however, he did smoke marijuana the day before. He does not use marijuana or other drugs or alcohol regularly.

M. M. Brown · M. A. Brooks (✉)
Department of Orthopedics & Rehabilitation, University of Wisconsin–Madison School of Medicine & Public Health, Madison, WI, USA
e-mail: Brooks@ortho.wisc.edu

© Springer Nature Switzerland AG 2021
R. M. Schwend, W. L. Hennrikus (eds.), *Back Pain in the Young Child and Adolescent*, https://doi.org/10.1007/978-3-030-50758-9_17

Physical Exam

BP 122/66 | Pulse 86 | Temp 97.9F | Ht 6′0″ (1.83 m) | Wt 155 lb. (70.49 kg) | BMI 21.1 | SpO2 98% RA | RR 16/min. He is well-appearing, in no distress. Neck and upper thoracic spine with normal ROM; pain free to palpation and ROM. No chest wall deformities or asymmetries. Lungs are clear on the left, diminished breath sounds on the right, primarily at the base and laterally. No wheezes or rales. Heart with a regular rate and rhythm, normal S1 and S2 without murmurs, clicks, gallops, or rubs. Lower extremities are normal. Screening neurological exam is normal.

Imaging and Radiographic Studies *(Figs. 17.1 and 17.2)*

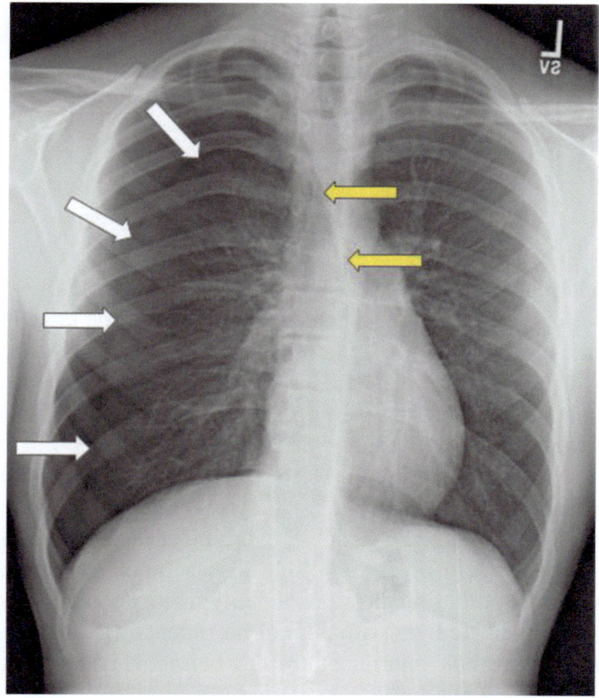

Fig. 17.1 AP chest radiograph. Notice the absence of lung markings at the periphery on the right in comparison to the left (*white arrows*) as well as the minimal leftward deviation of the mediastinum (*yellow arrows*). There are also subtle lucencies at the right apex suggesting blebs

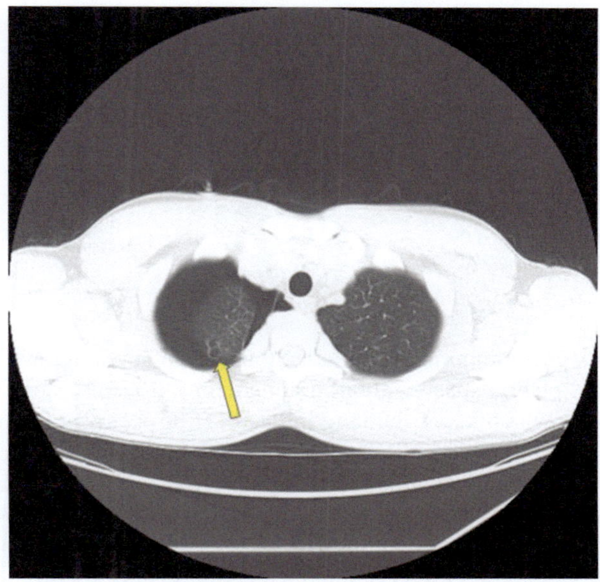

Fig. 17.2 CT scan demonstrating persistent pneumothorax as well as apical blebs (*yellow arrow*) which were later resected surgically due to pneumothorax recurrence

Questions About the Case the Reader Should Consider
1. Back or neck pain is not typically associated with shortness of breath. What is the reason for his dyspnea?
2. Pneumothoraces can occur as the result of trauma or can occur spontaneously. What are the risk factors for spontaneous pneumothorax?
3. How does a pneumothorax present and how is it diagnosed?
4. Small pneumothoraces can often be subtle on initial chest radiograph. What are the key features?
5. What is the appropriate referral after discovering a pneumothorax and what are important considerations?
6. What are possible initial treatments and what additional treatments are available for complex or refractory cases?

Discussion

While musculoskeletal back pain symptoms could be aggravated by deep respiration or cough, it would be unusual to be associated with true dyspnea or exercise intolerance. The presence of subjective shortness of breath should prompt further investigation into other causes or coexisting conditions involving the cardiorespiratory systems such as pneumothorax.

Short Differential Diagnosis
- Pulmonary embolism
- Pneumothorax
- Asthma exacerbation
- Pleural effusion
- Pericarditis
- Pleurodynia
- Pneumonia

Spontaneous pneumothorax is a relatively uncommon condition in which air is able to enter the pleural space without traumatic or iatrogenic cause, reducing the negative pressure which keeps the lung inflated [1]. It occurs at a rate of approximately 2.6–3.4 per 100,000 individuals ages 0–17 years, with a predominance in males (approximately 4–9:1) with a mean age range of 13.3–16.5 years when seen in children [1–3]. Those most commonly affected are between 15 and 22 years of age, but there is a bimodal distribution with increased rates also seen in older adults [2]. Furthermore, there does not seem to be a predominance by race [1]. While not definitive, it is believed that the development of spontaneous pneumothorax is related to the formation of subpleural blebs/bullae as the result of connective tissue changes which then leak air into the pleural space [1].

Spontaneous pneumothoraces are classified as primary or secondary. Primary pneumothoraces occur in those without any known lung disease [1]. Secondary pneumothoraces occur as the result of chronic lung diseases such as asthma, cystic fibrosis, or disorders affecting connective tissue. Asthma is the most common predisposing cause of pediatric pneumothorax; 16–47% of those with spontaneous pneumothorax have asthma [1]. It is believed that this relates to the chronic inflammation associated with asthma. Primary spontaneous pneumothorax tends to occur in tall, thin males, and there is suggestion that growth velocity may play a role in those who develop spontaneous pneumothorax [4]. There may be a genetic predilection for spontaneous pneumothorax, particularly for those with inherited conditions such as Marfan syndrome, alpha-1 antitrypsin deficiency, homocystinuria, or Birt-Hogg-Dube syndrome [1, 5, 6]. While adult smokers have higher risk of spontaneous pneumothorax (relative risk 22 for males and 9 for females), this risk is less for adolescents, suggesting a dose-response relationship [1]. Use of marijuana in conjunction with tobacco may increase the risk of primary pneumothorax; however, case-control studies have failed to show an isolated effect despite concerns about the deeper inhalation and Valsalva maneuvers often associated with marijuana use [7].

Onset of symptoms may occur at rest but also can be caused by Valsalva associated with lifting. Common symptoms are persistent dull or pleuritic chest or back pain/tightness, cough, and/or shortness of breath [1, 3]. Isolated back pain would be an unusual presentation. Typically symptoms are accompanied by diminished breath sounds, tachypnea, tachycardia, and hyper-resonant percussion although these are dependent on the pneumothorax size with small pneumothoraces having normal exam and vital signs [1]. Diagnosis of primary pneumothorax can be delayed due to the nature of slowly improving symptoms, and as such pneumothoraces may be noted in relatively asymptomatic patients who had imaging performed for other reasons. In a Japanese observational study, asymptomatic pneumothoraces were seen in 0.042% of patients who had chest radiographs performed as part of an annual physical examination [4].

Diagnosis of spontaneous pneumothorax is made with chest radiography. Sensitivity can vary based on severity of the pneumothorax; however, it has been reported to be about 40% with a specificity of 99% [8]. Key findings include absence of lung markings at the periphery of the thorax, but there may also be thoracic enlargement on the affected side as well as mediastinal displacement away from the affected side. Expiratory and lateral decubitus views may make small pneumothoraces more apparent via increasing the relative density of the lung and allowing gravity to pull the collapsed lung away from the chest wall; however, these have not been shown to improve diagnostic accuracy [9, 10]. Bedside ultrasound may also be utilized with 79% sensitivity and 98% specificity, particularly in critical care and emergency settings where it is more readily available [8]. CT scan can increase sensitivity for detecting small pneumothoraces in cases of high suspicion and can additionally better identify subpleural blebs that may impact management decisions. However, CT scans have 68 times the effective radiation dose of a chest radiograph, and therefore the decision to obtain advanced imaging should be made in conjunction with consulting cardiothoracic surgeons after considering the associated risks and benefits [1, 3].

Those identified to have a primary spontaneous pneumothorax require evaluation and monitoring for increasing size or worsening clinical status over subsequent hours, preferably in the emergency department or inpatient unit. A child with a small, minimally symptomatic pneumothorax that does not progress and who has ready access to emergency care should symptoms worsen can be discharged with close outpatient follow-up within 12–72 hours for repeat imaging and examination assessing for interval improvement [11]. Those who progress or those with a large pneumothorax or a symptomatic secondary pneumothorax require admission for management [1, 5, 6, 11, 12]. A small proportion (6.6%) of patients will present with a tension pneumothorax which is characterized by severe respiratory distress, hypoxia, and hemodynamic instability with possible tracheal deviation [1, 12]. This is a medical emergency diagnosed clinically that requires needle decompression immediately [5, 12].

Initial treatment for pneumothorax is often observation alone with cardiorespiratory monitoring and serial chest radiographs, although resolution can be sped up two- to fourfold with the continuous use of 100% high-flow oxygen via mask [1]. Small pneumothoraces with mild symptoms respond to noninvasive interventions [1]. The American College of Chest Physicians defines a small pneumothorax as <3 cm of intrapleural distance at the apex on upright chest radiograph, while the British Thoracic Society defines a small pneumothorax as <2 cm intrapleural distance at the level of the hilum [6, 11, 12]. There are many other methods of estimating size including Light, Rhea, and Collins methods, although they may underestimate size and there is often disagreement in classification between methods [1, 6]. For larger pneumothoraces or those that do not improve with observation alone, simple needle aspiration, pleural catheters, or chest tubes can be used. Simple aspiration results in recurrence in as many as 60% of pediatric cases [13]. Outpatient management can be considered in stable inpatients following placement of a pleural catheter with one-way Heimlich valve [5, 6, 11, 12].

In this case, the boy was noted to have a large right-sided pneumothorax. Initial therapy was conservative, with clinical monitoring and serial chest radiographs while on 100% high-flow oxygen via a non-rebreather mask. Unfortunately, after this failed to improve his symptoms, a pleural catheter was placed which led to improvement and resolution of his symptoms over the next 2 days. The catheter was then removed and he was discharged to home. One month later he had a recurrence of symptoms and was readmitted. He ultimately underwent surgical blebectomy and mechanical pleurodesis via a video-assisted thoracoscopic surgery (VATS) without further recurrence.

How to Approach the Case

Back pain should not be associated with dyspnea or exercise intolerance, which should lead to suspicion of cardiopulmonary causes. Careful history, physical examination, and chest radiographs are essential to diagnosis. Advanced imaging is typically only considered when deciding on treatment options and often is not necessary at all. Be aware of tension physiology which requires immediate intervention before imaging.

Final Diagnosis

Primary spontaneous pneumothorax.

Natural History and Treatment Considerations

Recurrence rates following cases of primary spontaneous pneumothorax are typically around 20% but range from 16% to 61%. Recurrence is more common for younger, taller patients and typically occurs within 4 years [1–3]. Those who have recurrent symptoms can be considered for surgical intervention in the form of VATS with stapling of blebs, which are found in 90% of cases, and/or mechanical or chemical pleurodesis [1, 5, 6, 11, 12].

Referral – Emergency, Urgent, or Routine: And to Whom?

Primary spontaneous pneumothoraces need emergency department evaluation due to risk of cardiorespiratory compromise, but can be managed by emergency physicians and generalists in the inpatient or outpatient environment after proper evaluation. Referral to a surgeon for operative management should be made for a recurrence with second ipsilateral pneumothorax, first contralateral pneumothorax, bilateral pneumothorax, spontaneous hemopneumothorax, failure of lung expansion, or persistent air leak for >48 hours despite chest tube/pleural drain placement [5, 6, 12]. Given higher rates of recurrence in nonoperative versus operative management, some advocate shared decision-making about more aggressive management at initial presentation, particularly for those at higher risk of recurrence or complications such as frequent divers or air travelers [3, 5, 12, 13].

Indications for Surgical Referral [5, 6, 12]
- Second ipsilateral pneumothorax
- First contralateral pneumothorax
- Bilateral pneumothorax
- Spontaneous hemopneumothorax
- Failure of lung expansion or persistent air leak >48 hours despite chest tube/catheter
- Secondary pneumothorax or high likelihood of recurrence
- High-risk patient (divers, frequent air travelers, pregnant women)
- Patient preference

Brief Summary

Back pain can be caused by a number of non-musculoskeletal causes including pneumothorax. When pain is accompanied with other symptoms such as dyspnea, other causes should be considered. Spontaneous pneumothorax presents most commonly in tall, thin adolescent males and is characterized by pain and dyspnea. In addition to history and physical examination, diagnosis is made with plain radiographs which demonstrate the absence of lung markings at the periphery of the thorax. Management is determined by the specific clinical picture, but treatments can span from close observation in a controlled setting to invasive surgery.

> **Key Features and Pearls**
> - Back pain should not be associated with pulmonary symptoms such as dyspnea which necessitates further workup.
> - Spontaneous pneumothorax is diagnosed with history, physical examination, and chest radiograph and typically is managed initially by observation or pleural catheter placement.
> - Clinicians should be aware of tension pneumothorax in those with significant respiratory features and hemodynamic compromise. Decompression treatment with a large bore needle in the 2nd intercostal space at the midclavicular line should not be delayed by further workup in those with appropriate clinical features.

Editor Discussion

All back pain does not stem from the spine. Although many cases of spontaneous pneumothorax will present with chest pain and dyspnea, some cases, as in this case, present with back pain. Consider this diagnosis in tall, thin high school athletes with atraumatic sudden-onset thoracic back pain that occurs at rest. Spontaneous rupture of a sub-pleural bleb allows air to leak into the pleural space causing pain. A chest x-ray is the key diagnostic test and an emergency room evaluation is prudent.

W.L. Hennrikus

As is true with so many conditions, not thinking about the diagnosis is one of the most common pitfalls, especially when it comes to conditions related to the back. This case illustrates how a properly done history and physical examination can lead to the chest as the source of the problem and not the spine. Everyone should be facile with a stethoscope. If you suspect a spontaneous pneumothorax, make sure to either look at the chest radiograph yourself or communicate to the radiologist what you suspect so there is no chance of missing the diagnosis. Since CT scanning involves such a much larger dose of radiation (5–10 mSv compared to 0.1 mSv for chest film and 3.0 mSv/year background radiation), following the principles of ALARA (as low as reasonably achievable), CT is more of an elective procedure, so the parents should have shared decision-making when CT is recommended.

R.M. Schwend

References

1. Dotson K, Johnson LH. Pediatric spontaneous pneumothorax. Pediatr Emerg Care. 2012;28(7):715–23.
2. Huang YH, Chang PY, Wong KS, Chang CJ, Lai JY, Chen JC. An age-stratified longitudinal study of primary spontaneous pneumothorax. J Adolesc Health. 2017;61(4):527–32.
3. Soler LM, Raymond SL, Larson SD, Taylor JA, Islam S. Initial primary spontaneous pneumothorax in children and adolescents: operate or wait? J Pediatr Surg. 2018;53:1960–3.
4. Mitani A, Hakamata Y, Hosoi M, et al. The incidence and risk factors of asymptomatic primary spontaneous pneumothorax detected during health check-ups. BMC Pulm Med. 2017;17(1):177.
5. Wong A, Galiabovitch E, Bhagwat K. Management of primary spontaneous pneumothorax: a review. ANZ J Surg. 2019;89(4):303–8.
6. Bintcliffe OJ, Hallifax RJ, Edey A. Spontaneous pneumothorax: time to rethink management. Lancet Respir Med. 2015;3:578–88.
7. Olesen WH, Katballe N, Sindby JE, et al. Cannabis increased the risk of primary spontaneous pneumothorax in tobacco smokers: a case-control study. Eur J Cardiothorac Surg. 2017;52(4):679–85.
8. Alrajab S, Youssef AM, Akkus NI, Caldito G. Pleural ultrasonography versus chest radiography for the diagnosis of pneumothorax: review of the literature and meta-analysis. Crit Care. 2013;17(5):R208.
9. Seow A, Kazerooni EA, Pernicano PG, Neary M. Comparison of upright inspiratory and expiratory chest radiographs for detecting pneumothoraces. Am J Roentgenol. 1996;166:313–6.
10. Beres RA, Goodman LR. Pneumothorax: detection with upright versus decubitus radiography. Radiology. 1993;186(1):19–22.
11. Baumann MH, Strange C, Heffner JE, et al. Management of spontaneous pneumothorax. Chest. 2001;119(2):590–602.
12. MacDuff A, Arnold A, Harvey J. Management of spontaneous pneumothorax: British Thoracic Society pleural disease guideline 2010. Thorax. 2010;65(Suppl 2):ii18–31.
13. Yeung F, Chung PHY, Hung ELY, Yuen CS, Tam PKH, Wong KKY. Surgical intervention for primary spontaneous pneumothorax in pediatric population: when and why? J Laparoendosc Adv Surg Tech A. 2017;27(8):841–4.

Chapter 18
Back Pain Associated with Discitis in a 5-Year-Old Boy

James F. Mooney III and Robert F. Murphy

Brief Case Presentation

Chief Complaint

A 5-year-old boy with a history of abdominal pain and limp for 3 weeks.

History

The patient is a 5-year-old otherwise healthy boy who presents to his primary care physician with an approximately 3-week history of vague back and abdominal pain, lethargy, and limp. He has had no other recent illnesses, no weight loss, and no nausea or vomiting. He has no medical allergies and takes no medications. There is no history of trauma or injury. His parents report a progressive decrease in his oral intake over the past few weeks, but his voiding patterns are generally unchanged. He has been seen twice in a local urgent care facility without any specific diagnosis being made. The only treatment recommended was symptomatic use of anti-inflammatories and activity limitations. To date, no laboratory tests or imaging studies have been performed.

J. F. Mooney III (✉)
Shriners Hospital for Children – Springfield, Springfield, MA, USA

R. F. Murphy
Department of Orthopaedics and Physical Medicine, Medical University of South Carolina, Charleston, SC, USA

© Springer Nature Switzerland AG 2021
R. M. Schwend, W. L. Hennrikus (eds.), *Back Pain in the Young Child and Adolescent*, https://doi.org/10.1007/978-3-030-50758-9_18

Physical Examination

He is developmentally normal. His height, weight, and BMI are all at approximately the 50th percentile for age. He is afebrile and does not appear to be clinically ill. He stands with mild flexion at the hips and knees. His gait is slow and appears a little unsteady. He has full passive range of motion of the hips, knees, and ankles when examined in a supine position. There are no abnormalities on his neurologic examination. He has no skin changes or lesions over his spine or lower extremities. Abdominal exam reveals normal bowel sounds, and there is no tenderness on palpation. Examination of his spine when upright shows some loss of lumbar lordosis and moderate midline tenderness to palpation over the lumbar spine. There is no evidence of scoliosis, but he has limitation on lumbar flexion/extension due to apparent discomfort. He refuses to touch his toes when encouraged. Gower's sign is abnormally present, and the physician currently examining the patient documented that it was not present at a well-child visit 6 months earlier.

Questions About the Case the Reader Should Consider
1. What is the reason for back tenderness and pain with movement?
2. What is Gower's sign and why is this sign positive?
3. Why can't he touch his toes?
4. What is the next diagnostic test to consider?
5. What is the appropriate referral?

Discussion

While complaints of back pain are not uncommon in children, persistence of such complaints, particularly in combination with other physical findings, may be a sign of significant underlying pathology. Back pain that limits activity and is associated with abnormal findings on physical exam, including limp or abdominal complaints, is a cause for concern [1]. In this patient, it is important to note any evidence of tenderness to palpation, as well as limitations of extremity and/or spinal range of motion. The presence of a Gower's sign, which was documented as absent previously, has been associated with specific types of spinal abnormalities in pediatric patients [2]. In this case flexion or extension of the spine may indicate a disease process in the disc, which receives pressure when the spine moves. Likewise, to arise from the floor requires spine motion, which could cause pain in an inflamed disc area.

At this point, based solely on the clinical picture, the primary care clinician should be concerned that there is some level of underlying pathology. Further evaluations utilizing both laboratory and radiographic studies are indicated. The fact that this has been a long-standing, non-progressive problem should indicate that, while additional evaluation should be performed expeditiously, it is not necessarily a medical emergency.

An appropriate evaluation includes serological/hematological studies consisting of a complete blood count (CBC) with differential, erythrocyte sedimentation rate (ESR), and C-reactive protein (CRP) and a blood culture. In light of positive Gower's sign, a serum creatine phosphokinase (CPK) assay may be appropriate as well. Baseline radiographic studies should be obtained, and these should include full-length upright PA (posterior-anterior) and lateral radiographs of the thoracic, lumbar, and sacral spine. More complex imaging, such as MRI, CT, or radionucleotide scans, should not be the initial modes of radiographic evaluation.

Laboratory results demonstrate moderate elevations of both the ESR and CRP, and the CPK level is normal. The results of the spinal radiographs (Fig. 18.1) are reviewed with a radiologist. The PA image shows no apparent abnormalities. However, there is evidence of irregularity and narrowing of the L1/L2 disc space on the lateral radiograph.

Based on the results of these studies, referral to an orthopedic surgeon with pediatric subspecialty training is indicated. Information regarding the laboratory and radiographic studies, along with copies of all imaging, should be sent either with the patient or preferably directly to the specialist for review. Advanced imaging should be ordered at the discretion of the consultant physician.

After complete clinical evaluation by the pediatric orthopedic surgeon, a magnetic resonance imaging (MRI) study of the area without contrast is obtained. Due to the child's young age, the MRI also required a general anesthetic. These images

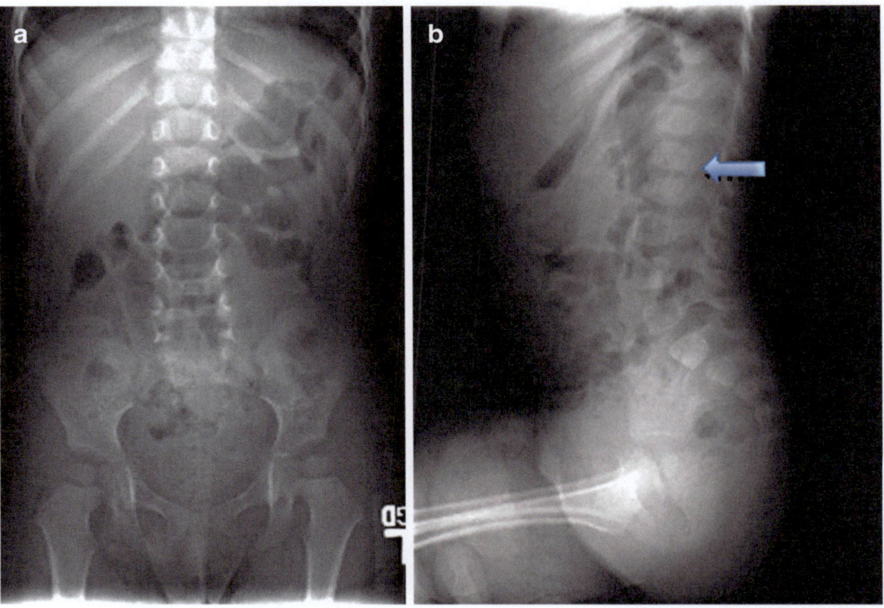

Fig. 18.1 (a) Postero-anterior radiograph of the thoracic and lumbar spine. (b) Lateral radiograph of the thoracic and lumbar spine demonstrating vertebral endplate irregularities at L1-L2. These changes are consistent with a diagnosis of discitis

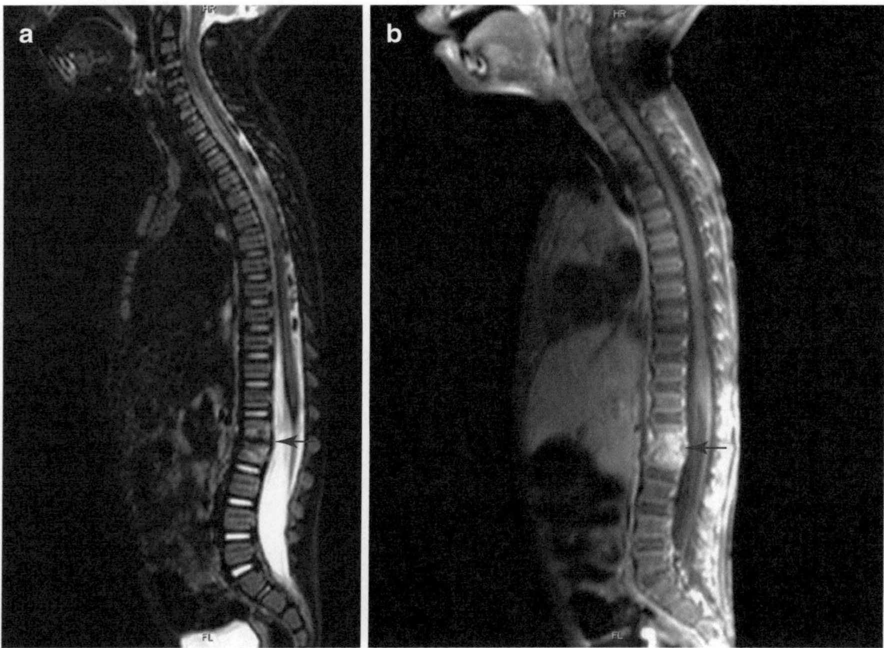

Fig. 18.2 (**a**) Sagittal T2 MR imaging. Note the signal change present within the L1-L2 disc space. (**b**) Sagittal T1 MR imaging. Note extensive signal changes involving not only the L1-L2 disc but also the adjacent vertebral bodies

(Fig. 18.2) further demonstrate abnormalities of the L1/L2 disc, as well as signal change within the L1 vertebral body. The combination of clinical, radiographic, and laboratory findings is felt to be consistent with a diagnosis of a disc space infection (discitis, also termed spondylo-discitis since the adjacent vertebrae are frequently involved). The patient is admitted to the hospital briefly and started on IV antibiotics that are broad spectrum and cover *Staphylococcus aureus*. On the third day, the blood culture grew *Staphylococcus aureus*. A thoraco-lumbar orthosis is recommended for comfort when the patient is upright during the day. He was transitioned to oral antibiotics once responsiveness to antibiotic therapy is demonstrated by an increased level of activity, decreased back discomfort, and the CRP returning to normal. The symptoms gradually resolved, and he returned to full baseline function and activity. The oral antibiotics were stopped once the ESR returned to normal.

How to Approach the Case

Always be suspicious of back pain in a young child. Stiffness is a red flag. A careful history, physical examination, and review of the plain radiographs are the essential first three aspects of making an accurate diagnosis. In this case, the blood culture was very helpful. The MRI confirmed the diagnosis but also required a general anesthetic due to the child's young age.

Red Flags for Back Pain, Stiffness, and a Limp in a 5-Year-Old
- Overall stiffness and caution with walking
- Inability to touch his toes
- Loss of lumbar lordosis
- Irregularity and narrowing of the L1-L2 disc space on the lateral x-ray
- Tenderness of the lumbar spine

Short Differential Diagnosis
- Infection
- Tumor – osteoid osteoma, osteoblastoma, ABC, malignant bone tumor, tumors of the neural elements, metastatic tumor
- Fracture – traumatic spondylolysis

Final Diagnosis

Discitis L1-L2 disk

Natural History and Treatment Considerations: Pediatric Discitis

Discitis in children accounts for approximately 2% of all pediatric musculoskeletal infections [3, 4]. The exact etiology of discitis remains unclear, as there has traditionally been controversy as to whether this is truly an infection or simply an inflammatory process. In addition, questions remain regarding the primary site (disc space or vertebral endplate) of the primary pathologic process [5].

A pediatric patient with discitis will often present with non-specific complaints, and these may include intermittent back and/or abdominal pain, alterations in gait or limping, and limited spinal or truncal range of motion. Patients are often afebrile and rarely appear toxic or systemically ill. The non-specific nature of the child's complaints and physical findings often leads to a delay in diagnosis. One study reported an average delay of 42 days to final diagnosis [3], although a more recent study showed an average delay of 22 days from onset of symptoms to diagnosis [4].

Laboratory findings in patients with possible discitis are similarly non-specific. While the ESR may be elevated in up to 80–90% of patients [5], other studies have demonstrated elevated ESR and CRP values in less than 20% of patients [4]. The WBC is generally normal to slightly elevated. Blood cultures are rarely positive.

The lumbar spine is the most common area involved in children with discitis. Plain radiographic findings include irregularity of the disc space and loss of intra-discal height compared to adjacent levels. These changes may not be evident on standard roentgenograms for 2–3 weeks after the onset of symptoms. MRI is the most sensitive study for demonstrating changes within the disc and adjacent verte-bral bodies and is the diagnostic method of choice at this time [5].

In most cases, antibiotics are the initial treatment of choice for pediatric patients with a presumed diagnosis of discitis. Antibiotic therapy generally targets *Staphylococcus aureus*, as in those patients with a positive bacteriological diagnosis, either from blood culture or biopsy, *Staphylococcus aureus* is the most common organism identified [5]. Historically, treatment has been primarily empirical, as most patients have negative blood cultures, and at this time most do not undergo biopsy. There is some recent evidence, however, that highlights the use of modern bacterial identification techniques in this patient population. Utilizing polymerase chain reac-tion (PCR) assays in patients with discitis, multiple authors have reported an increas-ing ability to diagnose organisms, particularly *Kingella kingae*. This organism appears to be associated with a large percentage of the pediatric discitis diagnosed in patients less than 4 years of age [6–8]. How the availability of this technology will affect the principles of medical management of discitis in the future is unclear at this time.

Antibiotic therapy for pediatric discitis generally consists of intravenous delivery for a period of time, followed by oral dosing. There is no formally recommended timeline for mode of treatment, and the length of intravenous versus oral therapy may vary widely. At this time, recommendations for biopsy are limited to those patients who do not show symptomatic improvement with intravenous anti-staphylococcal therapy, and in these cases may lead to changes in antibiotics based on the results of local tissue cultures. In some cases, a removable spinal orthosis may be recommended as part of the treatment program. The biomechanical benefit of a brace or external support is uncertain, and the brace may function primarily to limit activity and painful motion.

There is minimal long-term follow-up of pediatric patients with discitis, with little evidence of any functional sequelae [9, 10]. Disc space narrowing that is pres-ent on plain radiographs and MRI during the phases of diagnosis and treatment may progress to spontaneous fusion (Fig. 18.3) in some patients, but the true incidence and possible consequences of this as an adult are unknown.

Referral – Emergency, Urgent, or Routine: And to Whom?

Discitis is an urgent referral to an orthopedic surgeon or a pediatric orthopedic sur-geon depending on the availability of a pediatric orthopedic surgeon in your community.

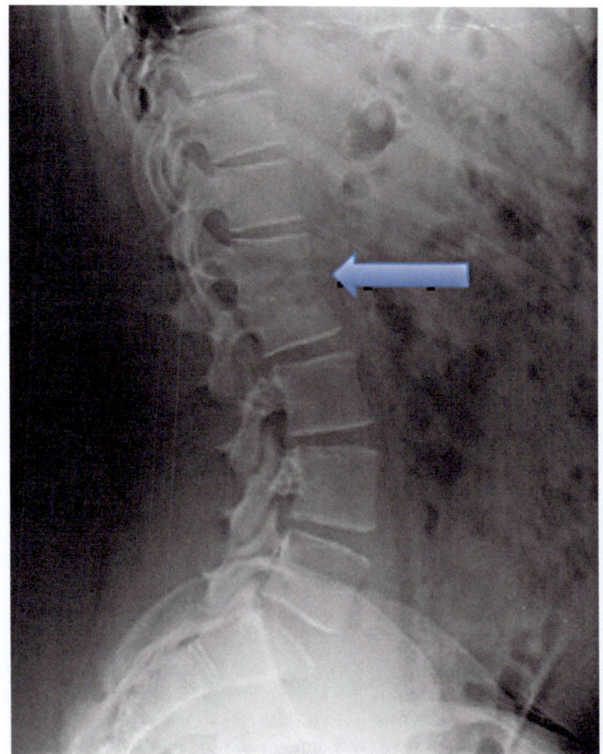

Fig. 18.3 Lateral radiograph demonstrating early spontaneous interbody fusion associated with discitis in a pediatric patient

Brief Summary

Back pain in children is not rare, but discomfort that is persistent and associated with a diagnosed abnormality is unusual. Discitis, most frequently involving the lumbar spine, is an unusual cause of such discomfort. Due to its relative rarity, and non-specific presentation, the diagnosis of discitis is often delayed. Management generally consists of antibiotic therapy, and external immobilization and/or activity limitations may be indicated for some patients. Long-term sequela is not well described.

> **Key Features and Pearls**
> - As in this case, discitis can often present without a fever.
> - The MRI is indicated if uncertainty exists and is confirmatory.
> - Don't forget to get a blood culture.
> - Biopsy is rarely needed.
> - In addition to a pediatric orthopedic surgeon, a pediatric ID specialist is another helpful consultant if available in your community.

Editor Discussion

The presentation of discitis can be obscure and result in a delayed diagnosis. The young child may complain of more belly pain than back pain. Discitis is one cause of refusal to walk in a young child.
W.L. Hennrikus

Discitis presents in a different manner in the young child compared to the adolescent. An adolescent is typically able to localize the pain to the spine. Despite this, even in the adolescent the diagnosis may be delayed since pain and stiffness are so often considered to be such common symptoms and signs. Discitis is even more difficult to diagnose in the young child since they may not complain of back pain. Abdominal pain, difficulty walking or limping, stiffness, and hip pain may lead to family and physician to believe that the problem is coming from a different source. Spine radiographs obtained early in the course can also be distracting since they are typically normal. The key to diagnosing discitis is to keep an open mind about the possibility and not be fooled by "negative spine radiographs." A child who appears stiff and guarding or walks in a stiff manner should be evaluated for discitis if another diagnosis is not determined.
R.M. Schwend

References

1. Tyagi R. Spinal infections in children: a review. J Orthop. 2016;13:254–8.
2. Mirovsky Y, Copeliovich L, Halperin N. Gowers' sign in children with discitis of the lumbar spine. J Pediatr Orthop B. 2005;14:68–70.
3. Garron E, Viehweger E, Launay F, Guillaume JM, Jouve JL, Bollini G. Nontuberculous spondylodiscitis in children. J Pediatr Orthop. 2002;22:321–8.
4. Spencer SJ, Wilson NI. Childhood discitis in a regional children's hospital. J Pediatr Orthop B. 2012;21:264–8.
5. McCarthy JJ, Dormans JP, Kozin SH, Pizzutillo PD. Musculoskeletal infections in children: basic treatment principles and recent advancements. Instr Course Lect. 2005;54:515–28.
6. Fernandes Machado SA, Ferreira Freitas JM, Alegrete da Silva NP, Coutinho Costa Moreira JM, Peixoto Pinto RA, de Melo Costa FG. Spondylodiscitis by Kingella Kingae: an emerging pathogen in an older pediatric population. Pediatr Infect Dis J. 2017;36:1096–7.
7. Spyropoulou V, Dhouib Chargui A, Merlini L, et al. Primary subacute hematogenous osteomyelitis in children: a clearer bacteriological etiology. J Pediatr Orthop. 2016;10:241–6.
8. Principi N, Esposito S. Infectious discitis and spondylodiscitis in children. Int J Mol Sci. 2016;17:539.
9. Song KS, Ogden JA, Ganey T, Guidera KJ. Contiguous discitis and osteomyelitis in children. J Pediatr Orthop. 1997;17:470–7.
10. Kang HM, Choi EH, Lee HJ, et al. The etiology, clinical presentation and long-term outcome of spondylodiscitis in children. Pediatr Infect Dis J. 2016;35:e102–6.

Chapter 19
Case of Limping – A Symptom of Spondylodiscitis in the Toddler

Jefferson W. Jex

Brief Case Presentation

Chief Complaint

A 3–4 week history of limp

History

This 2-year-old girl had been limping with a waddling gait for 3–4 weeks. She has been afebrile. The past several days she has stopped walking and prefers to crawl. She does not even tolerate sitting in chair and has been unable to stand from seated position. She has not gained weight over the last 3 months. On physical examination, she is afebrile and thin and has a nontoxic appearance. There are no bruises. Her hips have minimal pain with range of motion. She is able to walk but with a waddling/listing gait, and she will not bend to pick up an object off the floor. Laboratory values show ESR-43 mm/min, CRP 2.7, and WBC-14,300/mm3. AP pelvis (see Fig. 19.1), bilateral femur, and tib-fib radiographs are normal. Rheumatoid factor and antinuclear antibody (ANA) labs were negative.

She was diagnosed with hip transient synovitis and treated with NSAIDs. Two days later, her mother reported that she was 25–50% improved. A sedated MRI of bilateral hips was obtained the next day, which revealed spondylodiscitis at the L4 L5 level (see Fig. 19.2). She was admitted for IV antibiotics, and lumbar spine

J. W. Jex (✉)
Department of Orthopaedic Surgery, Walter Reed National Military Medical Center, Bethesda, MD, USA
e-mail: Jefferson.w.jex.mil@mail.mil

© Springer Nature Switzerland AG 2021
R. M. Schwend, W. L. Hennrikus (eds.), *Back Pain in the Young Child and Adolescent*, https://doi.org/10.1007/978-3-030-50758-9_19

"

Fig. 19.1 AP pelvis radiograph. Hips appear normal and there is no deformity of lumbosacral spine

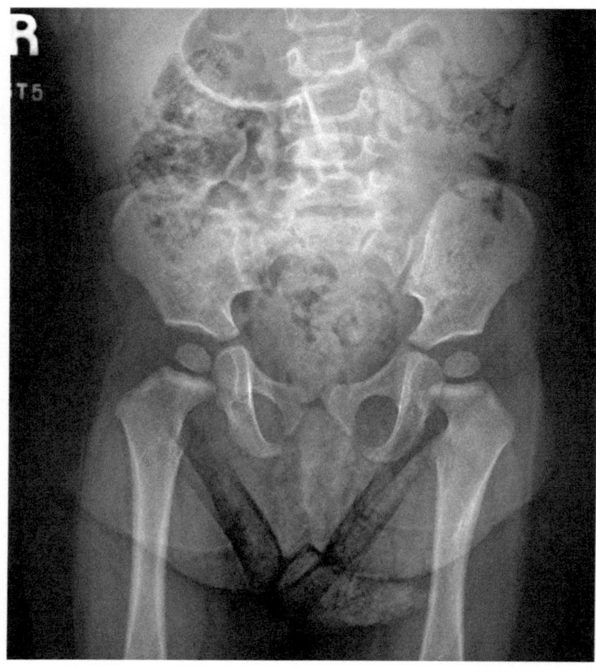

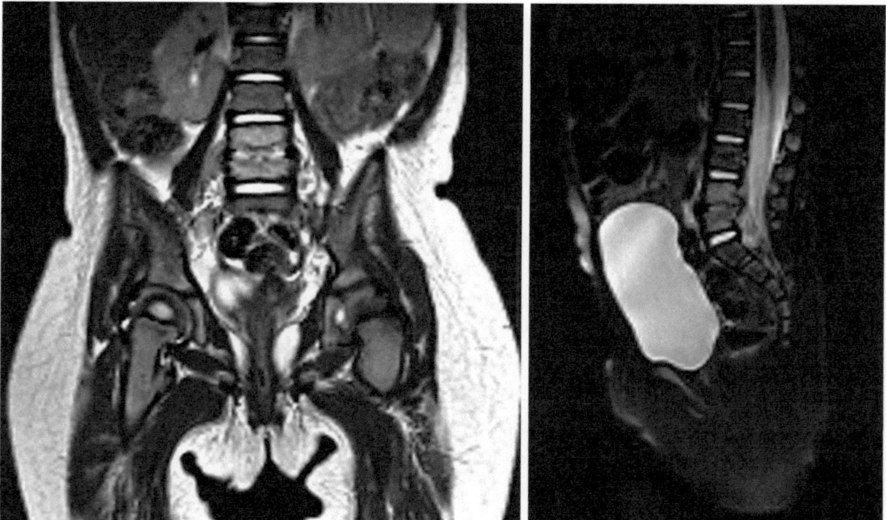

Fig. 19.2 MRI bilateral hips reveals no pathology related to the hips or pelvis. L4 and L5 show increased T2 signal and loss of L4/5 disk height consistent with spondylodiscitis

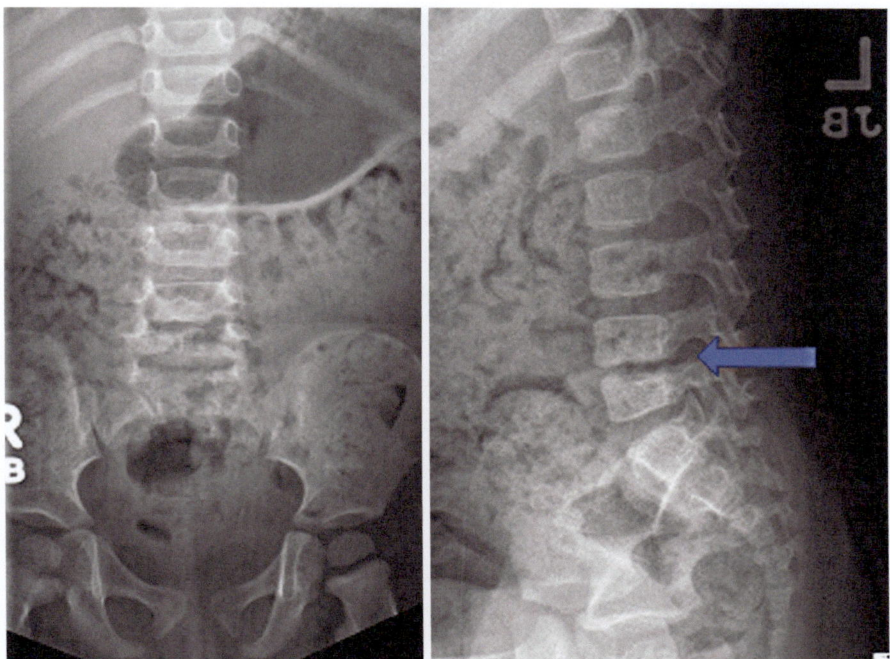

Fig. 19.3 AP/lateral lumbar spine radiographs. Decreased disk space between L4 and L5 is noted (arrow). Note the loss of lumbar lordosis, which is common with spine pathology

radiographs were obtained (see Fig. 19.3). She improved clinically, and an MRI was ordered to evaluate response to treatment (see Fig. 19.4).

Imaging and Radiographic Studies (Figs. 19.1, 19.2, 19.3, and 19.4)

Questions About the Case the Reader Should Consider
1. What is the differential diagnosis of a pediatric limp?
2. What is the benefit of examination of a joint above and below the suspected diagnosis?
3. How could no weight gain for 3 months in a 2 year old be explained?
4. What are indications for repeat MRI lumbar spine during treatment?

Fig. 19.4 Follow-up MRI of the lumbar spine shows persistent T2 signal and disk changes (arrow) despite clinical improvement on antibiotics. An MRI to evaluate response to treatment is *not* indicated in patients who are improving clinically. T2 changes of the involved vertebrae persist beyond resolution of the infection

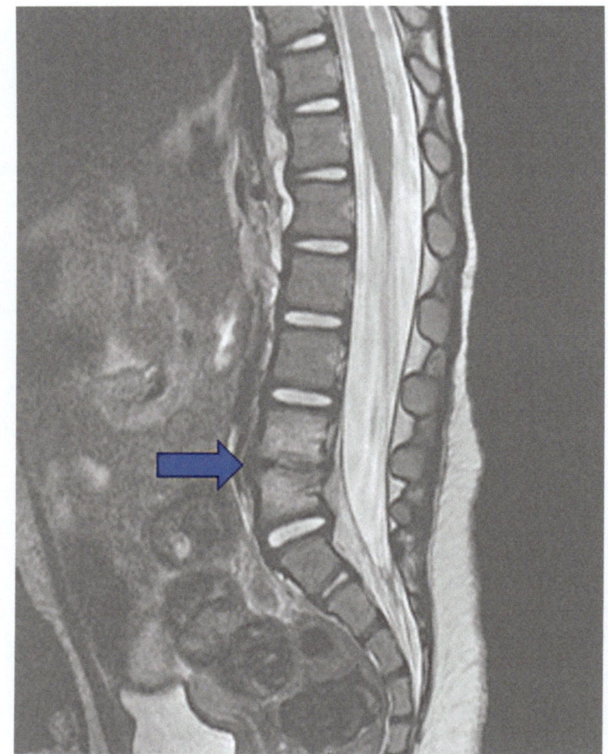

Discussion

Spondylodiscitis, which is often referred to as discitis, is an uncommon cause of back pain in children. Young children with discitis do not always complain of pain, although older children may. The insidious onset coupled with its rarity often leads to a delay in the correct diagnosis. Many children present without a complaint of back pain. Often, they refuse to walk or do not tolerate upright sitting in a chair. Approximately 50% will present with back pain, but this is more typical in older children. A loss of lumbar lordosis may be noted [1]. Children may have a prodromal illness [2] yet be afebrile, and inflammatory markers may not be elevated early in the illness. The only finding that the parent notices may be a limp. Children with discitis will typically list to the side to avoid motion of the back. They may be hesitant to pick something off the floor, or need to bend the knees and hips to do so on the floor (AKA, the coin sign, a sign of back stiffness). Since the spine infection can be associated with abdominal symptoms in young children and creates a large systemic load, generalized malaise, loss of appetite, and failure to thrive may occur. In this case, the differential diagnosis in a young child who is refusing to walk includes hip pathology such as septic hip arthritis, transient synovitis, osteomyelitis, or myositis. Other diagnoses to consider include tumor such as leukemia spine tumor, intra-abdominal etiology, or JIA. Trauma, including child abuse, should always be considered in a young child who refuses to walk.

Plain radiographs should be done and include the joints above and below the area of concern. In this case, a lateral radiograph of the lumbar spine would have shown the loss of disc height, even though transient synovitis was the suspected diagnosis. Radiographs may show decreased disk height; an MRI will show inflammation about the disc with or without involvement of the vertebral body. Blood culture and disk aspiration may yield a culture; however, many are negative. The vertebral apophyseal ring with its associated vasculature is similar to the metaphysis of long bones. The vessels that traverse these endplates disappear by age 7 years [3].

If there are no neurologic symptoms, presumptive treatment with an antistaphylococcal antibiotic is indicated. The response to antibiotics should be clinically apparent. For patients with continued or worsening symptoms, a repeat MRI is indicated to determine if there is an abscess to be drained or if amount of involvement is increasing. In this case, there was no indication for additional advanced imaging in a patient who was responding to antibiotics, especially since an MRI examination in a 2 years old requires anesthesia sedation.

Historically, patients were often treated with immobilization and no antibiotics [3, 4]. Antibiotic treatment with or without bracing has been shown to decrease the duration of symptoms and risk for recurrence [5]. A brace may be used for comfort.

Some have described reconstitution of vertebral defects and reconstitution of the disc height; however, most reports indicate that intervertebral fibrosis with eventual fusion is common.

How to Approach the Case

Always be concerned about spine stiffness in a toddler. Most children with discitis are not overtly sick. Findings may be subtle. Very often the child with discitis is first diagnosed with transient synovitis of the hip, since that is much more common. The psoas muscle may be irritated in lumbar discitis, causing some discomfort and guarding with passive hip range of motion. An ultrasound examination of the hips will indicate that the pathology is elsewhere. Obtain plain radiographs of the spine to further evaluate the stiff spine in a toddler. However, the initial radiograph may appear normal or only show some flattening of the normal lumbar lordosis or mild scoliosis. If suspicion persists despite negative radiographs, obtain an MRI of the spine. As a general principle, when an MRI of the spine is ordered in a young child, talk with the radiologists first, since a screening MRI can often be obtained with fewer sequences that require less time under anesthesia and without IV contrast. Generally, when ordered for a child, an MRI is done of the entire cervical to sacral spine.

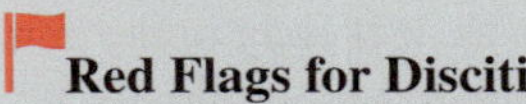

Red Flags for Discitis
- Younger child usually <5 years old, often a toddler
- Does not localize to hip/leg/back
- Has stopped walking or has listing gait
- Neural symptoms
- Neurological findings
- Loss of lumbar lordosis
- Does not tolerate sitting
- Stiff spine

Short Differential Diagnosis
- Infection – Whenever tumor is suspected, always suspect infection.
- Spine tuberculosis – It may occur in immigrant children. It more typically involves collapse of the vertebra and may involve several vertebral, leading to kyphosis and late myelopathy.
- Osteoid osteoma – These lesions are also painful at night, but are <1 cm in diameter and not typically associated with neurological signs.
- Osteoblastoma – Night pain, usually >2 cm in diameter, and as such can have associated neural symptoms and pain. It is often seen in the spine, typically in the posterior elements.
- Appendicitis – These children may appear to have abdominal pain and pain with back and hip motion.
- Langerhans cell histiocytosis – It can cause vertebra plana (flattened vertebra body) which can be confused with infection. Vertebra plana has several possible causes including tumor, as well as infection.
- Other infection – Hip infection, psoas abscess, septic knee, and Lyme disease can present with similar symptoms. These children generally appear less well.

Final Diagnosis

L4/L5 discitis

Natural History and Treatment Considerations

Making the correct and timely diagnosis is the key for this case. Look for the subtle clues that an insidious process is affecting the spine in a patient who cannot localize the pain. IV antibiotic treatment, typically without immobilization, will lead to resolution. Repeat MRI is indicated for patients who have persistent symptoms or develop neurologic findings. Long term, children recover well with no residual symptoms. However, warn the parents that the disc space may be narrow or even fused. Similar to a congenital fusion of a single level, long term there are minimal if any symptoms.

Referral – Emergency, Urgent, or Routine: And to Whom?

Patients with radiographic or MRI findings of discitis should be admitted to pediatrics for IV antibiotic therapy. If there are neurologic findings such as objective weakness or bowel or bladder symptoms, urgent consultation with pediatric spine specialists is necessary.

Brief Summary

Toddlers have difficulty in communicating the location of discomfort. Children who limp and have a stiff spine should be evaluated with plain spine radiographs. Laboratory tests may be normal, with the exception of ESR and CRP. Typically, there is a delay of 2–3 weeks between the onset of symptoms and a diagnosis of spondylodiscitis. In the pre-antibiotic era, these were treated with immobilization alone. Recent studies have shown faster resolution and reduced rates of recurrence with IV antibiotics. Long term, there is typically fibrosis of the disc and even vertebral fusion at the affected level.

Editor Discussion

Spine rigidity and lack of motion are key exam findings of a spine infection in a young child. Some children will refuse to walk or walk bent over with their hands on their knees. They may be reluctant to pick objects off the floor. Most cases are caused by MSSA; therefore, biopsy should be done selectively – most cases do not need a biopsy. Empirical treatment with antibiotics for MSSA remains the standard of care. A biopsy is indicated if the patient's symptoms worsen while on antibiotics or an unusual organism is suspected. Always get a blood culture during the initial workup. Keep treating with antibiotics until the ESR returns to normal.

W.L. Hennrikus

Spondylodiscitis (also termed discitis) is frequently missed in toddler since the focus in a limping child or one who refuses to walk is more typically on the hip. Early in the course of discitis, the disc space is preserved on plain radiographs, and diagnosis needs to be confirmed by MRI examination, which requires anesthesia sedation in the young child. In late cases, the plain radiograph can show loss of disc height. If there is minimal abscess or no abscess, which is typically the case, surgical drainage is not necessary. Since the organism is usually staphylococcus aureus, biopsy of the lesion is not necessary, unless there is lack of responsiveness to antibiotic therapy. For this 2-year-old girl responding to treatment, the second MRI was not needed and was an additional sedation and expense.

R.M. Schwend

References

1. Brown R, Hussain M, McHugh K, Novelli V, Jones D. Discitis in young children. J Bone Joint Surg Br. 2001;83(1):106–11.
2. Chandrasenan J, Klezl Z, Bommireddy R, Calthorpe D. Spondylodiscitis in children: a retrospective series. J Bone Joint Surg Br. 2011;93(8):1122–5.
3. Song KS, Ogden JA, Ganey T, Guidera KJ. Contiguous discitis and osteomyelitis in children. J Pediatr Orthop. 1997;17(4):470–7.
4. Menelaus MB. Discitis. J Bone Joint Surg Br. 1964;46(1):16–23.
5. Ring D, Wenger DR. Pyogenic infectious spondylitis in children: the convergence of discitis and vertebral osteomyelitis. J Pediatr Orthop. 1995;15(5):652–60.

Chapter 20
Delayed Osteomyelitis Diagnosis and Treatment in a Teenager

Jesse Galina and Wojciech L. Czoch

Brief Case Presentation

Chief Complaint

Lumbar back pain

History

A 14-year-old boy presented for evaluation of chronic low back pain of approximately 1-year duration. The onset of pain was insidious without any known trauma. Initially, the pain was described as sharp and localized to the lower back without radiculopathy. He initially presented to his primary care physician and chiropractor for evaluation. Some families and children use chiropractic for primary care [1]. He underwent several months of chiropractic manipulation/treatment. Additionally, he took occasional over-the-counter pain medications with some relief of his symptoms. His pain occurred at any time; however, approximately 1 year after initial onset, he experienced an acute worsening of his symptoms while at school. He described a sharp stabbing pain localized to his low back and sacrum. The severity of the pain hindered his ability to walk and sleep. At that time, he presented to the emergency department for evaluation. He received a radiograph and was given NSAIDs for the pain. Not satisfied, he then presented to the primary care clinic. History revealed no recent illnesses, fevers, chills, or night sweats. He noted exacerbating factors of rising from a seated or supine position, prolonged standing, or

J. Galina (✉) · W. L. Czoch
Pediatric Orthopaedics, Cohen Children's Medical Center, New Hyde Park, NY, USA

© Springer Nature Switzerland AG 2021
R. M. Schwend, W. L. Hennrikus (eds.), *Back Pain in the Young Child and Adolescent*, https://doi.org/10.1007/978-3-030-50758-9_20

ambulating longer distances. Low back pain was rated as 8/10 in severity and constant in nature. He related a "history of travel and cave exposure." There was no family history of back pain.

Physical Examination

He needed to be taken to the clinic on a stretcher. The vital signs were within normal limits: height 175.3 cm, weight 74.4 kg, and BMI 26.7. He was awake, alert, and in no acute distress, although he did appear generally uncomfortable. He did not appear diaphoretic. Neurological exam was unremarkable. He exhibited full and symmetric strength among all major upper and lower extremity muscle groups. There was no limitation in range of spine motion, instability, or exacerbation of pain with passive/active range of motion of all major joints. Reflexes were 2+ and symmetric. Sensation was fully intact throughout. Clinical alignment of the spine was unremarkable. He ambulated with a normal and steady heel-to-toe gait bearing equal weight across bilateral lower extremities.

Imaging and Radiographic Studies *(Figs. 20.1, 20.2, and 20.3)*

Questions About the Case the Reader Should Consider
1. What is the typical presentation of a child with vertebral osteomyelitis?
2. Is it normal that the patient was afebrile?
3. Are radiographs necessary and were the correct radiographs used?
4. How is vertebral osteomyelitis confirmed?
5. Were the lab results consistent with osteomyelitis?
6. When should antibiotic treatment begin? And for how long?
7. Are there any alternative treatments? Should surgery have been performed?
8. Was the postoperative course normal?
9. How do you know if treatment has failed? If failure occurs, what should the next steps be?

Discussion

Symptoms for vertebral osteomyelitis are noticeably broad. The most common symptom is back pain; however, early examination can produce broad and nonfocal, nonspecific pain. Largely for this reason, the diagnosis for osteomyelitis, especially in children, is often delayed [2].

This boy began experiencing symptoms approximately 1 year prior to initial consultation. Initially, his symptoms were mild and very nonspecific. As the disease

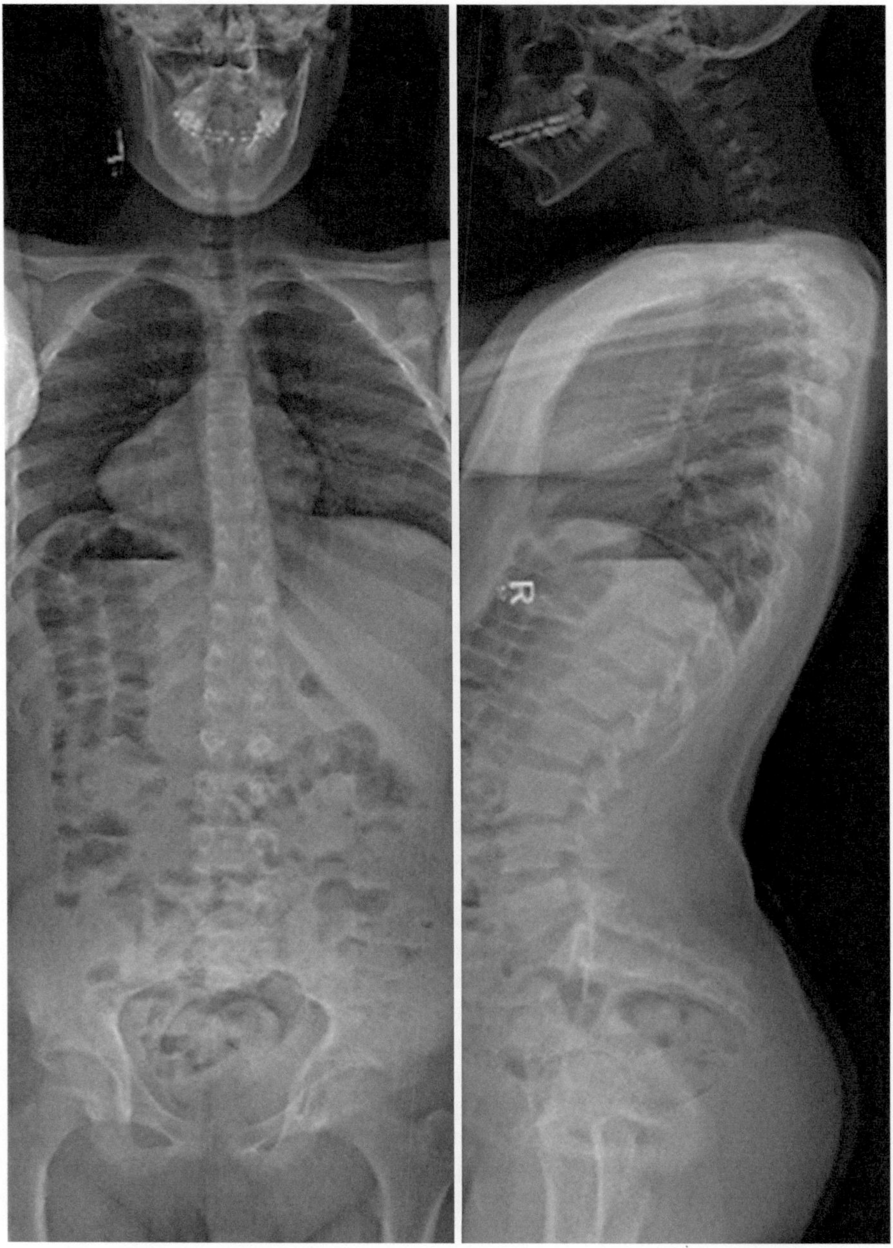

Fig. 20.1 Initial PA and lateral spine radiographs. These were taken to compare vertebral heights, look for bone erosion/soft tissue damage, and check for idiopathic deformity and spondylolisthesis. These were ruled out as the study was unremarkable. Therefore, the patient was indicated for MRI evaluation. Review of these initial radiographs suggested that the L3 L4 disc space was narrow

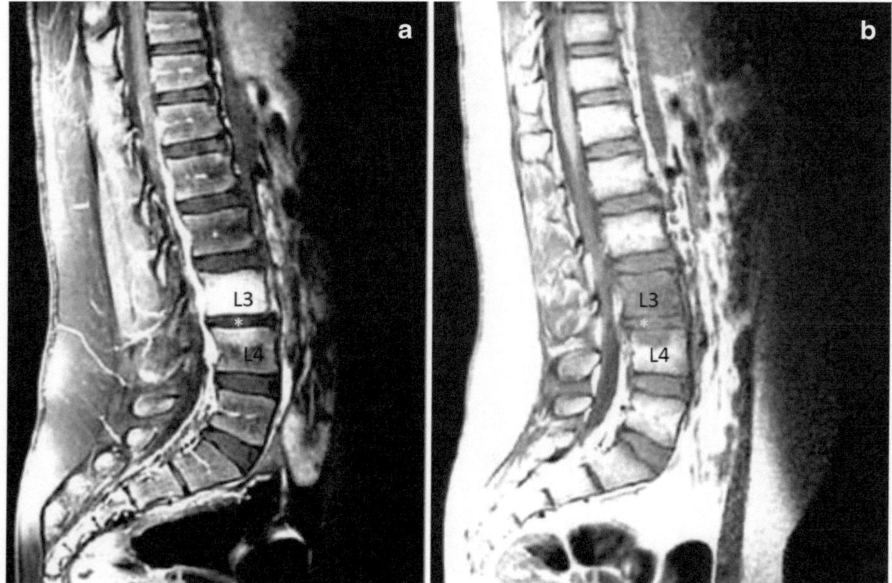

Fig. 20.2 Initial sagittal MRI images. There is moderate loss of intervertebral disc (*) height between the L3 and L4 vertebra. Disc heights between the remainder of the vertebra are normal. (**a**) Shows a STIR sequence with increased signal at L3 and upper part of L4. (**b**) Shows a decreased T1 signal in the same locations. These are tell-tale signs of vertebral osteomyelitis. Osteomyelitis should be confirmed using lab results

process progressed, the pain began to more reliably localize to the infected vertebrae. Although osteomyelitis can affect any portion of the spine, the lower 5 lumbar vertebrae are the most commonly affected [3]. Moreover, despite having an active infection, he was consistently afebrile. Fever has been shown to be an inconsistent measure of vertebral osteomyelitis [3]. Zimmerli speculated that one of the more probable reasons for this was related to the use of analgesics/anti-inflammatories for the back pain [4], which is consistent with this patient, who had been taking acetaminophen and NSAIDs intermittently for symptomatic improvement.

Therefore, the level of suspicion for osteomyelitis should remain high. Children who present with progressive and unremitting back pain should be subjected to further investigation and rigorous radiographic imaging. AP and lateral standing spine radiographs should be used for initial evaluation of coronal or sagittal plane deformity, loss of lumbar lordosis, disc space narrowing, vertebral body fracture, or density changes.

However, radiographs are a screening tool and do not exclude the diagnosis. At times, the presentation of osteomyelitis can be misrepresented as a compression fracture [5]. For this reason, MRI is often used as the most sensitive technique for identification of osteomyelitis, with a sensitivity of 97%, specificity of 93%, and accuracy of 94% [6, 7]. MRI findings consistent with osteomyelitis are most

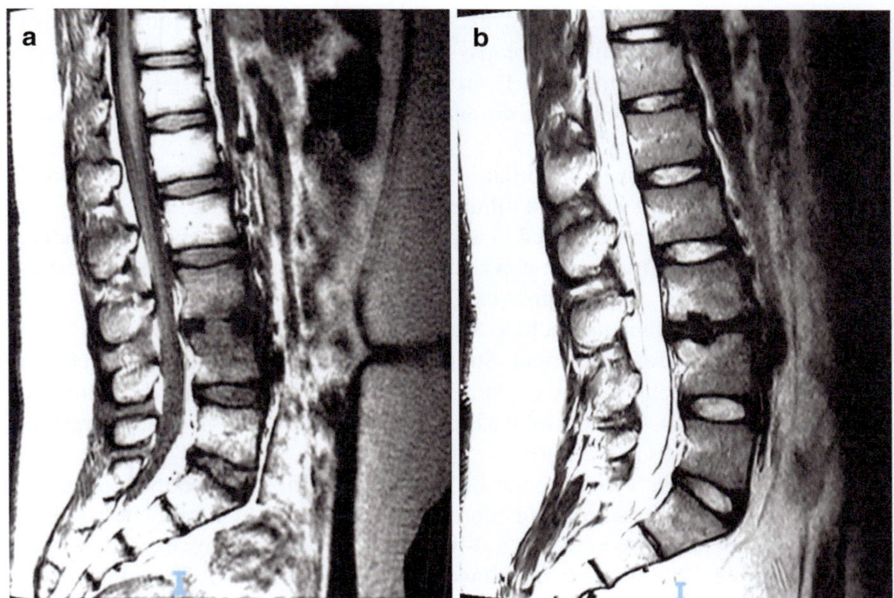

Fig. 20.3 (**a**) Follow-up MRI 2 months postdiagnosis. Image shows T2 hyper intensity in the L3–L4 vertebral bodies and the disc space between the two. When enhanced, a small edema can be seen in the L4–L5 interspinous region. However, when compared to the initial MRI, there has been marked improvement in T2 signal and inflammation of soft tissue. (**b**) Follow up MRI 1-year post-diagnosis. There is still shortening of the disc between L3 and L4. Additionally, there are Schmorl's nodes present on the inferior endplate of L3 and some endplate of L4. The signal intensity for the image is normal and no inflammation is noticeable, indicating recovery

commonly decreased signal intensity at the site of the infected vertebral body using T1-weighted images. Additionally, disc and endplate hyperintensity can be seen on T2 images. Later findings are consistent with disc space narrowing and bony erosions. Carragee reviewed 103 patients who were diagnosed with osteomyelitis and underwent MRI. The results of their study showed that 96% of patients were correctly diagnosed at or after 2 weeks of symptoms [8].

This boy had a normal appearing spine radiograph, although in retrospect the L3–L4 disc space appeared slightly narrow. Given his persistent symptoms, a spine MRI was ordered which revealed loss of L3–L4 disc height with a mild disc bulge but no evidence of spinal stenosis. There was a low T1 signal at these levels, which was associated to an endplate edema. The initial impression was highly suspicious for discitis or vertebral osteomyelitis of pyogenic or tuberculosis origin. This was significant given his history of travel, which should raise suspicion when evaluating a patient with generally vague but progressive symptoms. Should tuberculosis be a confirmed diagnosis, a chest radiograph and a complete TB workup should be performed.

Most cases are due to MSSA and are started on empiric antimicrobial therapy to cover MSSA without obtaining a biopsy specimen and culture. Blood cultures and serum studies are recommended. If an unusual organism is suspected or if the patient's symptoms worsen while on antibiotics, then an image-guided biopsy is indicated.

If a biopsy is done, it is important to have a skilled surgeon or interventional radiologist perform this step to minimize any complication risk. The biopsy and resulting cultures will then be used to adjust antibiotic selection. Hallmark findings of vertebral osteomyelitis are an elevated leukocyte levels, erythrocyte sedimentation rate (ESR), and C-reactive protein (CRP) [9].

Common microorganisms include Staphylococcus aureus and MRSA [10]. On initial blood cultures for this patient, Streptococcus viridans was isolated in culture; however, this was thought to be a contaminant. Because the finding did not match the possible diagnosis, he underwent a biopsy which then confirmed MSSA positive vertebral osteomyelitis and discitis.

He was started on a 6-week course of intravenous antibiotic treatment. At times, organism-specific treatment may be more prolonged due to high virulence or resistance [11]. This patient completed a 6-week course of clindamycin, and his pain improved from 8/10 to 0/10 by the 4th week.

Although antibiotic therapy is the mainstay of treatment for vertebral osteomyelitis/discitis, there is a role for surgical intervention in selected cases. Surgery is recommended for osteomyelitis patients if neurological deficits are present, distinct encapsulated fluid collections are seen, and there is any evidence of spinal cord compression or compromise, or in recurrent or resistant infection [11]. This patient had an excellent response to medical management and did not display any neurologic deficits or concerning lesions requiring surgical intervention.

For additional symptomatic improvement during therapy, soft rigid spinal braces have been proposed. Generally, the braces are worn for comfort, when the patient is out of bed to provide additional support and minimize low back motion. For severe pain, bed rest can be used along with initial therapy and weaned as symptoms improve.

According to clinical guidelines, medical treatment should be viewed as a failure if neurological deficits appear or persist, laboratory studies show continued elevation of inflammatory markers, the patient's clinical condition is noted to deteriorate, or there is a recurrence of infection [11]. A multispecialty team including pediatrics, orthopedics, radiology, and infectious disease doctors is often needed to treat such a case.

How to Approach the Case

Anytime a pediatric patient arrives supine because of back pain, there should be a high level of clinical suspicion for a serious condition. Additionally, pain characteristics such as nighttime pain should be of particular concern for infections or tumors.

If the pain is localized on presentation, this will allow for a more focused examination and radiographic evaluation. However, we recommend entire radiographic spine evaluation if concern is high for infection. Initial screening radiographs will be able to determine any structural damage such as a deformity, disk/vertebral height loss, bone erosion, or spondylolisthesis. If they are unremarkable, advanced imaging, such as MRI, may be indicated.

In all cases, CBC, ESR, CRP, and blood cultures should be obtained. Most cases can be treated empirically for MSSA infection. If an unusual organism is suspected or the patient fails to improve with IV antibiotics, then an image-guided biopsy is indicated.

Surgical intervention may be warranted in cases of neurological deficits, spinal cord compression/compromise, local vertebral body compromise and deformity, unstable spine, epidural abscess, or failure to respond to appropriate antibiotic. Surgery is accompanied by continued antimicrobial management.

Red Flags for Back Pain with Osteomyelitis
- Severe back pain
- Fever
- Chills
- Rapid, unexpected weight loss
- Numbness
- Radiculopathy
- Spine stiffness (decreased ROM). Difficult to pick an object off the floor
- Fatigue
- Tenderness at infection site

Short Differential Diagnosis
- Herniated disc – these are associated with significant back pain and radiculopathy
- Vertebral fracture – pain localized to one area
- Degenerative disc – associated with back pain, however generally in the older population
- Spinal epidural abscess – signs include back pain, neurological limitations, and fever
- Osteomyelitis – subtle, localized disc pain that worsens over time and with movement. Neurological damage is possible, and MRI will show a low T1 signal intensity at the height of the infection. Blood work generally will reveal elevated erythrocyte sedimentation rate and elevated C-reactive protein

Final Diagnosis

L3–L4 vertebral osteomyelitis with spondylodiscitis

Natural History and Treatment Considerations

Back pain in adolescent patients should be a cause for concern. Because of the many possible diagnoses, patients should be carefully examined for possible abnormal symptoms that will allow for an early detection for vertebral osteomyelitis. Definitive steps should be taken with clinical examination, radiographic imaging, and laboratory testing before prescribing a treatment. Clinical evaluation can be used to cast a wide net over possible diagnoses; MRI and CT can be used for further indication. Cultures should be used to confirm the diagnosis before treating with antibiotics.

Referral – Emergency, Urgent, or Routine: And to Whom?

Children with back pain that does not clearly fit into musculoskeletal strain/sprain and poor posture, or is accompanied by constitutional symptoms, should be urgently referred to a pediatric orthopedic spine surgeon. Following a careful history and physical examination, further routine workup will be pursued (radiographs, blood work, advanced imaging). In select cases, a biopsy may be indicated. In rare cases in which neurological symptoms or deficits are present (weakness, numbness, asymmetric reflexes, bowel/bladder dysfunction), patients should *immediately* be seen for evaluation as evolving spinal cord compression/compromise could be present.

Brief Summary

Although rare, vertebral osteomyelitis is an infection of the vertebra, usually involving the adjacent disk. Because adolescent back pain has a broad range of possible diagnoses, it is imperative to determine the cause. As the infection progresses, pain in the older child will often become more localized to a specific part of the spine. It is important to remember that lumbar spine is the most common site of osteomyelitis in children. A fever may be present; however, an afebrile patient may also have osteomyelitis. While extremely rare, the patient may also present with neurological compromise which requires immediate attention and surgical treatment. In summary, vertebral osteomyelitis highlights an interdepartmental diagnostic and treatment approach, utilizing clinical examination, radiographs, advanced imaging, blood studies, and medical (possibly surgical) intervention.

Key Features and Pearls

- Spinal pain has the potential for many diagnoses. Possible diagnoses can be herniated disc, vertebral fracture, a degenerative disk, or a tumor. For this reason, treatment for osteomyelitis is generally delayed due to the ambiguous symptoms. This delay is the most common for osteomyelitis and is known for its subtlety. With time, pain can begin to localize to the affected vertebrae.
- Vertebral osteomyelitis has similar symptoms to discitis and should be kept in mind. These can be differentiated through different diagnostic techniques. However, typically, vertebral osteomyelitis and discitis commonly occur together when viewed on MRI.
- Fevers may be indicative of osteomyelitis but are not always present. Advanced cases of osteomyelitis are at risk for neurological deficit, which should be subject to immediate intervention.
- Initial radiographs are generally inconclusive, especially early in the course. An MRI is then necessary to further examine the spine. Low T1–T2-weighted image signals may show an abnormal disk. Bone biopsy can be done to further confirm diagnosis. Laboratory blood work generally shows elevated leukocyte levels, erythrocyte sedimentation rate, and the presence of C-reactive protein.

Editor Discussion

Spine rigidity and lack of motion are key exam findings of a spine infection. Some children will refuse to walk or walk bent over with their hand on their thighs. Most cases are caused by MSSA; therefore, biopsy should be done selectively – most cases do not need a biopsy. The cost, morbidity, and low yield of a biopsy reinforce that empirical treatment with antibiotics for MSSA remains the standard of care. Biopsy is indicated if the patient's symptoms worsen while on antibiotic or an unusual organism is suspected. Do not forget to get a blood culture during the initial workup, and keep treating with antibiotics until the ESR returns to normal.

W.L. Hennrikus

Spondylodiscitis is believed to start in the end-arterioles of the vertebral endplate and spread to the adjacent disc, adjacent vertebral body, and through the disc to the other endplate and into the adjacent vertebral body. As this case demonstrates, what initially appears to be vertebral osteomyelitis is really the more typical spondylodiscitis, involving both the disc and the adjacent vertebral bodies. The adjacent endplates and the disc are the area of primary infection, but the surrounding soft tissue may also become involved. In more extreme cases, a psoas or epidural abscess can occur (see Chap. 21). In contrast to the toddler (see Chap. 19), the older child with spondylodiscitis is able to localize the painful area, which helps in the evaluation. MRI imaging is very sensitive for making the diagnosis. A child with typical symptoms and typical MRI findings of discitis may not need a biopsy of the lesion if there is an appropriate clinical response to IV antibiotic. If the *patient* is atypical (unusual travel, immunocompromised, implants present), if the *MRI findings* are atypical (large abscess, bone destruction resembles TB, lesion appears to be tumor), or if the *suspected organism* is atypical (history of MRSA, unusual travel), then interventional radiology-obtained biopsy may be useful. Whenever a biopsy is being considered, the surgeon who may need to perform a more extensive surgical drainage should be consulted, and discussion occurs with the interventional radiologist. For all biopsies, tissue should always be sent for both culture and for pathology. Culture should include a request for TB and fungal processing. In this case, since the response to antibiotic therapy was appropriate, the two follow-up MRI examinations were not necessary, even though they are interesting to visualize the natural history of recovery.

R.M. Schwend

References

1. Awwad AB, Hennrikus WL, Armstrong DG. Pediatric orthopaedic consults from chiropractic care. J Surg Orthop Adv. 2018;27:58–63.
2. Wheeless CR. Wheeless' textbook of orthopaedics. 2012. Duke University Medical Center's Division of Orthopaedic Surgery. Brooklandville, MD: Data Trace Internet Publishing, LLC; 2011.
3. Mylona E, Samarkos M, Kakalou E, Fanourgiakis P, Skoutelis A. Pyogenic vertebral osteomyelitis: a systematic review of clinical characteristics. Semin Arthritis Rheum. 2009;39(1):10–7.
4. Zimmerli W. Vertebral osteomyelitis. N Engl J Med. 2010;362(11):1022–9.
5. Abe E, Yan K, Okada K. Pyogenic vertebral osteomyelitis presenting as single spinal compression fracture: a case report and review of the literature. Spinal Cord. 2000;38(10):639.
6. An HS, Seldomridge JA. Spinal infections: diagnostic tests and imaging studies. Clin Orthop Relat Res. 2006 Mar;444:27–33.
7. Ledermann HP, Schweitzer ME, Morrison WB, Carrino JA. MR imaging findings in spinal infections: rules or myths? Radiology. 2003;228(2):506–14.
8. Carragee EJ. The clinical use of magnetic resonance imaging in pyogenic vertebral osteomyelitis. Spine. 1997;22(7):780–5.
9. Carragee EJ, Kim D, van der Vlugt T, Vittum D. The clinical use of erythrocyte sedimentation rate in pyogenic vertebral osteomyelitis. Spine. 1997;22(18):2089–93.
10. Livorsi DJ, Daver NG, Atmar RL, Shelburne SA, White AC Jr, Musher DM. Outcomes of treatment for hematogenous Staphylococcus aureus vertebral osteomyelitis in the MRSA ERA. J Infect. 2008;57(2):128–31.
11. Berbari EF, Kanj SS, Kowalski TJ, Darouiche RO, Widmer AF, Schmitt SK, et al. Infectious Diseases Society of America (IDSA) clinical practice guidelines for the diagnosis and treatment of native vertebral osteomyelitis in adults. Clin Infect Dis. 2015;61(6):e26–46.

Chapter 21
Case of a Child with a Spinal Epidural Abscess

John T. Anderson

Brief Case Presentation

Chief Complaint

Abdominal and right buttock pain

History of Present Illness

The patient is a 4-year-old healthy male who presented to the emergency department (ED) with a 1-week history of abdominal pain. The pain was located in the epigastrium and right lower quadrant. The pain has been worse at night and wakes him from sleep. He was recently evaluated by his primary care physician who thought he was constipated. A urinalysis was obtained, which was normal. He was treated with a stool softener and enema with only minimal hard stool output. His parents report that he has not been eating or drinking much. He has been tired and prefers to rest most of the time. There has been recent "low-grade fever." An abdominal radiograph revealed a nonobstructive bowel gas pattern. The abdominal ultrasound was negative. He was discharged from the ED with plans to follow-up with his primary care physician and instructions on constipation management.

Because of continued symptoms believed to be related to chronic constipation, he was referred to a gastroenterologist who started lactulose and hyoscyamine.

J. T. Anderson (✉)
Orthopaedic Surgery, University of Missouri – Kansas City School of Medicine, Kansas City, MO, USA

Orthopaedic Surgery, Children's Mercy – Kansas City, Kansas City, MO, USA
e-mail: Jtanderson@cmh.edu

© Springer Nature Switzerland AG 2021
R. M. Schwend, W. L. Hennrikus (eds.), *Back Pain in the Young Child and Adolescent*, https://doi.org/10.1007/978-3-030-50758-9_21

Erythrocyte sedimentation rate (ESR) was obtained which was 44 mm/hr. Despite having normal soft stools, his abdominal pain did not improve. He came back to the emergency department, complaining of continued abdominal and right buttock pain. His pain was so severe, he stopped walking. According to his parents, he would cry for hours in the fetal position grasping his abdomen and right buttock. His mother reports that he has not gained weight in 2 months. He has not had any recent documented fevers. His immunizations are current. There has been no foreign travel, insect or animal bites, exposure to tuberculosis, or unpasteurized dairy products. There is no significant family medical history.

Physical Examination

Blood pressure: 110/63; heart rate: 120/minute; respiratory rate: 32/minute; temperature: 36.6 °C.

The boy was writhing in pain in fetal position with his right hand grasping his right buttock. His abdomen was mildly distended with tenderness and guarding to palpation of all 4 quadrants. There was no organomegaly or rebound tenderness. The neurological examination was very difficult due to his young age and severe pain; however, he was moving all limbs appropriately. There was no clonus, negative Babinski's sign, and the reflexes were all normal. There was positive right straight leg raise test. Rectal tone was normal.

Laboratory Values

CBC with differential was normal, ESR was 39 mm/hr., and C-reactive protein (CRP) was 2.4 mg/dl. A blood culture was obtained that grew methicillin-sensitive staphylococcus aureus.

Imaging and Radiographic Studies

Abdominal ultrasound was negative. An abdominal radiograph revealed a nonobstructive bowl gas pattern.

Other than AP abdominal films, spine films were never obtained as they were focused on an abdominal problem. A CT scan with and without contrast of the abdomen was obtained by the emergency department physician (Fig. 21.1) that revealed abnormal spine findings at L1–2. The on-call spine surgeon was notified who ordered an MRI with and without contrast (Fig. 21.2).

Fig. 21.1 CT scan of the abdomen and pelvis with contrast revealed normal abdominal findings but sclerosis and areas of lucency in the L1 and L2 vertebral bodies. The L1–L2 disc is narrowed relative to T12–L1 and L2–L3 discs. Note the soft tissue density extending into the spinal canal (*green arrow*)

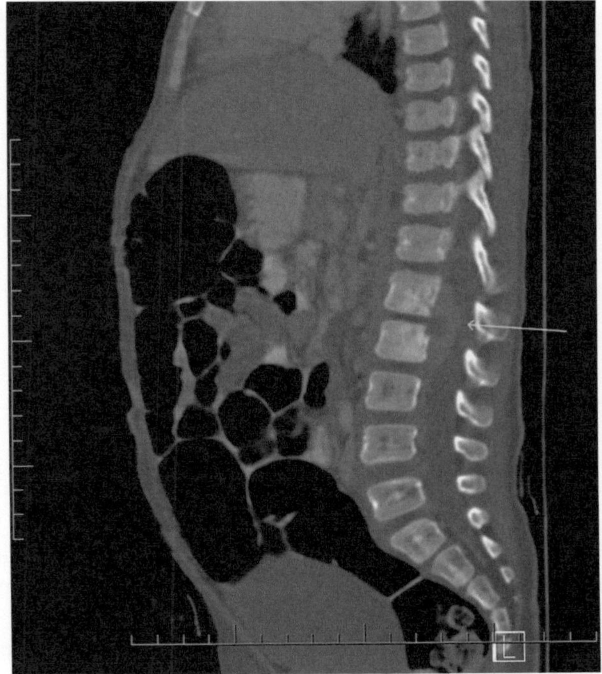

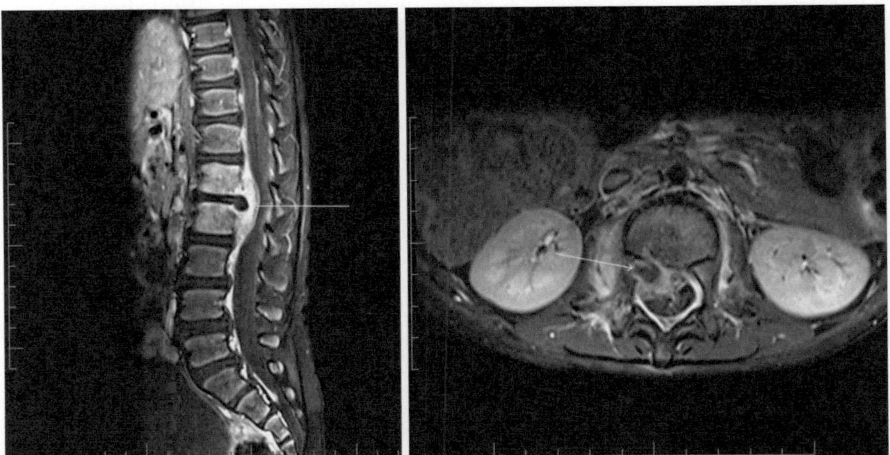

Fig. 21.2 MRI performed with and without gadolinium contrast revealed hyperintense post-contrast T1 signal in the L1–L2 vertebrae as well as a rim enhancing abscess causing significant compression centrally, the right lateral recess and foramen

Questions About the Case the Reader Should Consider
1. Are epidural abscesses common in children?
2. Why did this boy have abdominal pain?
3. Why did this boy have buttock pain?
4. What processes should be considered when a child is having pain that wakes them from sleep or is worse at night?
5. What processes should be considered when a child is having pain associated with malaise/lethargy and failure to gain weight or loss of weight?
6. What are the treatment options for this boy?

Discussion

Epidural abscesses are rare in adults and even rarer in children, with a reported incidence of 0.2 to 1.2 per 10,000 hospital admissions [1]. In adults, 50% of cases are thought to be secondary to hematogenous spread [2]. In children, hematogenous spread is thought to be very rare with most cases resulting from contiguous spread from a nearby infection [3]. In this particular case, the patient had L1–2 discitis. It is extremely rare for a child to have an isolated epidural abscess [3].

The classic triad of epidural abscesses is back pain, fever, and neurologic deficit; however, this triad is commonly not found in affected patients [4, 5]. This boy's primary complaint was abdominal pain and then later right buttock pain. Epidural abscesses can also cause abdominal and/or chest wall pain [6]. While cervical and lumbar level abscesses may present with neck pain radiating into an arm(s) and lower back pain radiating into the buttock(s) and or lower extremity(s), abscesses located in the thoracic level may present with chest or abdominal pain [6]. Likewise, patients with discitis in the area of T8–L1 may present with mostly abdominal pain [7]. This boy had both abdominal and buttock pain because the lower thoracic nerves and the lumbar and sacral nerves were being irritated by the abscess centered at the L1–L2 disc level.

Given that most affected children lack risk factors, and frequently present without classic findings, it is easy to understand why many cases are diagnosed in a delayed fashion. In this particular case, an infectious or neoplastic process could have been considered in light of the reported low-grade fever, night pain, malaise, failure to gain weight, and an ESR of 44 mm/hr. The patient's diagnosis was established by contrast-enhanced abdominal CT scan that was ordered by the ED physician to rule out an intra-abdominal etiology. After the L1–L2 abnormality was identified, the on-call spine surgeon was notified. He ordered an MRI with and without gadolinium administration, the imaging of modality of choice, which more clearly revealed the epidural abscess. It should also be stressed that radiographs not obtained for the purpose of spinal imaging, i.e., abdominal radiographs, should be closely scrutinized for abnormalities such as disc space narrowing, lack of a psoas shadow, or a missing pedicle, all subtle radiographic features suggestive of spinal or paraspinal destructive processes.

Typically, an epidural abscess is a surgical emergency, especially if the patient is neurologically impaired, as a delay in neural decompression can lead to permanent disability. The debate between surgical and medical management is still ongoing, particularly in the adult population [8–11], and cases of medical management alone have been described in the pediatric literature [12]. This decision should be made in collaboration between the spinal surgery and infectious disease teams. This boy underwent surgical decompression via a laminectomy. A laminotomy was initially performed but converted to a laminectomy as there was an abundant amount of firm phlegmon present that required more access than was provided by the laminotomy. Surgical intervention was also favored due the patient's severe radicular symptoms (buttock pain) and the inability to perform a reliable neurological assessment. The cultures grew methicillin-sensitive Staphylococcus aureus that was treated initially with intravenous antibiotics and then transition to oral antibiotics. He received antibiotic therapy for a total of 6 months and made an uneventful recovery.

How to Approach the Case

This case represented a diagnostic dilemma as a spinal infection would most likely not have been on top of most physicians' differential diagnosis. However, infection and/or a neoplastic process should be considered in any child presenting with pain that is worse at night and is associated with fever, malaise, and failure to gain weight or weight loss. Additionally, pain referred to the buttock(s) or leg(s) should raise suspicion of neural compression, and conditions of the spinal column should be considered in children presenting with abdominal pain, just as abdominal conditions should be considered in children with back pain.

Red Flags for Epidural Abscess
- Abdominal pain of unknown origin or failure to respond to treatment of common disorders
- History of fever, night pain, and malaise
- Pain so severe causes inability or reluctance to walk
- History of right buttock pain
- Elevated ESR
- No weight gain for 2 months

> **Short Differential Diagnosis**
> - Appendicitis – right lower quadrant pain, fever, malaise, loss of appetite
> - Intussusception – common age, abdominal pain, lethargy, loss of appetite
> - Constipation – common, abdominal pain, loss of appetite
> - Mesenteric lymphadenitis – right lower quadrant pain, malaise, loss of appetite
> - Malignancies – malaise, night pain, failure to gain weight
> - Discitis – not walking, abdominal pain, malaise, radicular pain, stiff spine, fever, spinal pain, night pain. Can be confused with hip pathology, such as transient synovitis, but more chronic
> - Epidural abscess – abdominal/chest wall pain, fever, radicular pain, neurological deficit, spinal pain

Final Diagnosis

Spinal epidural abscess secondary to contiguous spread from L1 to L2 discitis/osteomyelitis

Natural History and Treatment Considerations

With prompt diagnosis and treatment, the prognosis is good. However, if left untreated or inadequately treated, epidural abscesses can lead to permanent neurological impairment and even death [13, 14]. The most common organism cultured is Staphylococcus aureus, with methicillin resistance being fairly common [12, 13]. Compared to adults, children typically have more favorable outcomes [13].

Referral – Emergency, Urgent, or Routine: And to Whom?

An epidural abscess is an emergency, especially if the patient has a neurological deficit or is medically unstable. These patients should be referred to an orthopedic surgeon or neurosurgeon with expertise in treating pediatric spinal pathology. It is also imperative that the facility caring for the patient has a pediatric intensive care unit. If no such surgeon or facility exists in your community, prompt transfer should be arranged.

Summary

Children with epidural abscesses often present with symptoms that are not intuitively linked to an epidural abscess such as abdominal and/or chest wall pain. The classic triad of back pain, fever, and neurological deficit is actually not that common. Epidural abscesses, other spinal infections, or neoplasms should be considered in any child with a change in gait pattern or refusal to bear weight, abdominal pain/chest wall pain, neck or back pain, pain radiating to the upper/lower extremities, abnormal neurological findings, pain that is worse at night, fevers, lethargy or malaise, and/or weight loss or failure to gain weight. Epidural abscesses and spinal infections should especially be considered when atypical pain, febrile illness, sepsis, or hemodynamic instability cannot be explained by more common etiologies. Plain radiographs of the spine should initially be obtained since a narrow disc space or soft tissue findings may be noted. MRI with and without gadolinium administration is the imaging modality of choice. Blood cultures should be sent. Surgical decompression combined with appropriate antibiotics is considered the standard of care, especially if neurological deficits are present. The role of medical management without surgical intervention is controversial but can be done on a case-by-case basis after review of the case with the spine specialist and the infectious disease specialist.

> **Key Features and Pearls**
> **Epidural abscesses can manifest as abdominal or chest wall pain.**
> - Pain that is worse at night or wakes a child from sleep is suspicious for infection or malignancy.
> - Pain that radiates to the buttock and/or extremity is suspicious for neural compression.

Editor Discussion

This patient is sick and in severe pain. Think about infection or tumor and admit and work up the child immediately. This patient did not demonstrate the classic triad of back pain, fever, and neurologic deficit for an epidural abscess highlighting the fact that atypical presentations such as belly pain, chest wall pain, and buttock pain can also occur. This patient had both abdominal and buttock pain because the lower thoracic nerves and the lumbar and sacral nerves were being irritated by the abscess centered at the L1–L2 disc level. An epidural abscess with a neurologic deficit is a surgical emergency. In patients without a neurological deficit, some cases can be treated with medical management alone. This decision should be made on a case-by-case basis with input from the pediatric spine surgeon and the infectious disease specialist. Do not forget to order blood cultures if a spine infection is suspected.

W.L. Hennrikus

Discitis (spondylodiscitis) is a more common and likely diagnosis than epidural abscess in a child. This can be a very difficult diagnosis to make, since the clinical findings can be subtle – back stiffness, limp, reluctance to walk, or mild general symptoms such as night pain, abdominal pain, and weight loss. Discitis is occasionally confused with the more common diagnosis of transient synovitis of the hip since both may cause reluctance to walk, a limp, and pain. Pain in the psoas muscle from an adjacent discitis or adjacent hip infection can create pain with hip motion in either condition. When a child is in so much pain that he cannot be examined properly, think of serious conditions such as a neoplasm or infection in the spinal canal irritating the spinal cord or spinal nerves. Because these lesions are relatively rare, it is possible not to consider in the typical presentation of a child in pain. However, these children often have atypical clinical presentations such as seen with this boy, so think of these atypical conditions.

R.M. Schwend

References

1. Rubin G, Shalom M, Ashenasi A, Tadmor R, et al. Spinal epidural abscess in the pediatric age group: case report and review of the literature. Pediatr Infect Dis. 1993;12:1007–11.
2. Darouiche R. Spinal epidural abscess. N Engl J Med. 2006;355:2012–20.
3. Tay B, Deckey J, Hu S. Spinal infections. J Am Acad Orthop Surg. 2002;10:188–97.
4. Rigamonti D, Liem L, Sampath P, et al. Spinal epidural abscess: contemporary trends in etiology, evaluation, and management. Surg Neurol. 1999;52:189–97.
5. Davis D, Wold R, Patel R, et al. The clinical presentation and impact of diagnostic delays on emergency department patients with spinal epidural abscess. J Emerg Med. 2004;26:285–91.
6. Bremmer A, Darouiche RO. Spinal epidural abscess presenting as intra-abdominal pathology: a case report and literature review. J Emerg Med. 2004;26:51–6.
7. Ginsburg G, Bassett G. Back pain in children and adolescents: evaluation and differential diagnosis. J Am Acad Orthop Surg. 1997;5(2):67–78.
8. Kim S, Melikian R, Ju K, et al. Independent predictors of failure of nonoperative management of spinal epidural abscesses. Spine J. 2014;14:1673–9.
9. Arko L, Quach E, Nguyen V, et al. Medical and surgical management of spinal epidural abscess: a systematic review. Neurosurg Focus. 2014;37:E4.
10. Spernovasilis N, Demetriou S, Bachlitzanaki M, et al. Characteristics and predictors of outcome of spontaneous spinal epidural abscesses treated conservatively: a retrospective cohort study in a referral center. Clin Neurol Neurosurg. 2017;156:11–7.
11. Wang TY, Harward SC, Tsvankin V, et al. Neurological outcomes after surgical or conservative management of spontaneous spinal epidural abscesses: a systematic review and meta-analysis of data from 1980 through 2106. Clin Spine Surg. 2019;32:18–29.
12. Hawkins M, Bolton M. Pediatric spinal epidural abscess: a 9-year institutional review and review of the literature. Pediatrics. 2013;132:1680–5.
13. Auletta J, John C. Spinal epidural abscesses in children: a 15-year experience and review of the literature. Clin Infect Dis. 2001;32:9–16.
14. Enberg R, Kaplan R. Spinal epidural abscess in children: early diagnosis and immediate surgical drainage is essential to forestall paralysis. Clin Pediatr. 1974;13:247–8.

Chapter 22
The Pain Is "Knot" Getting Better: Case of a Girl with a "Knot in the Back". Back Pain Due to an Aneurysmal Bone Cyst

Matthew E. Oetgen and Shannon M. Kelly

Brief Case Presentation

Chief Complaint

Acute back pain after a motor vehicle collision and a preceding 1-month history of mid-back pain and a "knot in the back"

History

The patient is a 7-year-old girl who presents to the emergency department complaining of lumbar back pain after a car accident that evening. She was a backseat restrained passenger with a lap belt and shoulder harness involved in a motor vehicle collision. The car she was in that was traveling at approximately 40 mph struck the rear of a car that was traveling at a lower speed. No airbags deployed and moderate front-end vehicle damage was noted. She does not remember hitting her head, there was no loss of consciousness and no vomiting, and she has been behaving at baseline per family since the event. She was evaluated by the Emergency Medical Services at the scene, walked away from the car, and was brought to the emergency department by family members. Her main complaint is acute, sharp pain in the mid-lumbar portion of her back without radiation into her legs.

Upon further discussion with the patient, she describes having ongoing moderate dull achy pain in the mid-lumbar spine that has been worse with flexion and

M. E. Oetgen (✉) · S. M. Kelly
Division of Orthopaedic Surgery and Sports Medicine, Children's National Health System, Washington, DC, USA
e-mail: Moetgen@Childrensnational.Org

© Springer Nature Switzerland AG 2021
R. M. Schwend, W. L. Hennrikus (eds.), *Back Pain in the Young Child and Adolescent*, https://doi.org/10.1007/978-3-030-50758-9_22

associated with intermittent left anterior thigh pain for about 1 month before the collision. She recalls no inciting incident or trauma for the pain. Additionally, she noted swelling in the left mid-lumbar region that she describes as a "knot in her back," which has gotten more pronounced over this time. Her pain wakes her from sleeping around 3 AM most nights. Her pain improves somewhat with acetaminophen. She has not been able to play as much because of this back and thigh pain. She reports no paresthesias or weakness, but her mother has noticed a limp after more vigorous activities. She has not noticed bowel or bladder incontinence or perianal anesthesia.

Physical Examination

Weight 34.3 kg, height 131.8 cm, body mass index 19.75

Appearance: No acute distress healthy appearing patient when lying in bed. Her skin is normal. Gait and station: She stands with a level pelvis and walks with a slight limp on the left, with a shortened stride on that side due to limited left hip flexion. Balance and coordination: Patient can heel walk and toe walk without difficulty. There is no ataxia. Upper extremities: Both upper extremities, on inspection, show no deformities or contractures. On palpation, there are no areas of tenderness on either upper extremity. She has full range of motion of all joints from the shoulders to hands without pain or instability. There is normal motor strength sensation in both upper extremities in the C5-T1 distributions. Back: The patient stands with a level pelvis, and overall she is well balanced. The shoulders are level. The waist is symmetric without a trunk shift. There is a subtle mass in the left paraspinal region of the lumbar spine. On Adams forward bend test, there is no rotational prominence, but the left para-spinal mass is more noticeable. There is tenderness to palpation over this left paraspinal mass, but no other tenderness or muscle spasms noted. She has limited range of motion of the back, with flexion limited by pain. There is normal back strength and sensation. The skin is normal with no cutaneous manifestations of dysraphism.

Lower extremities: Both lower extremities, on inspection, show no deformities or contractures. On palpation, there is tenderness to the left distal medial thigh that is worse with knee and hip extension. Otherwise, there are no areas of tenderness on either lower extremity. She has full range of motion of all joints in both lower extremities without instability. There is normal motor strength in all muscles and normal sensation to light touch in both lower in the L1-S1 distributions. The skin is normal in both lower extremities. Reflexes: The patient has 2+ reflexes in the triceps, biceps, brachioradialis, patella, and Achilles. She has no beats of clonus in either lower extremity, and the toes are down going with the Babinski test. Vascular: She has 2+ dorsalis pedis and radial artery pulses with regular rate and rhythm. There is no distal extremity edema in any extremity.

Imaging and Radiographic Studies (Figs. 22.1, 22.2, 22.3, and 22.4)

Questions About the Case the Reader Should Consider

1. Why did this patient have these underlying baseline symptoms of back pain and what is the "knot in the back?"
2. Why the acute change in symptoms after the motor vehicle collision?

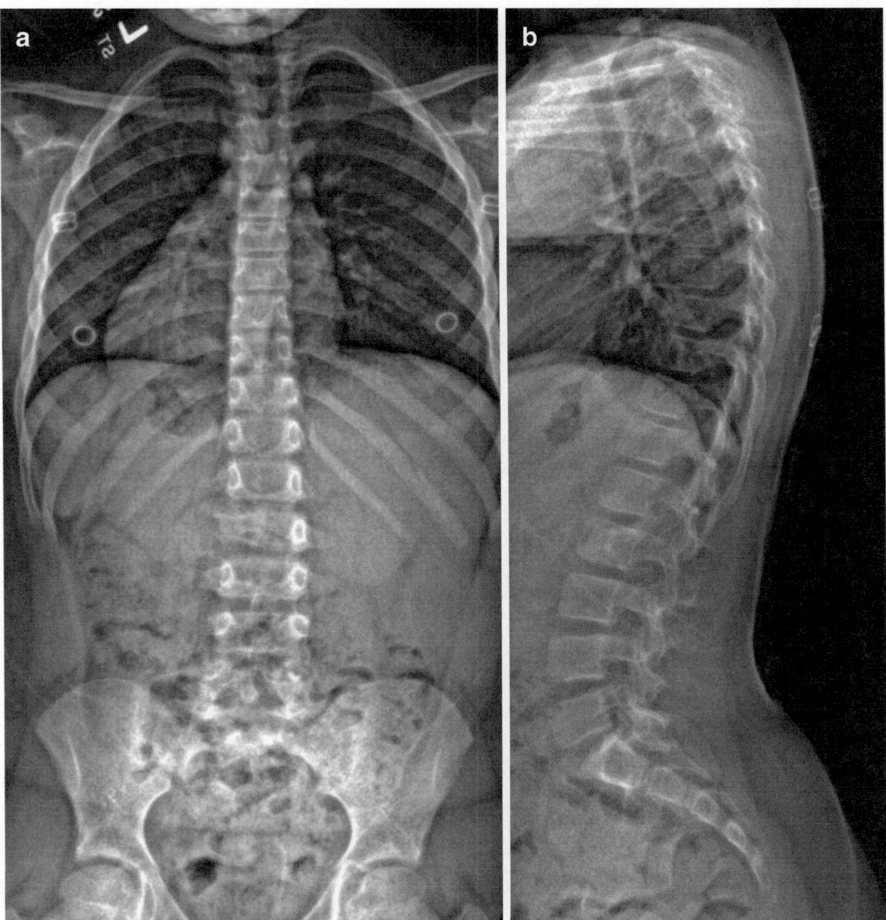

Fig. 22.1 (**a, b**) PA and lateral standing radiographs. The standing scoliosis radiographs, on first inspection, do not show any malalignment or deformity. There are 12 rib-bearing thoracic vertebrae and 5 lumbar vertebrae. No evidence of scoliosis is seen, and no abnormal kyphosis or lordosis is noted on the lateral image. The triradiatae cartilages are near closed, and the patient has a Riser sign of 0

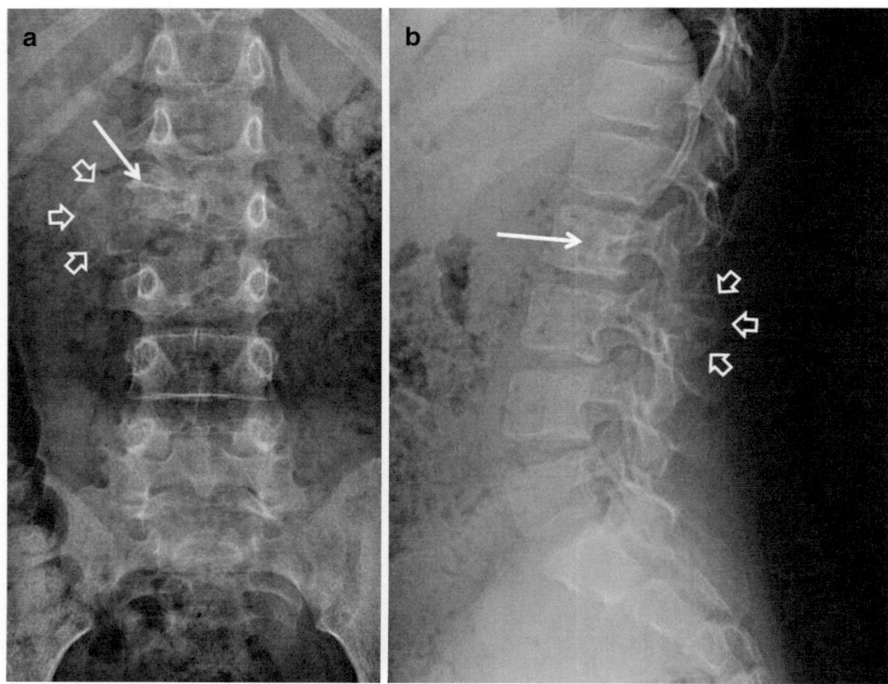

Fig. 22.2 (**a**, **b**) Magnified view of the lumbar spine PA and lateral standing radiographs. Upon closer inspection of the lumbar spine, there is obliteration of the left L2 pedicle (*solid arrow*) with evidence of an expansile mass centered in this area (*open arrows*). Additionally, there appears to be mild compression of the left portion of the L2 vertebral body compared to the right side. The lateral view shows the L2 vertebral body to have a mixed sclerotic/lytic lesion in the posterior half of the body (*solid arrow*), and a subtle overlying soft tissue mass extending into the posterior aspect of the spine with an expanded spinous process of L2 (*open arrows*)

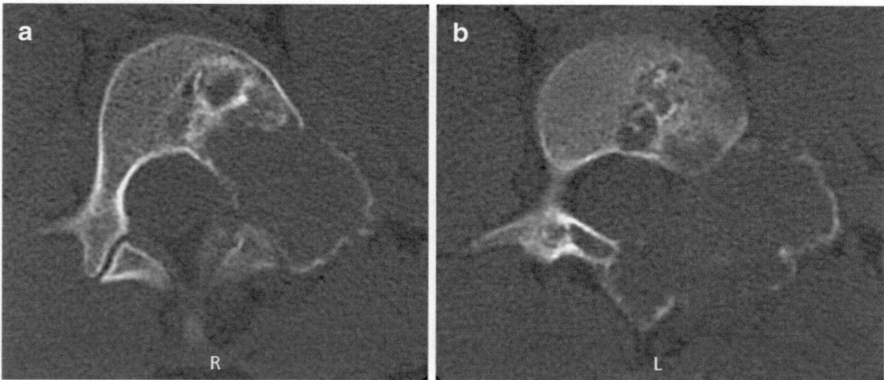

Fig. 22.3 (**a**, **b**) A CT was ordered to better define the lesion noted on pain radiographs. Axial CT demonstrates a lytic expansile lesion in the left posterior elements of L2 with extension down the left pedicle into the left side of the L2 vertebral body. The entire posterior structure of the L2 vertebrae (spinous process, lamina, facet joints) on the left side of this vertebral body is expanded and thinned by this bony process. The right-sided posterior elements are normal as are the surrounding vertebral bodies

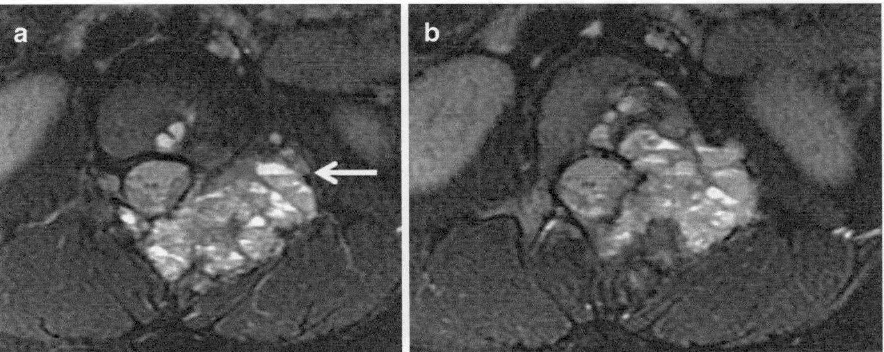

Fig. 22.4 (a, b). An MRI was ordered to assess the lesion in the L2 vertebral body. This MRI further demonstrates this expansile lesion in the posterior and anterior elements of L2 with distinct fluid-fluid levels within the lesion (*solid arrow*), a pathognomonic finding for an aneurysmal bone cyst

3. Why did the patient have limited spine flexion, a limp, and complain of night and left thigh pain?
4. How are the radiographs best interpreted?
5. What is the appropriate referral?
6. What is the next diagnostic test that should be considered?

Discussion

The radiographs demonstrate a relatively normally aligned spine, with a destructive lesion centered in the left side of the L2 vertebral body. Further imaging with the CT scan demonstrates this to be an expansile bony lesion in the posterior elements of L2 with extension into the pedicle and vertebral body. Given the extremely thinned cortex in the posterior elements, especially the facet joints and the mixed lytic lesion in the vertebral body, it is likely this lesion has led to some micro-instability of the spine at this level. As the facet joints in the posterior aspect of the spine experience a significant amount of bending force with motion, the extremely thinned cortex of the right-sided facets can lead to pain with activity as they are stressed beyond their compressive strength, resulting in micro-fractures in this area [1]. Given the expansile nature of the lesion and the thin body habitus of this child, it is not uncommon for these lesions to be palpable and visible as they grow. Forward flexion can accentuate the visibility of these masses.

As aneurysmal bone cysts enlarge in the vertebral column, these lesions are typically silent until they lead to a mass effect or instability of the spine. The instability initially is not frank structural instability but more of micro-instability, as the walls of the affected vertebral body become thinned. When this critical level of mass growth is reached, patients can have pain with motion [1–3]. In this case, while there were symptoms prior to the motor vehicle crash as discovered with the detailed history, she then had acute worsening of pain likely due to compression of the anterior vertebral body as a result of the accident. As can be appreciated on the imaging (Fig. 22.2a), there is mild height loss of the left side of the vertebral body compared to the right, indicating a compression fracture through the aneurysmal bone cyst from the collision.

Her symptoms are likely related to the mass affect from the expansile nature of this tumor and the micro-instability due to the thinning of the cortex of the vertebral body. The combination of the mobile nature of the spine (especially the lumbar spine) and the thinned cortical structures including the facet joints leads to some loss of structural integrity and thus pain with motion. In addition, the mass effect of the expanded vertebral elements causes pressure on the exiting nerve roots [4]. With this L2 vertebral lesion and the concomitant expansion of the L2 pedicle, the exiting nerve roots above and below this L2 pedicle are potential sources of compression. In this case, the pain in the anterior thigh is likely due to compression of the L2 nerve root. As is often the case, tumors can cause pain that is more significant at night. While it is unknown if there is a true physiologic reason for this, it is postulated the dull underlying pain caused by the tumor is more recognized at night as patients have fewer distractions from this pain.

Assessment of symmetry is important when interpreting radiographs of the spine in children. Alignment and the presence of bony landmarks in a normal cascade from superior to inferior is one standard method to approach the assessment of spine radiographs. With this in mind, as the radiographs in this case are reviewed, it is obvious there is a missing pedicle bony landmark on the left side at L2 (Fig. 22.1a). The pedicle is the bony channel that connects the posterior elements to the anterior elements of the spine. In this case, with growth of this aneurysmal bone cyst and expansion of this area of the vertebral column, the bony cortical boundaries of this pedicle are thinned and widened, leading to the apparent destruction of this landmark on the radiographs. This radiographic finding is sometimes called the "winking owl sign." In addition, when viewing the vertebral column from the lateral view, there should again be a normal cascade of the vertebral bodies, which should appear uniform. In this case, there is an obvious mixed sclerotic/lytic lesion in the vertebral body of L2 that is different from the surrounding normal vertebral bodies (Fig. 22.1b). Also evident, on close inspection, there is a bony mass extending into the posterior spine (corresponding to the "knot" described by the patient), which can be seen (Fig. 22.2b).

While back pain is common in adolescent, back pain associated with "red flags" in children requires further evaluation. In this case, back pain associated with radiating symptoms to the lower extremity, pain at night, and pain that limits children from normal activity is worrisome and should be more closely scrutinized [4]. In this case, given the concerns of a destructive lesion in the L2 vertebrae seen on radiographs associated with this back pain, referral to a pediatric spine specialist was done.

Further evaluation of this lesion in the L2 vertebrae is needed. The history and physical exam and basic radiographic assessment reveal the presence of this symptomatic expansile, mixed sclerotic/lytic lesion in the spine. More accurate characterization of the lesion can help narrow the differential diagnosis and suggest the next best course of action for treatment. In general, lesions that appear to be inherent bony lesions are best evaluated first with a CT scan. On the other hand, soft tissue lesions, lesions within the neural elements in the spinal canal, or those with significant neurologic symptoms are best evaluated with magnetic resonance imaging (MRI). In this case, there are elements of both bony involvement (expansile nature of this lesion and the vertebral body abnormality) and neurologic involvement (radiating pain in the anterior aspect of the left leg). Given this mixed picture, further evaluation of this lesion with both CT scan (Fig. 22.3) and MRI (Fig. 22.4) was appropriate [4, 5].

How to Approach the Case

This is an unusual case in that she presented with an acute exacerbation of back pain after a traumatic event. Back pain is common in children, and this complaint often is heard following minor accidents. The case illustrates the importance of a thorough history of the presenting complaints, a detailed physical exam, and careful inspection of spine radiographs. While back pain can result from being in a motor vehicle collision, the detailed history taken in this case revealed abnormal "red flags" that the patient was experiencing prior to the motor vehicle accident that had not yet been expressed to a physician [4]. A careful history and physical examination in children with back pain, focusing on "red flags" and the course of pain over time, even in the face of a traumatic event, can reveal abnormalities which require further evaluation.

Red Flags for This Case
- Pain at night
- Pain radiating into the extremities
- Child avoiding activities because of the pain
- Palpable mass – bone or soft tissue
- Painful scoliosis
- Radiographic destruction of bone such as missing pedicle or vertebral collapse
- Additional bone where it does not belong such as a sclerotic pedicle

> **Short Differential Diagnosis**
> - Infection – It may present as radiolucent spinal lesion associated with pain and fever/chills.
> - Osteoblastoma – Night pain, usually a lesion >2 cm in diameter. These typically are located in the posterior elements of the spine and are expansile lesions.
> - Leukemia/Lymphoma – This can present with diffuse pain and night pain. Typically seen as lytic lesions in the anterior vertebral body of the spine, usually without an associated soft tissue mass.
> - Ewing's sarcoma – Pain, radiographic vertebral body destruction with associated soft tissue mass.
> - Osteosarcoma – Pain, radiographic vertebral body destruction with neoplastic bone formation, associated soft tissue mass.

Final Diagnosis

Aneurysmal bone cyst of left L2

Natural History and Treatment Considerations

Aneurysmal bone cysts are benign lesions which can occur in the pediatric spine, typically arising from the posterior elements. They are described as cystic lesions of bone composed of blood filled spaces separated by connective tissue septa [1, 3, 6, 7]. While these are benign, they can be quite locally aggressive causing significant destruction of the encasing bone, leading to pathologic fractures and compromise of adjacent structures due to the rapid expansion of the bone. Typically, these are primary lesions, but can occur in association with other pathologic conditions [1, 6]. The usual course of these lesions is local growth and expansion and thinning of the bone from which they arise. This growth and bony destruction in the spine typically results in pain, deformity secondary to collapse of the bone, and in some cases neurologic deficits from the mass effect of the bony expansion or acute deformity. Given the local aggressiveness of these lesions and high likelihood of complications due to progressive structural compromise, surgical treatment is typically required [1, 2]. The vascular nature of these lesions often leads to large blood loss during surgical resection; thus preoperative selective arterial embolization of the lesion is recommended by some [1, 6]. The recommendations for surgical treatment vary, but recurrence rates are high (up to 30%) with incomplete resection of the lesion, so complete resection of the lesions is paramount [1–3, 6, 7] Intralesional curettage, burring of the lesion, electrocautery, and en-bloc resection are all recommended in

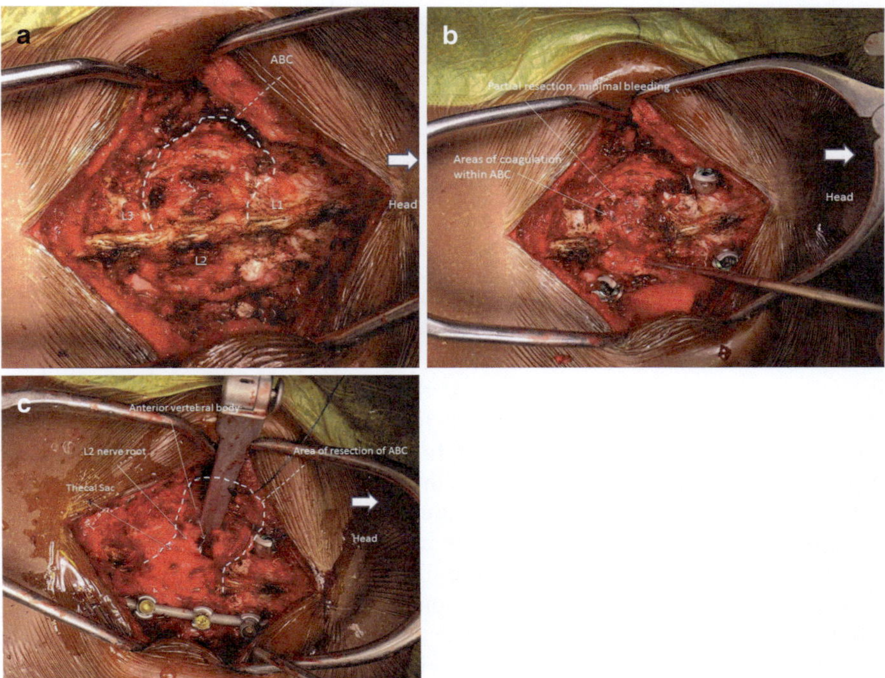

Fig. 22.5 (a) The appearance of left L2 posterior elements during surgery prior to resection. Note the expanded left-sided posterior elements at L2 (*outlined*). (b) Photo of partial resection of the posterior portion of the ABC. Note the areas of coagulation due to preoperative lesion embolization and blood filled caverns (*solid arrows*). (c) Photo of posterior spine post-resection of the ABC

the literature, alone or in combination. While the most reliable surgical approach has not been determined, complete obliteration of the lesion is required to prevent local recurrence. Given the underlying bony destruction, reconstruction of the spine and stabilization with implants are usually required after local resection (Fig. 22.5) [1, 2, 6, 7].

Referral – Emergency, Urgent, or Routine: And to Whom?

Back pain in a growing child is common and often does not need referral to a specialist. In cases like this one, when the back pain is associated with "red flags," more *urgent* referral to an orthopedic surgeon is needed. Pain at night is often a feature of a neoplastic process, and pain radiating to an extremity from the back is found in cases of mass effect irritating exiting spinal nerve roots. With acute changes in back pain after high energy trauma or cases with structural changes of the spine after trauma (such as this case with compression of the L2 vertebral body) or in cases demonstrating radiographic destruction of a vertebrae (obliteration of the L2 left pedicle), *emergent* referral to an orthopedic surgeon experienced in pediatric spine surgery is recommended given the evidence of an active process.

Brief Summary

Back pain in children is common and, although rare, can be associated with a number of pathologic processes. A detailed history of the back pain and careful physical exam can often reveal details that allow the physician to determine if the back pain is benign or possibly secondary to an underlying condition. While mild pain can be present for some time, it is not uncommon for children with back pain to present for the first time following a traumatic event. In these cases, it is especially important to determine the course of the back pain, as the history may reveal long-standing pain with an acute change after the trauma. Patients presenting with "red flag" signs and symptoms and those with acute changes in the back pain after a traumatic event require more urgent evaluation. Basic radiographic evaluation demonstrating changes in the vertebral body or destruction of the bony radiographic landmarks in the spine should lead to emergent further evaluation, as these issues often are caused by more aggressive processes associated with pathologic bone disease. Benign but locally aggressive bony spinal tumors, such as aneurysmal bone cysts, are uncommon in children and can lead to pain and eventually pathologic instability of the spine which are at risk for pathologic spine fractures with even minor trauma. As such, early detection of these lesions is imperative to avoid secondary spinal injury, and complete surgical resection is needed to avoid recurrence of the lesion.

Key Features and Pearls
- Local destruction of bony anatomy in the spine in association with back pain is abnormal and requires specific work-up or referral for complete evaluation.
- Bony lesions causing expansion of the bony cortex arising from the posterior elements of the spine are suspicious for aneurysmal bone cysts, which are very locally destructive and can lead to spinal deformity and neurologic compromise.
- Pediatric patients often present following trauma. A thorough history and physical is required to determine if back pain after trauma is due to the traumatic event, or if it was present prior to the event and due to an underlying pathologic process.

Editor Discussion

In teenagers, tumors of the spine are fairly uncommon and are generally benign except for Ewing sarcoma and osteosarcoma. A reasonable differential diagnosis can be developed for most spinal lesions on the basis of patient age, lesion location in the spine – body vs posterior elements – and radiologic appearance. Benign tumors with a predilection for the posterior elements include osteoid osteoma, osteoblastoma, osteochondroma, and ABC. Radiologic evaluation of a patient who presents with osseous vertebral lesions often includes plain films, computed tomography (CT), and magnetic resonance (MR) imaging. Because of the complex anatomy of the vertebrae, CT is often most useful for evaluating lesion location and analyzing bone destruction. Sometimes, the clinical presentation is so typical for a certain disorder that they allow the final diagnosis. For example, in a teenager, bone pain that occurs mainly at night and is promptly relieved with salicylates is highly suggestive of osteoid osteoma. In other cases, such as this case, spine trauma with resulting fracture reveals a spinal tumor – an ABC in this case. Although benign, ABC's are expansile, vascular, and destructive. In addition, every ABC should be biopsied because occasionally, lurking in the ABC is another more sinister tumor such as a telangiectatic osteosarcoma or a giant cell tumor. In general, the biopsy should be done by a pediatric spine specialist at the hospital where the child can also get a definitive cancer operation if needed.

W.L. Hennrikus

Aneurysmal bone cysts can affect any bone of the body, but have a propensity for the spine (15% occur in the spine, except the coccyx) and especially for the cervical spine. They have a peak incidence during the second decade. The key to diagnosing an aneurysmal bone cyst, which typically involve the posterior elements of the spine, is to meticulously evaluate each spinal level for absence of a pedicle on the AP radiograph, or surrounding expansion of bone in either view, as was seen in this patient. The presence of a sclerotic pedicle would suggest a bone-forming tumor such as osteoblastoma or osteosarcoma. If a benign lesion such as aneurysmal bone cyst is suspected, a CT scan is the next best test since it properly characterizes the lesion. When MRI is the initial advanced imaging study, the soft tissue involvement can inappropriately suggest a malignant tumor, an error that should be avoided for the sake of the patient. Although aneurysmal bone cysts are benign, they can be locally aggressive and recur unless they are completely resected. In unusual circumstances, an aneurysmal bone cyst represents a secondary reactive lesion and contains another underlying benign tumor such as chondroblastoma, non-ossifying fibroma, fibrous dysplasia, or osteoblastoma. In rare cases, a malignancy such as telangiectatic osteosarcoma is the underlying cause of the aneurysmal bone cyst. Thus, the tissue obtained during the surgical resection should be thoroughly examined by an experienced pathologist for malignancy. In this case, surgical resection and stabilization was appropriate. Because of the risk for recurrence, patients should be followed long term during their growing years.

R.M. Schwend

References

1. Zenonos G, Jamil O, Governale LS, Jernigan S, Hedequist D, Proctor MR. Surgical treatment for primary spinal aneurysmal bone cysts: experience from Children's Hospital Boston. J Neurosurg Pediatr. 2012 Mar;9(3):305–15.
2. Garg S, Mehta S, Dormans JP. Modern surgical treatment of primary aneurysmal bone cyst of the spine in children and adolescents. J Pediatr Orthop. 2005;25(3):387–92.

3. Sebaaly A, Ghostine B, Kreichati G, Mallet JF, Glorion C, Moussa R, Kharrat K, Ghanem I. Aneurysmal bone cyst of the cervical spine in children: a review and a focus on available treatment options. J Pediatr Orthop. 2015;35(7):693–702.
4. Garg S, Dormans JP. Tumors and tumor-like conditions of the spine in children. J Am Acad Orthop Surg. 2005;13(6):372–81.
5. Ropper AE, Cahill KS, Hanna JW, McCarthy EF, Gokaslan ZL, Chi JH. Primary vertebral tumors: a review of epidemiologic, histological, and imaging findings. Part I: benign tumors. Neurosurgery. 2011;69(6):1171–80.
6. Ozaki T, Halm H, Hillmann A, Blasius S, Winkelmann W. Aneurysmal bone cysts of the spine. Arch Orthop Trauma Surg. 1999;119(3–4):159–62.
7. Novais EN, Rose PS, Yaszemski MJ, Sim FH. Aneurysmal bone cyst of the cervical spine in children. J Bone Joint Surg Am. 2011;93(16):1534–43.

Chapter 23
A Girl with Lower Back Pain and Rapidly Progressive Atypical Scoliosis

Lorena V. Floccari and Kerwyn C. Jones

Brief Case Presentation

Chief Complaint

Low back pain

History

A 9-year-old girl presents with 9 months of nonspecific low back pain. She had no history of trauma or other inciting factors. The pain initially was mild and bothersome for several months and did not respond to a course of physical therapy with core strengthening and stretching. The pain slowly progressed and is now nearly constant in the midline and to the right side of her lower back.

Over the past 3–4 weeks, her pain has significantly worsened, becoming sharper and more severe in nature. She now awakens with pain, and daytime discomfort has caused her to miss several days of school. She requires daily nonsteroidal anti-inflammatory drugs (NSAIDs) to "take the edge off" of her pain, but they do not provide complete relief. Her parents have noticed that she stands with her trunk shifted toward the left, with a prominence on the left side of her mid-back. She denies any neurologic symptoms, including no change in her gait, strength, sensation, bowel, or bladder function.

Before the onset of this back pain, this child was healthy and active. She had normal development, with no chronic medical problems. Prior surgery included a

L. V. Floccari · K. C. Jones (✉)
Department of Orthopedic Surgery, Akron Children's Hospital, Akron, OH, USA
e-mail: kjones@akronchildrens.org

© Springer Nature Switzerland AG 2021
R. M. Schwend, W. L. Hennrikus (eds.), *Back Pain in the Young Child and Adolescent*, https://doi.org/10.1007/978-3-030-50758-9_23

tonsillectomy. She has no family history of scoliosis, spinal disorders, or other musculoskeletal conditions.

She is premenarchal, and a review of systems is negative for other complaints, including no lethargy, myalgias, polyuria, fevers, chills, rash, or weight loss/gain. She has had no recent travel outside of her home state.

Physical Examination

This 9-year-old girl appears healthy and size appropriate for her age. She is prepubertal and is normal intellectually and developmentally. Her gait is non-antalgic, but she has mild listing toward her left. The Adams forward bending test shows scoliosis with a left thoracic prominence. She has a left-sided trunk shift with waistline asymmetry, and her left shoulder is slightly higher than her right. She has tenderness to palpation on her right paraspinal musculature and along the midline of her lower lumber spine. There is limited forward flexion and cannot even touch her knees due to increased discomfort. Neurologic exam is negative for abnormalities, including normal sensation, motor function, reflexes, Babinski response, and no ankle clonus.

Imaging and Radiographic Studies (Figs. 23.1, 23.2, 23.3, and 23.4)

Questions About the Case the Reader Should Consider
1. What is the appropriate workup for progressive back pain with scoliosis?
2. What is the differential diagnosis of a bony lytic lesion with vertebral compression fracture (vertebra plana or wedged vertebra)?
3. What is the next diagnostic test that should be considered?
4. How is systemic involvement evaluated?
5. What is the appropriate referral?
6. What are possible treatments in this case?

Discussion

Back pain that is persistent for several months warrants AP and lateral spinal radiographs of the entire spine, taken in the upright position. In this case, the initial radiographs were interpreted as normal, so a course of physical therapy for core strengthening and stretching was appropriate. During this time, her back pain worsened to the point that she could not attend school, and she developed acutely progressive scoliosis. Scoliosis is not typically painful or acutely progressive; this signifies an atypical nature and requires repeat radiographs and advanced imaging such as MRI.

Vertebra plana ("flat vertebra") was previously thought to be pathognomonic for eosinophilic granuloma (EG) in children, but other causes now are recognized [1]. A careful history, physical exam, and review of systems should be conducted to evaluate for a malignancy, infection, or systemic disease process associated with the lytic lesion. Patients with a lytic lesion should have a complete blood count with a peripheral blood smear and inflammatory markers (C-reactive protein, erythrocyte sedimentation rate). After identification of a lytic lesion or vertebra plana/wedged vertebra on plain radiographs, the next step is advanced imaging with MRI to evaluate the extent of soft tissue involvement and marrow edema, as well as to rule out other conditions such as a sarcoma or other malignancies.

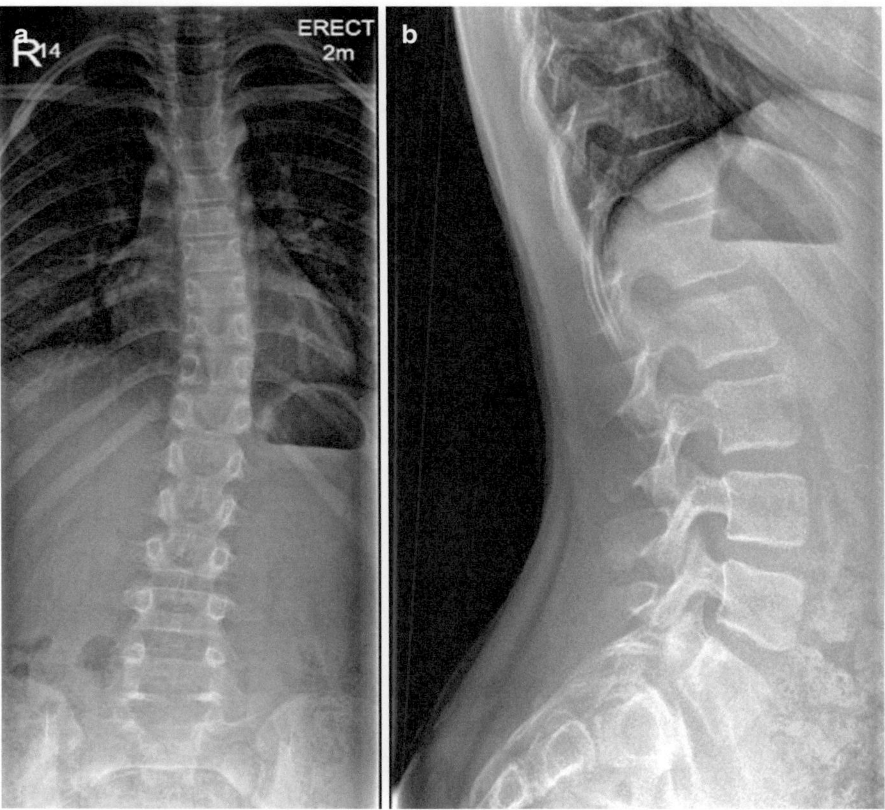

Fig. 23.1 Standing AP (**a**) and lateral (**b**) upright radiographs after this child initially presented with 8 months of low back pain. She had 6 lumbar segments with an L6 transitional vertebra at the lumbosacral junction and mild spine asymmetry. Otherwise, the radiographs were interpreted as normal. Repeat upright radiographs were obtained 1 month later, after her pain worsened in severity (**c–e**), revealing an L6 lytic lesion with vertebral body wedging and progressive scoliosis

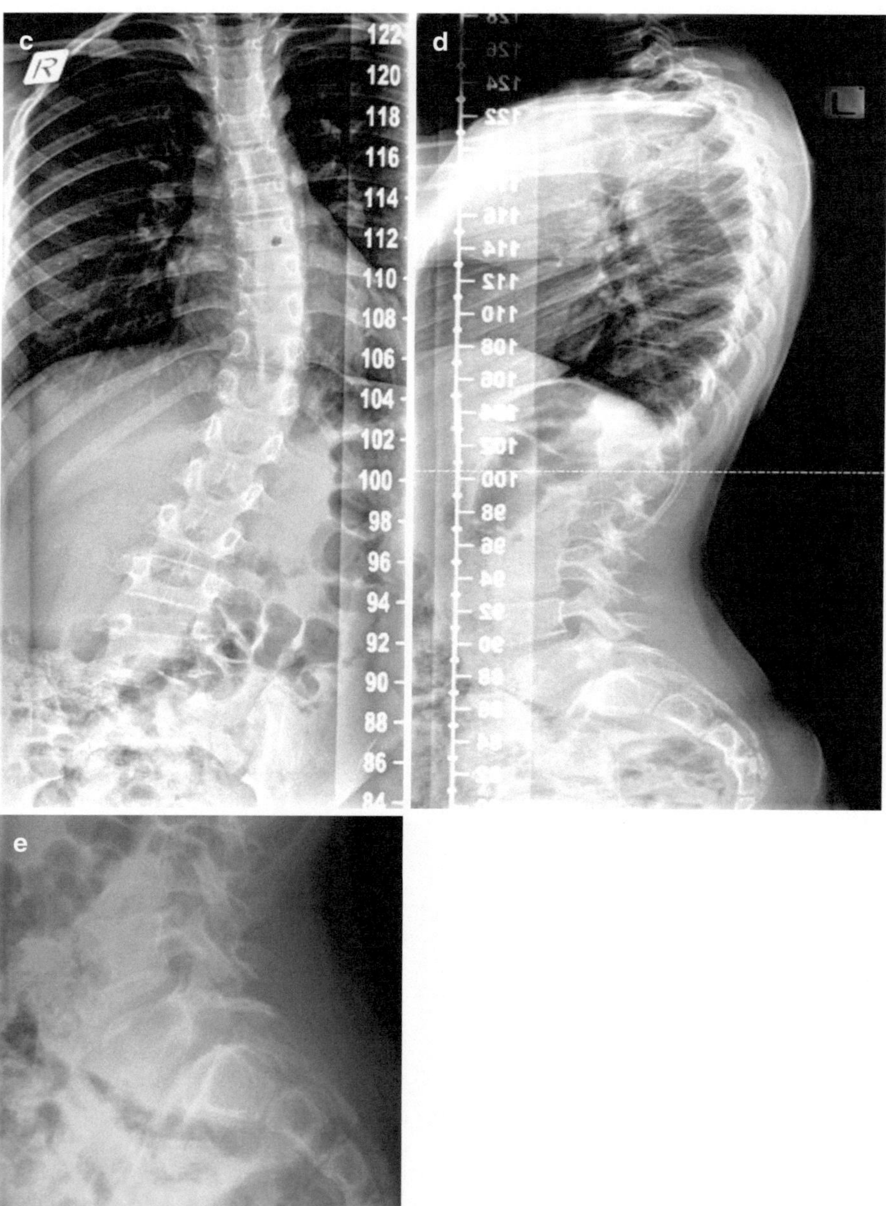

Fig. 23.1 (continued)

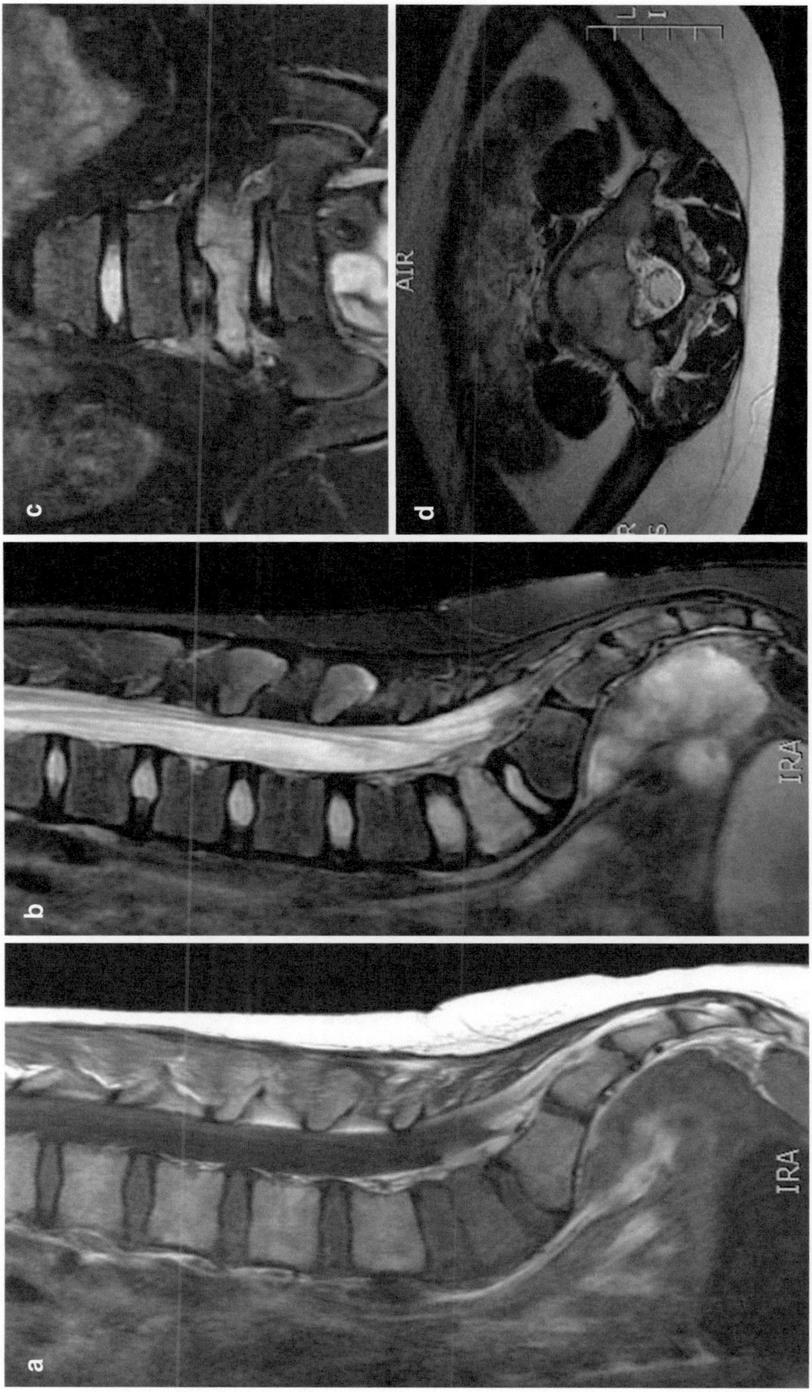

Fig. 23.2 Sagittal T1 (**a**), T2FS (**b**), coronal (**c**), and axial (**d**) slices of an MRI scan that reveals high T2 signal abnormality of the L6 vertebral body. There is associated compression fracture of the right side of the L6 vertebra with 40% height loss. The discs appear normal. There is only mild paravertebral edema and no paravertebral soft tissue mass. The spinal canal is widely patent

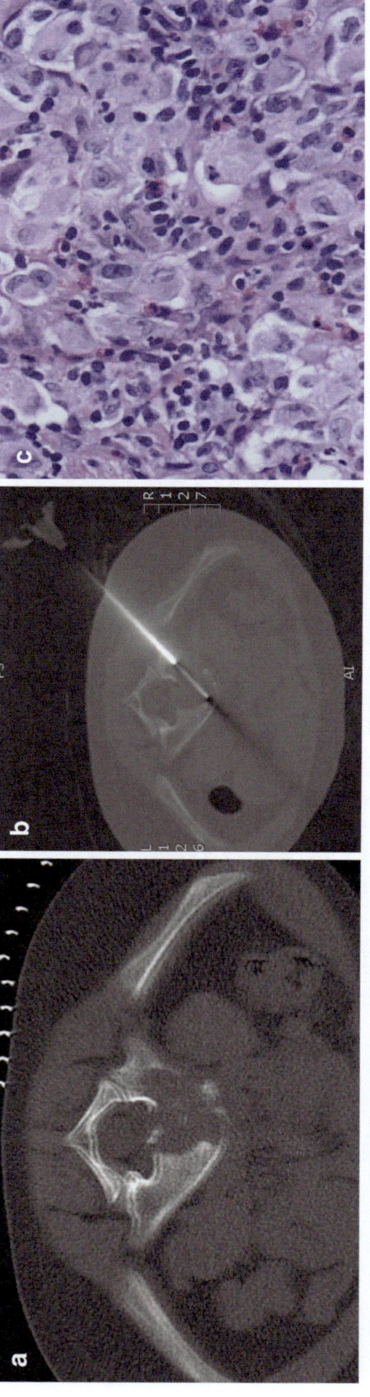

Fig. 23.3 CT-guided fine-needle aspiration and core needle biopsy (**a**, **b**) were obtained, including blood, sclerotic bone fragments, and inflamed fibrous tissue. Histologic evaluation revealed histocytic cells with nuclear grooving and associated inflammatory cell infiltrate rich in eosinophils. The appearance was consistent with Langerhans cell histiocytosis (**c**)

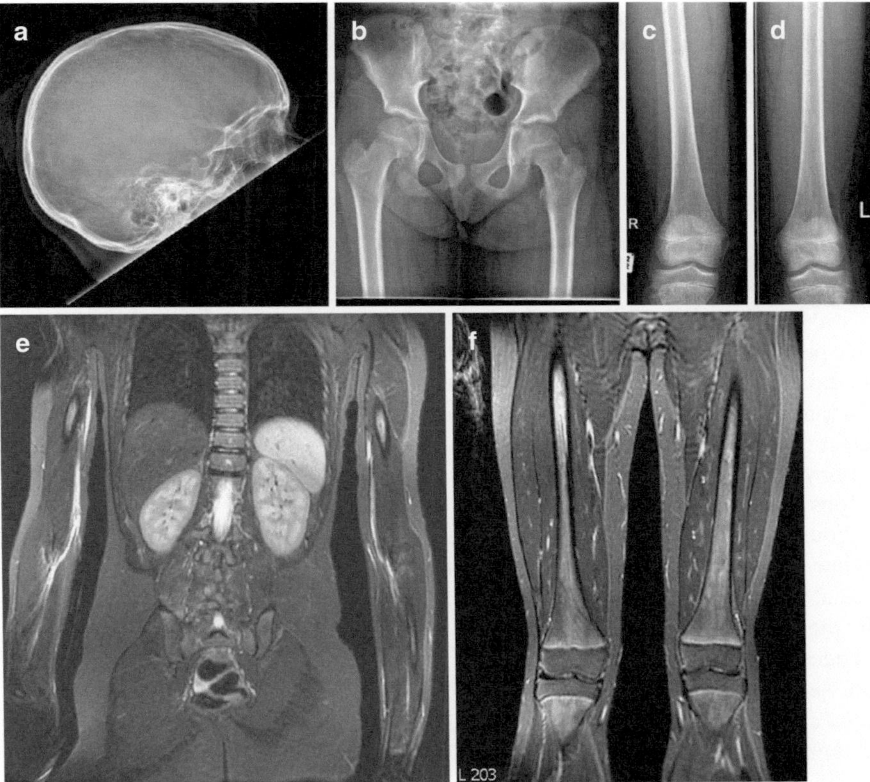

Fig. 23.4 Screening for other lesions with a skeletal survey (**a–d**) and whole-body MRI (**e, f**) were negative for associated bony or visceral involvement

Differential Diagnosis of Vertebra Plana
- Eosinophilic granuloma
- Osteomyelitis
- Tuberculosis
- Osteogenesis imperfecta
- Ewing's sarcoma
- Leukemia
- Lymphoma
- Metastatic neuroblastoma
- Gaucher's disease
- Spondylometaphyseal dysplasia
- Aneurysmal bone cyst

Children with a wedged or flattened vertebra should be referred to a pediatric orthopedic surgeon with experience caring for the spine. The imaging and clinical findings are not specific enough for diagnosis of EG, so tissue biopsy is recommended in most cases of suspected EG [2]. CT-guided percutaneous needle biopsy has >90% diagnostic accuracy and is the recommended first-line diagnostic approach [3]. Histology reveals a mixture of eosinophils and Langerhans cells, which are large, mononuclear cells with racket-shaped organelles (Birbeck granules) in the cell cytoplasm (Fig. 23.3c) [4].

After histologic diagnosis of EG, additional imaging should be performed to rule out associated bony and/or systemic disease. A skeletal survey should be performed to evaluate for additional bony lesions (Fig. 23.4a–d), as up to 40% of patients will have polyostotic disease [1, 5]. Bone scan has also been used to detect other lesions, but this inconsistently demonstrates EG, with 10–20% false-negative rate [5]. Alternatively, whole-body MRI scan (Fig. 23.4e, f) is being increasingly used to detect other foci of disease, as was performed in this case. CT can show the extent of bony involvement, but this typically is reserved for preoperative planning of bone lesions that require surgical intervention.

Young children with EG should have an abdominal ultrasound [6] and careful review of systems to guide other workup, after evaluating for pain, polyuria, polydipsia, respiratory symptoms, irritability, diarrhea, loss of appetite, fever, rashes, otorrhea, growth failure, poor weight gain, and behavioral and neurological changes [6]. While laboratory workup is often completely normal for EG, erythrocyte sedimentation rate can be slightly elevated [5, 7]. Complete blood count, blood chemistry, coagulation studies, and liver function studies should be obtained. Serum and urine osmolality also can be evaluated if the history suggests diabetes insipidus, which is the most common extraskeletal abnormality in patients with bone involvement and is a classic feature of Hand-Schuller-Christian disseminated disease [6].

The natural history of a solitary EG bony lesion is spontaneous resolution, regardless of whether the lesion is treated [1, 5, 8–10]. Therefore, treatment is limited to lesions that cause severe pain or neurologic deficit. In this case, the patient had incomplete response to NSAIDs, so she was prescribed a 4-week course of corticosteroids that provided near-complete pain relief. She also was placed into a custom-molded spinal orthosis that corrected her scoliosis and was positioned in slight hyperextension to prevent further vertebral collapse through the involved vertebral body. Repeat radiographs 9 months after diagnosis (Fig. 23.5) showed resolution of her scoliosis, while repeat MRI (Figs. 23.5 and 23.6) showed resolution of the bony edema and partial reconstitution of vertebral height, which is expected to continue reconstituting with time and growth.

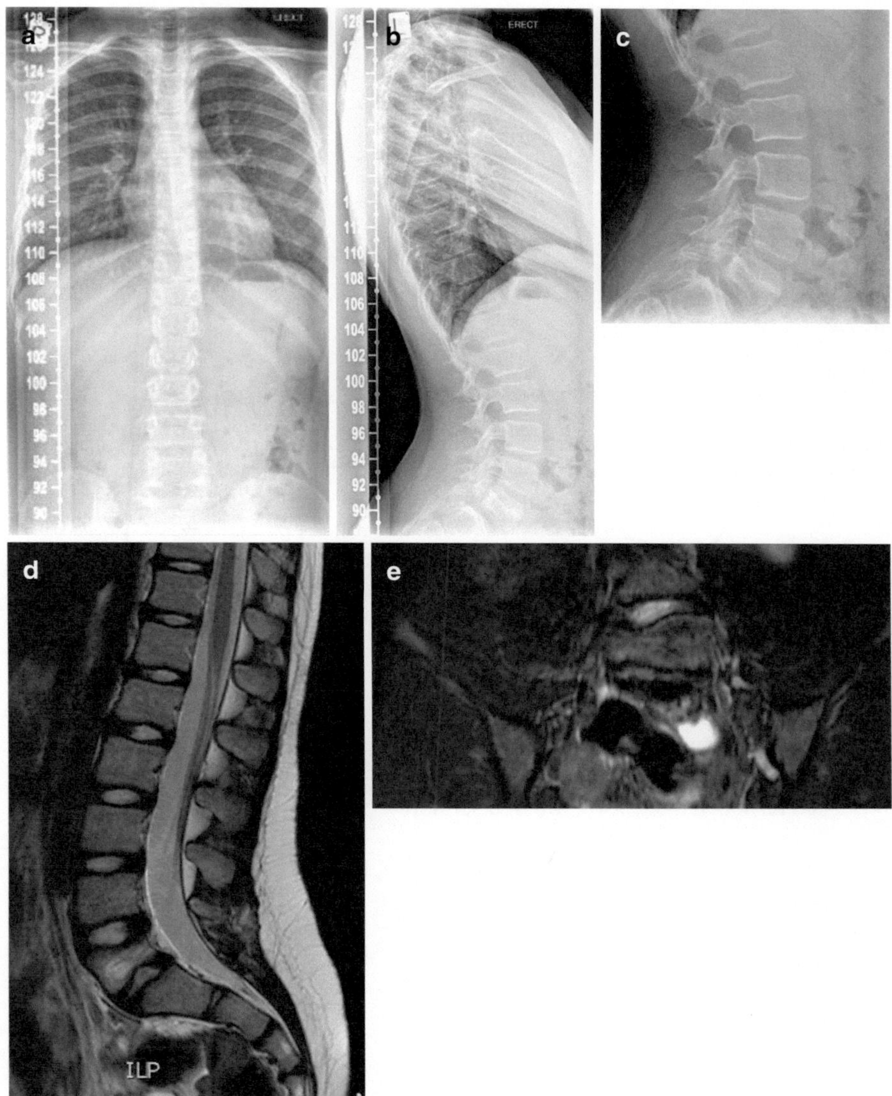

Fig. 23.5 Upright radiographs (**a–c**) and MRI (**d, e**) obtained 9 months after diagnosis reveal progressive healing of the lesion with gradual, partial reconstitution of vertebral height

How to Approach the Case

Always be suspicious of back pain in young children that persists despite conservative treatment, or is severe enough to limit school attendance or other activities. Loss of spine range of motion with inability to touch the knees is also an abnormal

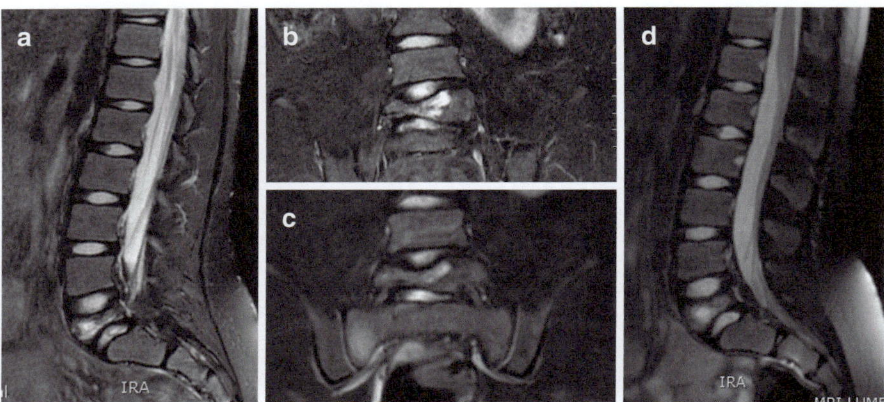

Fig. 23.6 Sequential MRIs obtained 2 months (**a**, **b**) and 4 months (**c**, **d**) after diagnosis, revealing gradual resolution of the bony edema without progression of the lesion nor with any further loss of vertebral height

finding. Be alert for painful or acutely progressive scoliosis, which is a marker of an atypical scoliosis. While a wedged vertebra or vertebra plana suggests the diagnosis, tissue biopsy is necessary for definitive diagnosis.

Red Flags for Eosinophilic Granuloma
- Back and/or neck pain, often <10 years old
- Decreased activity level, missed school
- Night pain
- Spine stiffness
- Acute torticollis
- Acute onset of scoliosis
- Atypical (left) scoliosis curves
- Neurologic symptoms or signs
- Vertebra plana or wedged vertebra

Referral – Emergency, Urgent, or Routine: And to Whom?

Consultation with a pediatric spine specialist is necessary; if there are neurologic findings, such as weakness or bowel or bladder dysfunction, referral should be urgent. CT-guided needle biopsy is typically performed by interventional radiology. For a confirmed diagnosis, patients should be referred to hematology-oncology.

Final Diagnosis

Eosinophilic granuloma involving L6 vertebral body

Natural History and Treatment Considerations

Eosinophilic granuloma (EG) refers to a bone lesion within the spectrum of conditions known as Langerhans cell histiocytosis (LCH), previously termed histiocytosis X. These conditions are characterized by proliferation of Langerhans cells, which are bone marrow-derived antigen-presenting cells in the dendritic cell family [4]. LCH disorders are highly variable, ranging from solitary, self-resolving bone lesions (eosinophilic granuloma) to life-threatening, disseminated disease (Letterer-Siwe, Hand-Schuller-Christian diseases).

LCH can manifest at any age, but occurs most frequently in pediatric and adolescent patients [1]. While the pathogenesis previously was debated, the World Health Organization now defines LCH and EG as a neoplasm, with clonal proliferation of Langerhans cells [11, 12]. Hematology-oncology consult is recommended for patients with Langerhans cell histiocytosis (LCH) . While involvement of nearly every organ system has been described, bone is the most commonly involved in 80% of cases. EG typically refers to a solitary bone lesion, but 10–15% of patients have polyostotic involvement. The skull is the most common site, followed by the spine, femur, pelvis, ribs, mandible, and other long bones [4, 5].

LCH also includes disseminated forms of the disease [4, 5]. Letterer-Siwe disease is an acute disseminated type found in children less than 2 years old. Severe, diffuse multisystem involvement can include hepatosplenomegaly, lymphadenopathy, anemia, polyostotic lesions, and bone marrow failure with a poor prognosis and high incidence of mortality. Hand-Schuller-Christian disease is the chronic disseminated type, diagnosed in children less than 5 years. The classic Hand-Schuller-Christian triad is diabetes insipidus, exophthalmos, and polyostotic lesions.

Back and/or neck pain is the most common presentation of a vertebral EG, often acute or subacute with pain duration <6 months [1, 2, 5, 9]. Pain can be mild and dull or severe and sharp in nature. On examination, patients frequently have localized midline tenderness to palpation with loss of spinal range of motion. Acute torticollis can develop from cervical lesions, while thoracic and/or lumbar lesions can cause acute onset of painful scoliosis and/or kyphosis. Neurologic signs are infrequent but have been previously reported [2].

The radiographic appearance of a lesion is highly variable, which is why LCH is often referred to as "the great imitator" and requires tissue biopsy for diagnosis [1]. Plain radiographs of the spine can initially be interpreted as negative for any abnormality early in the disease process, such as in this case (Fig. 23.1a, b). The first evidence is often a destructive lytic lesion, initially appearing aggressive with a moth-eaten appearance. Later in the process, it typically appears more sclerotic and well-defined, with variable amount of focal destruction and collapse. A wedged vertebra from partial collapse of the vertebral body is the most common manifestation of vertebral EG, while complete collapse causing the classic vertebra plana is actually seldom observed [1]. A characteristic feature is preservation of the disc spaces, which can distinguish EG from osteomyelitis.

The natural history of a solitary EG bone lesion is spontaneous healing with at least partial vertebral height restitution. Most lesions show partial or complete healing within 4 months, while nearly all lesions heal within 2 years [2, 5–10, 13]. The apophyses are spared, so the vertebrae gradually reconstitute a variable degree of vertebral height, typically 50–80%, over several years [7, 10, 13]. Therefore, the treatment of skeletal LCH is generally conservative and focuses on pain control, unless there is spinal instability or neurologic deficit. Pain management often begins with NSAID medication. Short-term immobilization in a hyperextension brace can relieve symptoms and potentially prevent vertebral collapse while awaiting healing [7]. Intralesional corticosteroid injection after histologic diagnosis has been shown to effectively relieve pain [3, 14], while a short course of oral steroids can also provide relief for uncontrolled pain.

Surgical decompression and stabilization is required for patients with neurologic deficit from spinal cord or nerve root compression. Curettage of the lesion is an option for patients with debilitating pain who do not respond to conservative treatment. Low-dose radiotherapy has also been used successfully for refractory pain, but the risk of secondary malignancy outweighs the benefit of radiation for solitary bone lesions. Chemotherapy can be used in disseminated disease, but is not typically recommended for a solitary EG [5].

Patients with a solitary EG without extraosseous LCH have an excellent prognosis, regardless of treatment [1, 2, 5, 7, 9]. While patients should be carefully followed for healing and reconstitution of the vertebral body, the recurrence rate is low, and long-term spine and neck problems from vertebral EG are uncommon.

Brief Summary

Eosinophilic granuloma is nonspecific and variable in clinical presentation and radiographic appearance. Patients with vertebral EG typically present with acute or subacute back or neck pain, but also can develop torticollis, kyphosis, and/or scoliosis. The most classic radiographic feature of vertebral EG is vertebra plana or a wedged vertebra due to compression fracture through a vertebral body lytic lesion. However, since the appearance is highly variable, LCH is often referred to as "the great imitator" and requires tissue biopsy for definitive diagnosis, typically with CT-guided needle biopsy. Other conditions can cause vertebra plana, which is not pathognomonic for EG. Systemic involvement of disseminated Langerhans cell histiocytosis must be ruled out with a careful history, physical exam, review of systems, imaging, and referral to hematology-oncology, especially in young children ≤5 years of age with multifocal bony disease. The natural history of a solitary EG is spontaneous resolution, so children are typically managed symptomatically with nonsteroidal anti-inflammatory medications, spinal orthoses, steroids, and/or CT-guided corticosteroid injections. The long-term prognosis is excellent with low recurrence rate.

> **Key Features and Pearls**
> - Eosinophilic granuloma can present in young patients with acute back pain, torticollis, kyphosis, and/or atypical scoliosis.
> - Radiographic findings of wedged vertebra or vertebra plana.
> - Tissue biopsy is required.
> - The natural history of solitary EG is spontaneous resolution with excellent prognosis; treatment is typically symptomatic.

Editor Discussion

Several features in this case are of concern. The character of the pain is atypical: night pain, pain so bad that the child misses school, acute worsening of the painful scoliosis, stiffness, and change in shape of a vertebra that suggests a fracture or collapsing lesion. Typical scoliosis has a convexity to the right, which in this case is to the left. Back pain and scoliosis are more typical after age 10 years or the onset of puberty. Her young age, prepuberty, rapidly progressive left apex scoliosis, and character of the pain are atypical and raise many red flags that there is a serious problem. The history, physical examination, and plain radiographs, although not giving the specific diagnosis, were sufficient to indicate the need for urgent referral to a pediatric spine specialist, who can then obtain the advanced imaging and biopsy.
  R.M. Schwend

Eosinophilic granuloma is a benign osseous tumor. Ten percent of lesions occur in the spine and affect the vertebral body. EG can cause back pain and scoliosis. Replacement of the vertebral body by tumor causes collapse into vertebral plana. The natural history of the majority of solitary EG lesions of the spine is spontaneous regression with reconstitution of the vertebral height. Management is supportive including bracing. There is no consensus on the need for chemotherapy. Radiation therapy is not recommended.
  W.L. Hennrikus

References

1. Arkader A, Glotzbecker M, Hosalkar HS, Dormans JP. Primary musculoskeletal Langerhans cell histiocytosis in children: an analysis for a 3-decade period. J Pediatr Orthop. 2009;29(2):201–7.
2. Ghanem I, Tolo VT, D'Ambra P, Malogalowkin MH. Langerhans cell histiocytosis of bone in children and adolescents. J Pediatr Orthop. 2003;23(1):124–30.
3. Yasko AW, Fanning CV, Ayala AG, Carrasco CH, Murray JA. Percutaneous techniques for the diagnosis and treatment of localized Langerhans-cell histiocytosis (eosinophilic granuloma of bone). J Bone Joint Surg Am. 1998;80(2):219–28.

4. Lieberman PH, Jones CR, Steinman RM, Erlandson RA, Smith J, Gee T, et al. Langerhans cell (eosinophilic) granulomatosis. A clinicopathologic study encompassing 50 years. Am J Surg Pathol. 1996;20(5):519–52.
5. Bollini G, Jouve JL, Gentet JC, Jacquemier M, Bouyala JM. Bone lesions in histiocytosis X. J Pediatr Orthop. 1991;11(4):469–77.
6. Haupt R, Minkov M, Astigarraga I, Schäfer E, Nanduri V, Jubran R, et al. Euro Histio Network. Langerhans cell histiocytosis (LCH): guidelines for diagnosis, clinical work-up, and treatment for patients till the age of 18 years. Pediatr Blood Cancer. 2013;60(2):175–84.
7. Robert H, Dubousset J, Miladi L. Histiocytosis X in the juvenile spine. Spine (Phila Pa 1976). 1987;12(2):167–72.
8. Womer RB, Raney RB Jr, D'Angio GJ. Healing rates of treated and untreated bone lesions in histiocytosis X. Pediatrics. 1985;76(2):286–8.
9. Levine SE, Dormans JP, Meyer JS, Corcoran TA. Langerhans' cell histiocytosis of the spine in children. Clin Orthop Relat Res. 1996;(323):288–93.
10. Nesbit ME, Kieffer S, D'Angio GJ. Reconstitution of vertebral height in histiocytosis X: a long-term follow-up. J Bone Joint Surg Am. 1969;51(7):1360–8.
11. Thacker NH, Abla O. Pediatric Langerhans cell histiocytosis: state of the science and future directions. Clin Adv Hematol Oncol. 2019;17(2):122–31. Review.
12. Badalian-Very G, Vergilio JA, Degar BA, MacConaill LE, Brandner B, Calicchio ML, Kuo FC, et al. Recurrent BRAF mutations in Langerhans cell histiocytosis. Blood. 2010;116(11):1919–23.
13. Alexander JE, Seibert JJ, Berry DH, Glasier CM, Williamson SL, Murphy J. Prognostic factors for healing of bone lesions in histiocytosis X. Pediatr Radiol. 1988;18(4):326–32.
14. Rimondi E, Mavrogenis AF, Rossi G, Ussia G, Angelini A, Ruggieri P. CT-guided corticosteroid injection for solitary eosinophilic granuloma of the spine. Skelet Radiol. 2011;40(6):757–64.

Chapter 24
A Hockey Player with Persistent Low Back Pain and Hamstring Inflexibility: Enthesitis-Related JIA

Melanie Kennedy and Kelsey Logan

Brief Case Presentation

Chief Complaint

Low back pain for 4 months after a noncontact injury during a game

History

A 17-year-old male hockey goalie presents with low back for 4 months that is worsening, despite over 3 months of physical therapy. He complains of pain that alternates between the left and right posterior gluteal muscles, sacroiliac joint pain, quadriceps and calf achiness, and occasional shooting pain down his left thigh to his posterior knee. Additionally, he developed pain that wakes him at night, morning stiffness of 1–2 hours, and 1–2 kg of unintentional weight loss. There has been no significant improvement since initial injury.

M. Kennedy
Division of Sports Medicine, Cincinnati Children's Hospital Medical Center, Cincinnati, OH, USA

Department of Pediatrics, University of Cincinnati College of Medicine, Cincinnati, OH, USA

K. Logan (✉)
Division of Sports Medicine, Cincinnati Children's Hospital Medical Center, Cincinnati, OH, USA

Departments of Pediatrics and Internal Medicine, University of Cincinnati College of Medicine, Cincinnati, OH, USA
e-mail: Kelsey.logan@cchmc.org

© Springer Nature Switzerland AG 2021
R. M. Schwend, W. L. Hennrikus (eds.), *Back Pain in the Young Child and Adolescent*, https://doi.org/10.1007/978-3-030-50758-9_24

His pain began after falling on his left side trying to make a save in hockey. Originally, he had pain in the left low back, with left-sided radiculopathy. He was unable to continue participation after the injury occurred. Lumbar spine radiographs obtained after this acute injury were normal. He then completed 8 weeks of physical therapy to address poor hamstring flexibility and weak core strength, with minimal improvement. He attempted to return to hockey, but this worsened his pain. At follow-up visits, he was noted to have bilateral ischial tuberosity pain and inflexibility of bilateral hamstrings. At 8 weeks after injury, pelvic radiographs were normal. He wanted to continue to try to return to sport and elected to continue with physical therapy, transitioning to functional rehabilitation with an athletic trainer. After an additional progression with functional rehabilitation, he began to have worsening low back and returned for reevaluation.

At this visit, 4 months after initial presentation, he recalled back pain, noting intermittent bilateral low back pain over the past several years, without injury or other acute cause known. These episodes were much less severe. Furthermore, he reports nocturnal pain and weight loss.

His past medical history is significant for mild intermittent asthma, allergic rhinitis, sacral dimple at birth, and patellar tendonitis.

Physical Examination

Weight: 58 kg; height: 167.7 cm; BMI: 21. He was developmentally normal and well appearing.

Back exam: Overall posture was normal and well balanced. There was tenderness to palpation over both posterior iliac crests and bilateral sacroiliac joints. ROM: limited lumbar flexion and extension of lumbar spine due to pain, pain with flexion, left and right rotation, and poor flexibility of bilateral hamstrings. Strength: 5/5 in lower extremities and symmetric. Neurologic exam: sensation intact and symmetric in all dermatomes, 2+ patellar and Achilles reflex and Babinski reflex were normal. Special tests: FABER positive bilaterally, negative straight leg test, negative slump test, and no clonus.

Imaging Studies (Figs. 24.1, 24.2, 24.3, 24.4, and 24.5)

Laboratory Studies

CBC, ESR, and CRP are all within normal limits.

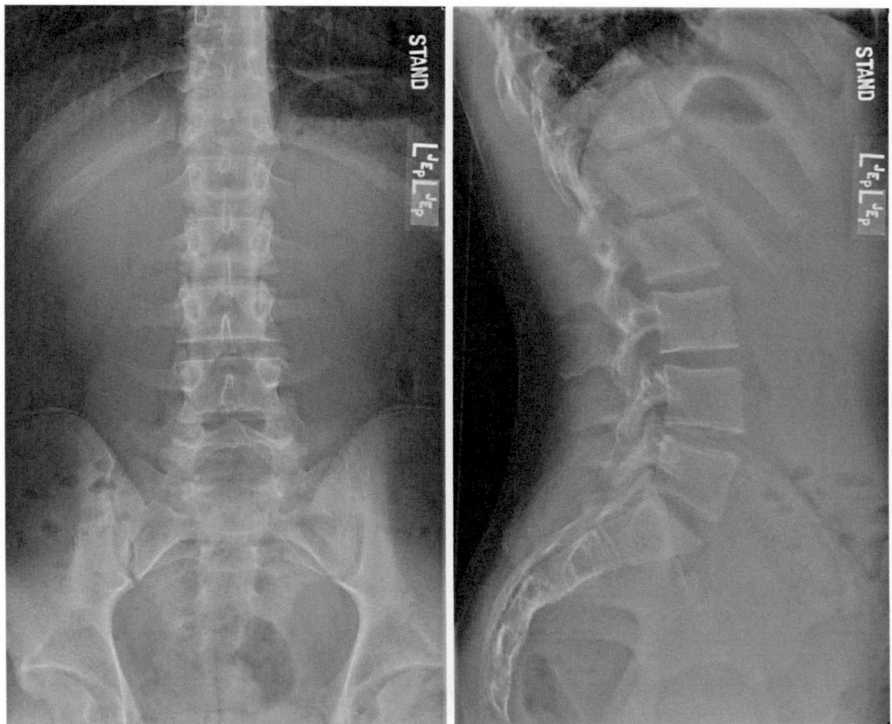

Fig. 24.1 Initial, normal lumbar radiographs with no fracture, spondylolysis, or spondylolisthesis

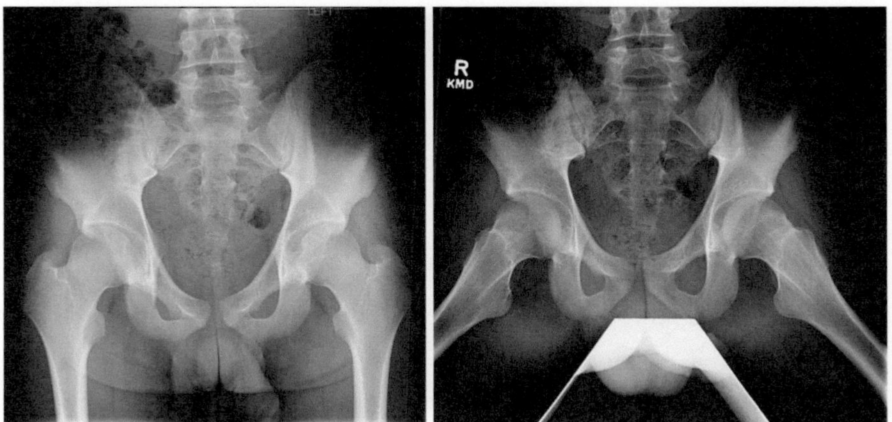

Fig. 24.2 Pelvic radiographs obtained 8 weeks into presentation. Normal with no bony abnormalities

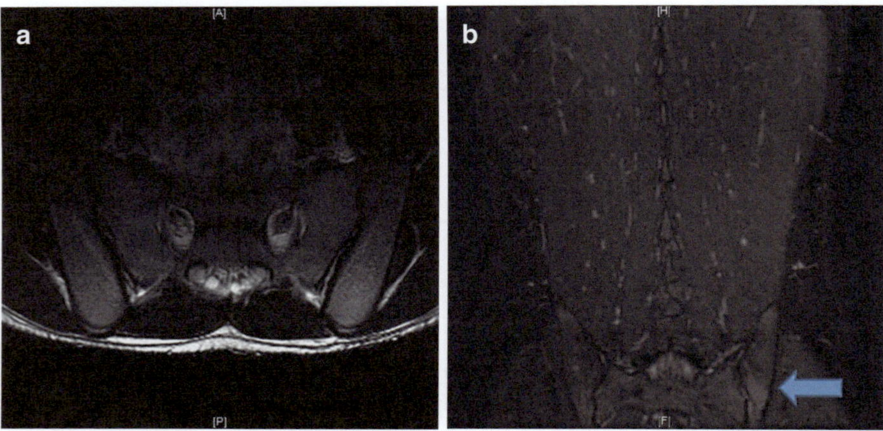

Fig. 24.3 (**a**) The consulting sports medicine physician ordered an MRI of his lumbar spine, including bilateral sacroiliac (SI) joints. It was read as normal, with no evidence of sclerosis or SI edema. (**b**) On subsequent review of the original MRI, one view did demonstrate mild SI joint edema (*arrow*)

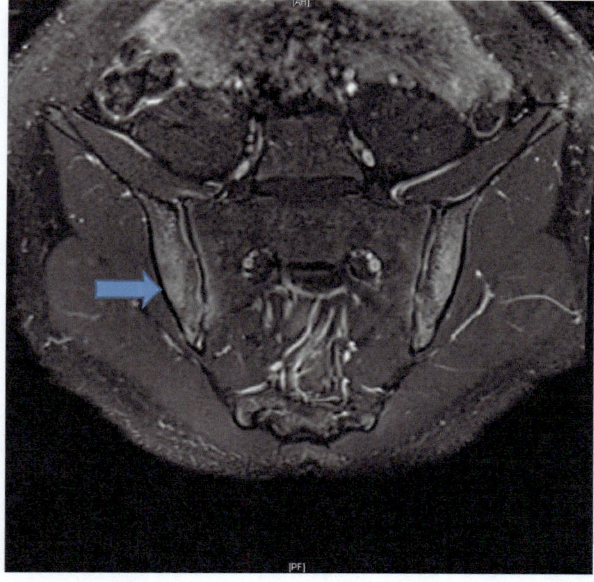

Fig. 24.4 MRI SI joint without contrast ordered by sports medicine physician: Note increased signal intensity in the left and right SI joints and edema in surrounding bone, more in ilia compared to sacrum (*arrow*)

Questions About the Case the Reader Should Consider

1. What clues in the history suggest that the back pain is more than muscular or mechanical low back pain?
2. What is enthesitis and how can it be diagnosed?
3. Why were the lumbar and pelvic radiographs and lab work normal?

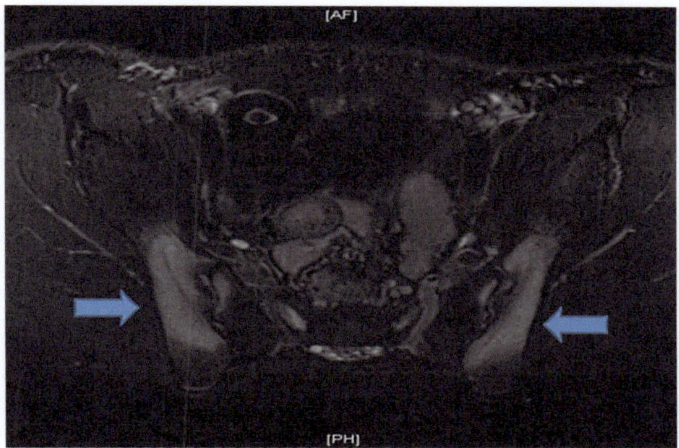

Fig. 24.5 MRI SI joints with contrast, with increased signal, amplified with contrast material, in bilateral ilia (*arrows*)

4. What are the next steps regarding diagnosis and management?
5. Is there additional diagnostic testing or imaging to consider?
6. What are the return-to-play recommendations for this athlete?

Discussion

This patient initially presents after an acute injury with no prior reports of pain, which lessens concern for underlying chronic condition. However, as his case progresses, there are key complaints that prompt need for additional evaluation. The patient developed worsening symptoms during treatment, which should encourage the physician to complete a new assessment and revisit the differential diagnosis. Additionally, the patient developed nocturnal pain and morning stiffness, which should cue evaluation with laboratory work and additional imaging. Lastly, decreased spinal motion despite significant physical therapy, combined with his weight loss and pain in other joints, raise suspicion for an underlying systemic process.

Additional history taking reveals that this patient has struggled with low back pain intermittently over the past few years. While this may be caused by biomechanical issues (weakness, abnormal sport motion mechanics), the pain should fully abate once those abnormalities are corrected. His lack of response to prolonged physical therapy is concerning, and the differential diagnosis needs to be widened.

One symptom he demonstrates on examination is enthesitis. An enthesitis is inflammation where a tendon or ligament inserts on bone in a patient with arthritis [1]. Common locations for enthesitis are in the lower extremities, such as the hip extensors at the greater trochanter, the patellar tendon on the patella, and the plantar fascia and Achilles tendon on the heel [2].

An enthesitis can be difficult to diagnose on physical exam, and additional imaging such as MRI or ultrasound is sometimes needed [3]. One study suggests that ultrasound with a skilled technician is better at diagnosing enthesitis [3]. A review of this patient's history relevant to inflammatory back pain noted several positive responses seen in patients younger than age 45 who have had back pain for at least 3 months [4]. Specificity for inflammatory back pain increases with each positive response:

- Morning stiffness of >30 minutes
- No improvement in back pain with rest
- Awakening because of back pain during the second half of the night
- Alternating buttock pain

Diagnosis of spondyloarthropathy, specifically enthesitis-related arthritics (ERA) with sacroiliitis, may be difficult as lab work and imaging can be equivocal. However, HLA-B27 testing is most often positive [5]. HLA-B27 is positive in 90% of patients with ankylosing spondylitis but only in 50% of patients with ERA [2, 6]. ESR and CRP may be normal or elevated; ANA and RF are negative [2]. Patients may or may not have anemia [7]. Plain radiographs are not good at detecting synovitis or early erosive changes in the sacroiliac joints of these patients [5]. If sacroiliitis is present on radiographs, ERA is more difficult to treat and is associated with a poorer prognosis [2]. MRI may detect inflammatory changes earlier in the disease course, but the changes may be subtle and overlooked, as evident in this case [6]. Contrast MRI is superior to noncontrast in detection of sacroiliitis [8].

The classification for enthesitis-related arthritis is shown below. Initial treatment for ERA is NSAIDs, typically naproxen, ibuprofen, meloxicam, or indomethacin [2]. When synovitis is present for more than 2 months, additional treatment should be considered. If there is true joint involvement in JIA, some patients respond to intra-articular corticosteroid injections for rapid reduction of inflammation [5]. Methotrexate, a folic acid analog, is often added for its ability to achieve disease control with low toxicity, but it has less effect on axial symptoms. When sacroiliitis is seen, especially on plain radiographs, additional biologic medication like antitumor necrosis factor (Anti-TNF) medications is added to the treatment regimen. Anti-TNF medication may not stop progression of spinal involvement but does help provide symptomatic relief [2].

Classification Criteria for Enthesitis-Related Arthritis [7]
- Arthritis and enthesitis, or arthritis, or enthesitis, with at least two of the following:

    - Presence/history of sacroiliac joint tenderness and/or lumbosacral pain
    - Presence of HLA-B27 antigen
    - Onset of arthritis in a male >6 years old
    - Acute anterior uveitis
    - History of one of the following in a first-degree relative: ankylosing spondylitis, enthesitis-related arthritis, sacroiliitis with inflammatory bowel disease, Reiter's syndrome, or acute anterior uveitis

Exercise and activity are important for patients with arthritis and should be a part of the treatment plan [9]. Participation in some sports is encouraged as long as patients have control/remission of the disease, full range of motion of the joint, full strength, and appropriate endurance [9]. Use caution with children with neck arthritis and contact sports, and evaluate for cervical instability radiographically prior to participation [9]. High-velocity and high-impact sports should be restricted as there is higher risk of spinal cord injury in those with ankylosing of the spine [6]. Individualized exercise programs designed with the aid of a sports medicine physician, rheumatologist, and physical therapist with knowledge of JIA are recommended [9].

How to Approach the Case

Any musculoskeletal pain that wakes patients up at night is a red flag. Night pain heightens concern for underlying infectious or inflammatory process, including malignancies, and warrants evaluation with additional imaging and lab investigation. This case also highlights the importance of a detailed history and review of systems to reveal his weight loss and morning stiffness, which may also suggest an underlying inflammatory process. Morning stiffness and low back pain relieved with NSAIDs or heat are characteristic of spondyloarthropathy. Finally, if the patient is not improving, the differential diagnosis must be revisited with each patient encounter and additional workup considered.

Short Differential Diagnosis
- Chronic, mechanical low back pain
- Sacral contusion, stress injury
- Discogenic low back pain with radiculopathy
- Inflammatory arthritis

Final Diagnosis

Enthesitis-related arthritis juvenile idiopathic arthritis (ERA JIA) with sacroiliitis

Natural History and Treatment Considerations

There are several classifications for JIA and spondyloarthropathy, and often distinguishing between subtypes has little impact on clinical management [1]. Typical symptoms of ERA are enthesitis, arthritis, and uveitis and can be treated with nonsteroidal anti-inflammatories and biologic agents [2]. If left untreated, sacroiliitis can lead to spontaneous fusion of the spine, chronic back pain, and stiffness.

The prognosis for this patient is fair. When compared to other types of JIA, those with ERA tend to have more pain, worse function, a lower quality of life, and lower remission rates [2].

Referral – Emergent, Urgent and Routine: And to Whom?

The majority of athletes with low back pain can be evaluated and treated by a primary care physician or a sports medicine physician. Patients with severe pain, weakness or decreased range of motion, signs of inflammatory arthritis, or enthesitis should be referred to a rheumatologist urgently for additional evaluation. If nocturnal pain is present, blood work including CBC, ESR, CRP, UA, ANA, RF, and HLA B27 is indicated and referral done. If the patient is otherwise well appearing without signs of neurologic deficit, imaging can be reserved for the subspecialty evaluation.

Brief Summary

This case of a hockey player with a back injury that is not improving illustrates the need to consider medical causes of musculoskeletal pain in athletes. The young athlete in this case presented for evaluation of low back pain 4 months after a fall in hockey; he was not improving with physical therapy. In addition, he is complained of symptoms such as morning stiffness, increasing pain, and weight loss that were inconsistent with a lingering musculoskeletal injury.

A diagnosis of enthesitis-related JIA was made by the consulting pediatric rheumatologist based on elements of his history and physical exam, combined with the MRI findings. The patient improved on methotrexate and returned to playing hockey.

Key Features and Pearls
- Back pain that is not improving as expected with time and correction of mechanical or strength deficits should be reevaluated for underlying inflammatory conditions.
- Normal plain radiographs and laboratory work do not rule out inflammatory disease.
- Athletes with enthesitis-related arthritis can often return to normal levels of physical activity.

Editor Discussion

Juvenile idiopathic arthritis (JIA) is an inclusive diagnosis and often a diagnosis of exclusion. The term "rheumatoid" has been omitted because most subtypes of JIA lack this factor. Some patients with JIA will have iridocyclitis – inflammation of the anterior uvea. Be sure to also refer to an ophthalmologist for a possible slit lamp examination. Enthesitis-related JIA is often HLA B27 positive. The former names for enthesitis-related arthritis (ERA) includes ankylosing spondylitis and Reiter syndrome.

W.L. Hennrikus

Enthesitis, mediated by pro-inflammatory cytokines, is an important feature of axial spondyloarthritis. Neuropathic-like pain is common in patients with psoriatic arthritis and is associated with greater disease activity, fatigue, depression, and anxiety [10]. Since ligaments and tendons attach at so many locations on the skeleton, pain can be located just about anywhere. For example, coccydynia has been seen as an enthesitis associated with ankylosing spondylitis. Besides enthesitis-related arthritis (ERA), chronic recurrent multifocal osteomyelitis, which may also be an autoimmune disease, can present as painful back and limb pain, with bone changes noted on MRI. In addition to medical treatment, it is important to maintain good weight and muscle strength, since obesity has been shown to be a risk factor for the overall response to treatment in conditions such as rheumatoid arthritis. The complexity of these conditions warrants referral and treatment with a pediatric rheumatologist.

R.M. Schwend

References

1. Deodhar A, Strand V, Kay J, Braun J. The term 'non-radiographic axial spondyloarthitis' is much more important to classify than to diagnose patients with axial spondyloarthritis. Ann Rheum Dis. 2016;75(5):791.
2. Weiss Pamela F. Diagnosis and treatment of enthesitis-related arthritis. Adolesc Health Med Ther. 2012;3:67–74.
3. Kaeley GS, Eder L, Aydin SZ, Gutierrez M, Bakewell C. Enthesitis: a hallmark of psoriatic arthritis. Semin Arthritis Rheum. 2018;48(1):35–43.
4. Braun J, Inman R. Clinical significance of inflammatory back pain for diagnosis and screening of patients with axial spondyloarthritis. Ann Rheum Dis. 2010;69(7):1264–8.
5. Giancane G, Consolaro A, Lanni S, et al. Juvenile idiopathic arthritis: diagnosis and treatment. Rheumatol Ther. 2016;3:187–207.
6. Harper BE, Reveille JD. Spondyloarthritis: clinical suspicion, diagnosis and sports. Curr Sports Med Rep. 2009;8(1):29–34.
7. Abramowicz S, Kim S, Prahalad S, et al. Juvenile arthritis: current concepts in terminology, etiopathogenesis, diagnosis, and management. Int J Oral Maxillofac Surg. 2016;45(7):801–12.
8. Alguin O, Gokalp G, Baran B, et al. Evaluation of sacroiliitis: contrast-enhanced MRI with subtraction technique. Skelet Radiol. 2009;38(10):983–8.
9. Philpott J, Houghton K, Luke A. Physical activity recommendations for children with specific chronic health conditions: juvenile idiopathic arthritis, hemophilia, asthma, and cystic fibrosis. Clin J Sport Med. 2010;20(3):167–72.
10. Ramjeeawon A, Choy E. Neuropathic-like pain in psoriatic arthritis: evidence of abnormal pain processing. Clin Rheumatol. 2019;38(11):3153–9.

Chapter 25
A Young Child with Activity-Limiting Back Pain for the Last 3 Months

Jefferson W. Jex and Richard M. Schwend

Brief Case Presentation

Chief Complaint

A 3-month history of daily thoracic back pain affecting activities

History

A 4-year, 9-month-old boy presented with daily back pain for about 3 months duration. The pain had been increasing and was affecting his daily activities. The pain increased with sitting. He demonstrated a decreased appetite, lethargy, and a less playful mood. The pain was centered at the mid-thoracic level without any radiation to the lower extremities. He has not had trouble falling asleep or staying asleep. NSAIDs help with the pain. He has had no fever, sweats, chills, weight loss, urinary incontinence, or extremity weakness.

His past history was unremarkable. He was full term at birth with normal birth weight and normal development. He had myringotomy tubes placed at age 3 years. There has been no history of trauma. He is doing well in pre-kindergarten. Family history was unremarkable.

J. W. Jex (✉)
Department of Orthopaedic Surgery, Walter Reed National Military Medical Center, Bethesda, MD, USA
e-mail: Jefferson.w.jex.mil@mail.mil

R. M. Schwend
Department of Orthopaedic Surgery, Children's Mercy Hospital, Kansas City, MO, USA

© Springer Nature Switzerland AG 2021
R. M. Schwend, W. L. Hennrikus (eds.), *Back Pain in the Young Child and Adolescent*, https://doi.org/10.1007/978-3-030-50758-9_25

Physical Examination

Weight 17 kg; height 111.8 cm. He had a normal growth chart and was healthy and developmentally normal with good nutrition. He was bright and cooperative on examination with normal lymph nodes. The spine is straight and balanced. He demonstrated mild tenderness in the mid-thoracic region in the midline. He was moderately stiff on forward bend able to touch just below his knees. Hyperextension was also mildly stiff and uncomfortable. Neurologic exam was normal.

Imaging and Radiographic Studies (Figs. 25.1 and 25.2)

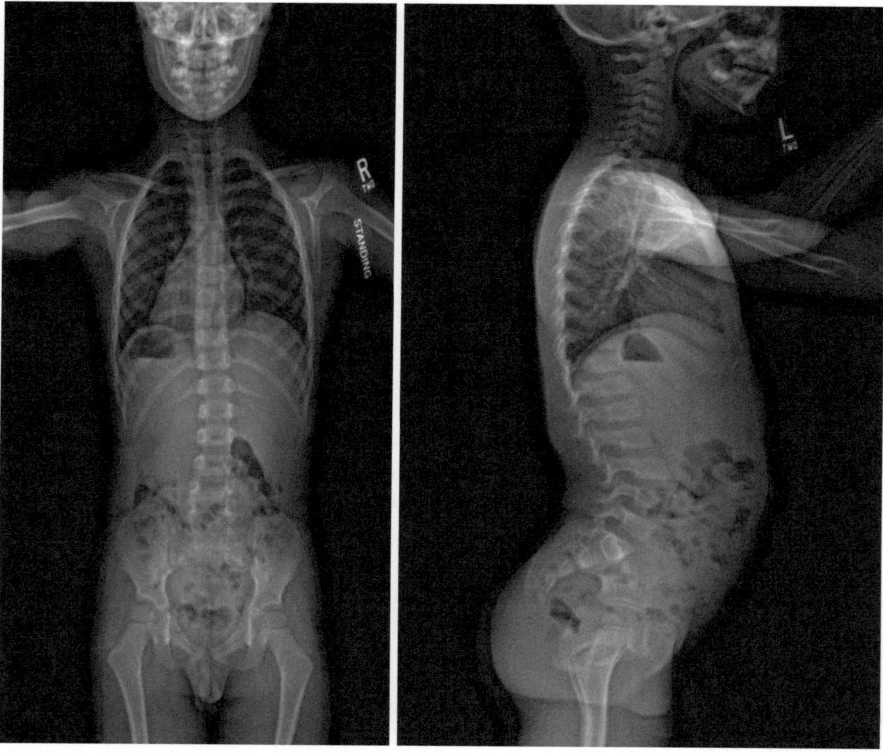

Fig. 25.1 Standing anterior/posterior and lateral radiographs of the spine. The spine is balanced with a mild scoliosis of 11 degrees. There are no soft tissue, disc space, or bony abnormalities. The boy's physician ordered a thoracic level MRI to evaluate for infection or tumor. Since the child was under 7 years of age and could not lie still, anesthesia was required

Fig. 25.2 Axial view MRI
T2 showing the edema and
inflammation surrounding
the left-sided posterior
elements at T6. The MRI
showed an enhancing T2
hyperintense signal within
the left posterior elements
at T5 and T6. There was
edema surrounding the
spinous processes at T5
and T6. Although there
was no well-defined mass,
there was periosteal
inflammatory soft tissue
surrounding the bone, with
an indistinct
posterior cortex

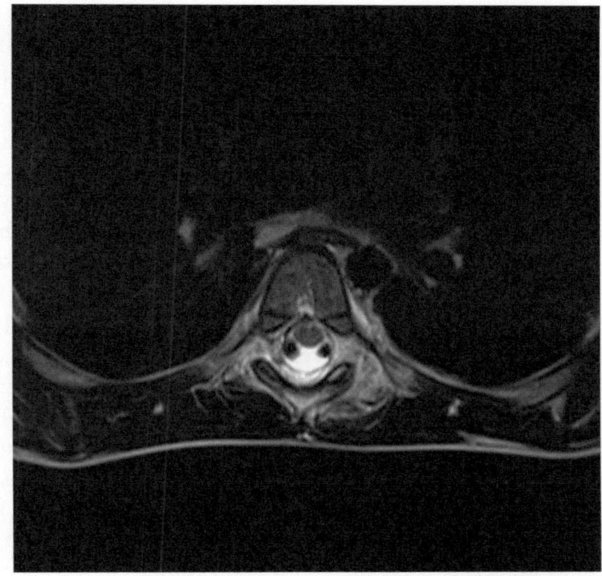

Questions About the Case the Reader Should Consider

1. Back pain is unusual in a child less than 5 years of age. What is the differential diagnosis for this patient?
2. Before advanced imaging is considered, what other studies are useful?
3. What are the advantages and disadvantages of using the MRI as the next imaging modality?
4. What other advanced imaging test is useful?
5. What are the treatment options?

Discussion

Progressive back pain in young children that leads to activity limitation is a red flag. This child experienced progression of symptoms over a 3-month period. Remember that the back pain is a symptom of the problem. Your task is to rule out the potentially catastrophic diagnoses including infection, neoplasia, leukemia, lymphoma, autoimmune disease, or trauma.

The workup begins with the history, physical examination, and radiographs of the painful location. The examination revealed a stiff spine, pain with motion, and a child who avoids spinal movement [1]. Plain radiographs are often normal but are quick and inexpensive and help to rule out some of the sinister causes of back pain. Young children with back pain may have secondary scoliosis that is noted on radiographs. Scoliosis secondary to osteoid osteoma typically lacks a rotational deformity that would be seen with most idiopathic scoliosis [2]. This lack of rotation would lead to a normal examination on Adam's forward lean test despite a radiographic appearance of scoliosis. Similarly, osteoid osteoma (OO) occurring in the cervical spine may present with a painful torticollis [3].

Laboratory analyses are important in ruling out infection and tumor. For example, CBC with manual differential will assist in evaluation of leukemia. About one-quarter of patients with leukemia present with bone pain. Atraumatic back pain of duration longer than 2 weeks with or without night pain should arouse suspicion and initiate further workup.

ESR and CRP are keys in evaluating for infection. The CRP has a high negative predictive value. The ESR responds more slowly to infection but can provide insight on the duration of infection and the success of treatment. Additionally, these studies may be elevated with autoimmune disease. ESR would also be elevated in leukemia.

Bone scan can be a helpful screening tool in cases such as this. Bone scan does not require sedation and can localize a bone-forming lesion such as OO. However, processes such as acute leukemia, infections, avascular necrosis, and cysts may be negative on bone scan as it is principally a measurement of bone formation.

In this case, MRI was not a good choice for advanced imaging. The lesion was smaller than what the MRI was able to visualize. MRI is better for soft tissue characterization and less effective for bony lesions. MRI is a very sensitive modality with false positives. MRI of osteoid osteoma may misleadingly appear as a more aggressive lesion and lead to the wrong diagnosis and overtreatment. Additionally, MRI is expensive and typically requires insurance preauthorization and can add to the family angst. In cases such as this, early consultation with a pediatric spine physician is helpful to guide advanced imaging recommendations.

CT scan was the best advanced imaging test for this patient (Figs. 25.3 and 25.4). CT scan provided excellent bony detail and resolution in the evaluation of an OO. CT does not typically require sedation for young children due to the speed of acquisition. CT is the study of choice for bone lesions. If the pain is easily localized

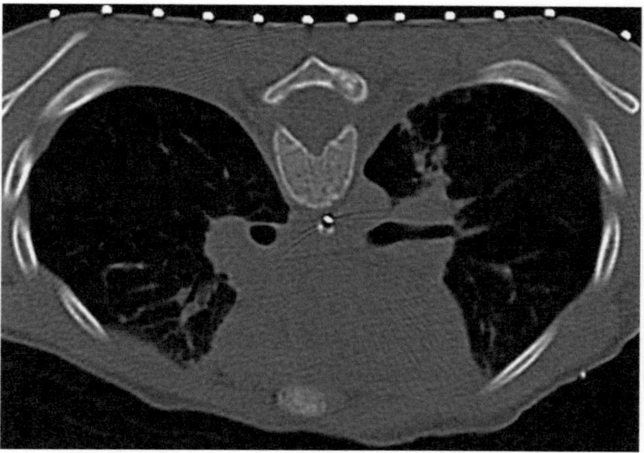

Fig. 25.3 Axial CT showing 1 cm radiolucent lesion with central calcified nidus located in the left hemilamina

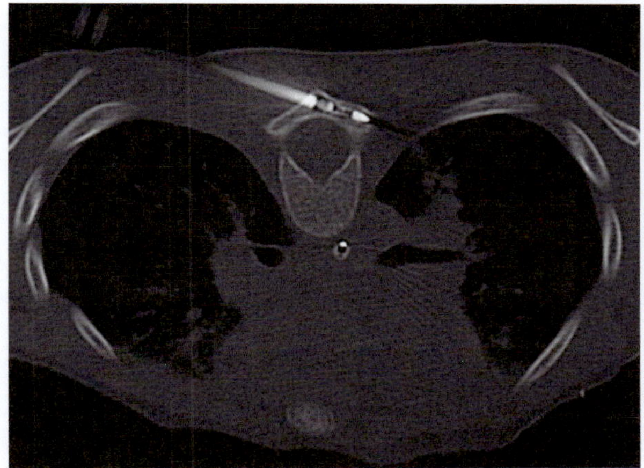

Fig. 25.4 Axial CT image showing the cryotherapy ablation tool coming in from the right side

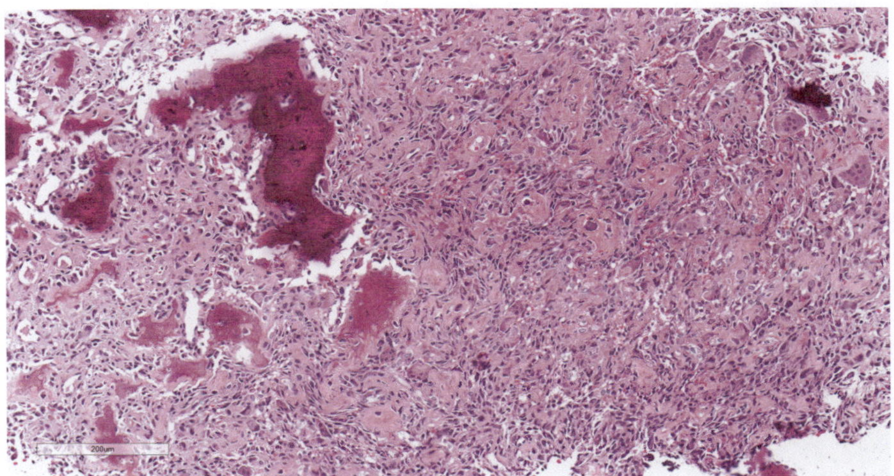

Fig. 25.5 A high-power micrograph of an osteoid osteoma showing a central nidus of bone with rimming osteoblasts surrounded by reactive fibrovascular stroma. (Courtesy of Alejandro Luiña Contreras, MD, Joint Pathology Center, Silver Spring, MD)

on physical examination, forego the bone scan and opt for a CT directly. If there is an associated soft tissue mass noted on CT that was not perceived on examination, MRI can be performed.

An osteoid osteoma is a small <1 cm benign lesion of bone. It consists of a central nidus of cells that produce cyclooxygenase 1 and 2 as well as prostaglandin E2 (Fig. 25.5). These compounds incite reactive bone formation about the nidus and produce the typical pain of an osteoid osteoma that responds to salicylates and NSAIDs.

How to Approach the Case

Back pain in a young child that is activity limiting is a red flag. The evaluation should be based on the clinical presentation and physical examination findings and radiographs. Longer duration of activity-limiting pain, night pain, or constitutional symptoms suggests diagnoses such as leukemia or lymphoma. Laboratory studies are indicated if these conditions are to be evaluated.

A history of night pain that is responsive to salicylates or NSAIDs is suggestive of osteoid osteoma. If the radiographs are normal and the location of the pain is difficult to determine, a bone scan may be obtained. If osteoid osteoma is suspected and the bone scan shows a lesion, further investigation with CT scan is indicated.

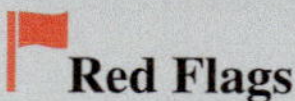

Red Flags
- Night pain
- Pain that is causing decreased activity
- Lethargy
- Decreased appetite enough to cause weight loss
- Stiffness on examination

Short Differential Diagnosis
- Spondylodiscitis
- Leukemia
- Lymphoma
- Osteoid osteoma/osteoblastoma
- Langerhans cell histiocytosis

Final Diagnosis

Osteoid osteoma of left T6 spine posterior elements

Natural History and Treatment Considerations

Osteoid osteoma is the third most common benign lesion of bone following non-ossifying fibroma and osteochondroma. It tends to present with pain that is worse at night. Salicylates or NSAIDs provide substantial pain relief. After obtaining an appropriate history and performing a physical examination, plain radiographs are ordered of the location of the back pain. Radiographs may document bony sclerosis associated with the reactive bone occurring adjacent to a nidus.

Advanced imaging with a bone scan for localization followed by a CT will confirm the diagnosis. An MRI is not ideal to confirm the presence of this lesion. Children must be sedated, and although the MRI does not expose them to ionizing radiation, the resolution is inadequate to accurately characterize a small lesion such as an osteoid osteoma. CT and bone scans may be performed without anesthesia.

Treatment of OO can be radiofrequency ablation or surgical excision. If the OO lesion is located near vital structures such as the spinal cord and/or nerve roots, surgical excision may be safer than radiofrequency ablation [4]. Both radiofrequency ablation and CT-guided surgical excision in select cases have been shown to provide excellent results [5]. Lastly, nonoperative management with long-term suppression of symptoms by oral NSAIDs can also be used with remission experienced at an average of 33 months [6].

Referral – Emergency, Urgent, or Routine: And to Whom?

A young child presenting with activity-limiting back pain that is atraumatic should be urgently evaluated by the primary care physician with early collaboration with a pediatric spine surgeon. Radiographic imaging and hematologic studies are a good start with further advanced imaging such as CT ordered by the subspecialist to confirm the diagnosis of OO. Shared decision making with the physicians and the family will facilitate the decision to treat the OO with excision, percutaneous ablation, or medical treatment.

Brief Summary

Activity-limiting back pain in a young patient, pain that interferes with sleep, and constitutional symptoms are red flags. Young children may have difficulty verbalizing the frequency, extent, and location of the pain. The examination may identify significant spinal stiffness. Although up to 30% of children with adolescent idiopathic scoliosis have reported pain, scoliosis does not typically present with severe pain or night pain. Children with painful scoliosis should receive greater scrutiny and not have their symptoms ascribed to the scoliosis alone. The scoliosis may be a manifestation of an underlying disease. In young children, back pain should not be attributed to secondary motives as can occur in teenagers or adults.

Key Features and Pearls
- Progressive, activity-limiting pain
- Significant pain relief with NSAIDs
- Pain worse at night
- Painful scoliosis that lacks rotational deformity
- Spinal stiffness/rigidity

Editor Discussion

The major clue to the diagnosis of an osteoid osteoma is the history of night pain relieved by aspirin or NSAIAs. The osteoid osteoma produces prostaglandins, and the salicylates or NSAIAs inhibit prostaglandins. It can be difficult to locate an osteoid osteoma of the spine on plain radiographs alone. The best advanced imaging test in this case is a CT rather than an MRI. The MRI can be misleading due to bone edema and lead one to misdiagnosis infection or a malignancy.

W.L. Hennrikus

Osteoid osteoma is notorious for being difficult to diagnose. The most challenging aspect is to even consider it as a diagnostic possibility. The lesion can hide out in unusual places, such as a rib, in the femoral neck, talus, tibia, and spine. Normal plain films or MRI should not exclude the diagnosis, which, once suspected, should be pursued with determination. I find that for such cases, calling your pediatric orthopedic surgeon directly can share some of the stress and uncertainty in working up this and other lesions. Having key pediatric consultants who are readily available in your "favorites" and willing to discuss a difficult case is one benefit of modern communication.

R.M. Schwend

References

1. Kirwan EO, Hutton PA, Pozo JL, Ransford AO. Osteoid osteoma and benign osteoblastoma of the spine. Clinical presentation and treatment. J Bone Joint Surg Br. 1984;66(1):21–6.
2. Keim HA, Reina EG. Osteoid-osteoma as a cause of scoliosis. J Bone Joint Surg Am. 1975;57(2):159–63.
3. Raskas DS, Graziano GP, Herzenberg JE, Heidelberger KP, Hensinger RN. Osteoid osteoma and osteoblastoma of the spine. J Spinal Disord. 1992;5(2):204–11.
4. Yu X, Wang B, Yang S, Han S, et al. Percutaneous radiofrequency ablation versus open surgical resection for spinal osteoid osteoma. Spine J. 2019;19(3):509–15.
5. Kadhim M, Binitie O, O'Toole P, Grigoriou E, De Mattos CB, Dormans JP. Surgical resection of osteoid osteoma and osteoblastoma of the spine. J Pediatr Orthop B. 2017;26(4):362–9.
6. Kneisl JS, Simon MA. Medical management compared with operative treatment for osteoid-osteoma. J Bone Joint Surg Am. 1992;74(2):179–85.

Chapter 26
A Case of a Boy with Neck Pain at Night Associated with Acute Torticollis and Kyphoscoliosis

Stephen D. Lockey, Michael DeFrance, Alicia McCarthy, Arun R. Hariharan, and Suken A. Shah

Brief Case Presentation

Chief Complaint

Neck pain and head tilt

History

This 10-year-old boy presents with persistent, dull neck pain for 3 months. His symptoms are worse with lying in a supine position and at night. He does not report any associated pain in other parts of his body or any radiating pain down his arms or legs. He complains of head tilt to the left and a stiff neck after basketball. He has

S. D. Lockey
Department of Orthopaedics, Medstar Georgetown University Hospital, Washington, DC, USA

M. DeFrance
Department of Orthopaedic Surgery, Rowan University School of Osteopathic Medicine, Stratford, NJ, USA

A. McCarthy · A. R. Hariharan
Department of Orthopaedics, Nemours/Alfred I. duPont Hospital for Children, Wilmington, DE, USA

S. A. Shah (✉)
Division of Spine and Scoliosis, Department of Orthopaedics, Nemours/Alfred I. duPont Hospital for Children, Wilmington, DE, USA
e-mail: Suken.Shah@nemours.org

© Springer Nature Switzerland AG 2021
R. M. Schwend, W. L. Hennrikus (eds.), *Back Pain in the Young Child and Adolescent*, https://doi.org/10.1007/978-3-030-50758-9_26

taken NSAIDs and diazepam, but with minimal relief. Otherwise, he has not had fever, chills, night sweats, weight loss, weakness, unbalanced gait, loss of manual dexterity, numbness in his extremities, or bowel/bladder symptoms.

He was previously evaluated 8 weeks before this clinic visit by another physician and had an otherwise normal physical exam, but with mild rotatory instability at C1/C2 on plain cervical spine radiographs (Figs. 26.1 and 26.2). A computed tomography (CT) scan was negative for bony abnormalities. He completed several sessions in physical therapy with neck stretching and strengthening but stated his symptoms, primarily the pain, had only worsened.

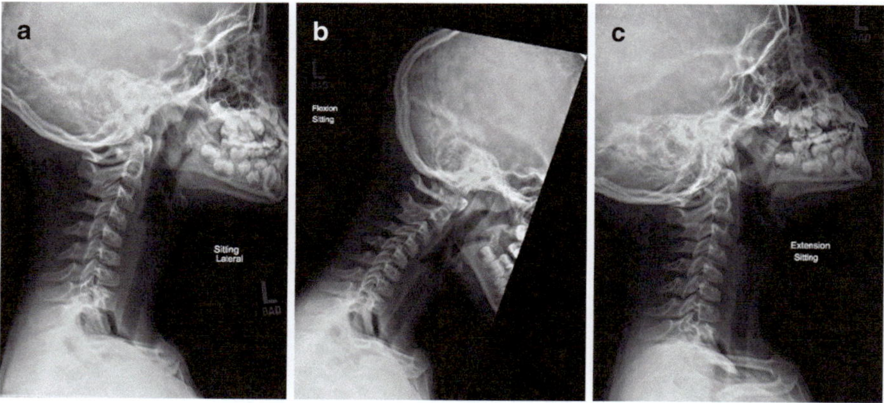

Fig. 26.1 Seated lateral views of the cervical spine positioned in neutral (**a**), flexion (**b**), and extension (**c**) used to assess for structural abnormalities including fracture and spondylolisthesis

Fig. 26.2 Open mouth odontoid view demonstrating mild rotatory deformity at C1/C2. Note the difference in distance between the odontoid process of C2 compared to the lateral masses of C1

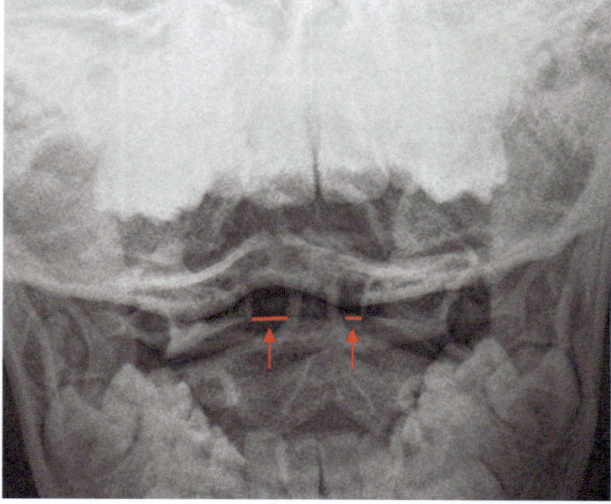

Medical History

His past medical history was significant for well-controlled asthma for which he takes an inhaler. His developmental history was unremarkable, and family history was negative for scoliosis or cancers.

Physical Examination

Weight 32.5 kg, height 146 cm, afebrile. He is well appearing and developmentally normal. He exhibits a left-sided head tilt and right shoulder elevation with right cervicothoracic scoliosis. Neck active range of motion is painless but significantly limited in all directions. There is no tenderness to palpation along his spinal-pelvic axis. His right hand grasp is weaker compared to the left, along with subjective sensory disturbance. The remainder of his strength, sensation and reflex testing was normal and symmetric.

Imaging and Radiographic Studies (Figs. 26.1, 26.2, 26.3, and 26.4)

Questions About the Case the Reader Should Consider
1. Neck pain is a common complaint in children. What features in the patient's presentation raise red flags?
2. How do spinal cord tumors typically present?
3. What is a possible explanation for his torticollis?
4. What is the next diagnostic test that should be considered?
5. What is the appropriate referral and treatment in this case?

Discussion

Neck pain is a common complaint with a variety of etiologies in the pediatric population. While many causes can be managed with reassurance and conservative therapy, it is important that the physician be familiar with presenting signs suggestive of more serious conditions. Examples of nontraumatic neck pain associated with significant morbidity include infection (meningitis, epidural abscess), vascular or congenital anomalies (berry aneurysm, Arnold-Chiari malformation), and central nervous system tumors. The presence of pain at night and the development of acute torticollis with progressive spinal deformity (cervicothoracic) and motor weakness should raise suspicion and prompt immediate workup with advanced imaging.

Fig. 26.3 Standing posterior-anterior (PA) scoliosis view demonstrates deformity with apex right scoliosis at the upper thoracic region

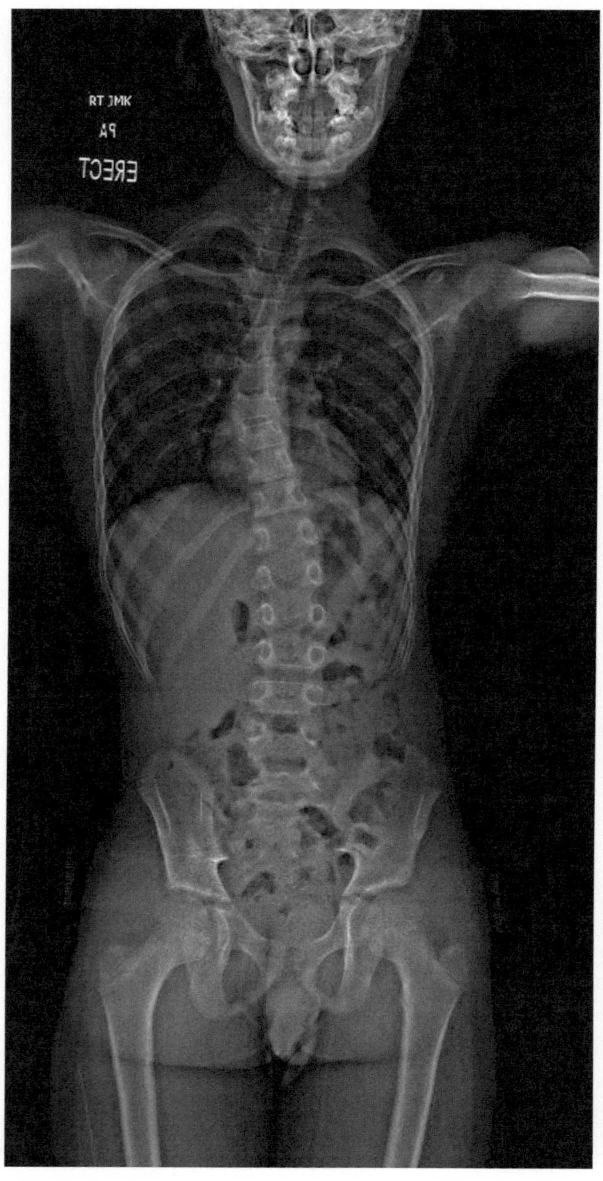

Central nervous system tumors represent the most common solid organ malignancy in children, with a variety of presenting signs and symptoms depending on the location of the lesion. Spinal cord tumors usually present with back pain (67%), gait or coordination disturbances (42%), and spinal deformity (39%). Other findings may include focal weakness (21%), sphincter disturbance (20%), decreased upper limb movement (17%), headache (7%), and head tilt (7%) [1]. The wide range of

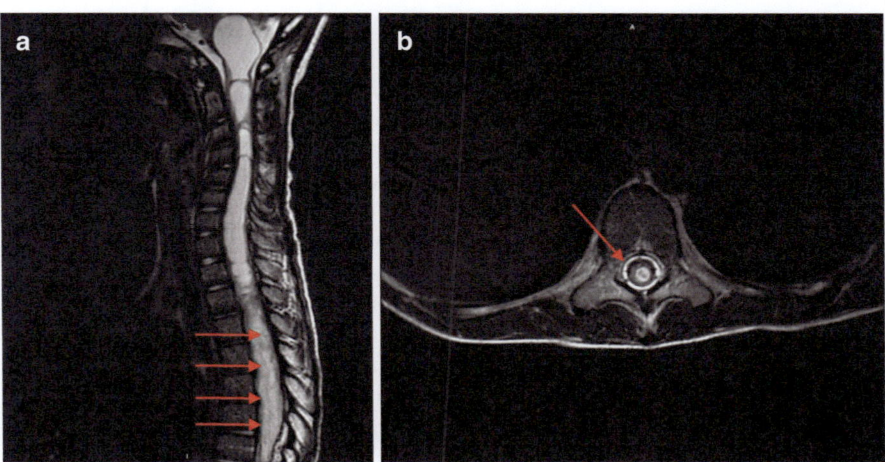

Fig. 26.4 (**a**) Sagittal T2-weighted MRI demonstrates the presence of a syrinx extending the entire length of the spinal cord. Additionally, note the presence of a nodular mass within the thoracic spine. (**b**) Axial T2-weighted MRI demonstrates the presence of a syrinx as well as nodularity adjacent to the spinal cord

nonspecific symptoms can often delay diagnosis, which may lead to disabling neurologic deficits that are partially or completely irreversible. The key to preventing unnecessary delays in treatment and morbidity is recognizing red flags in the presentation that warrant further immediate workup. Pain associated with spinal cord tumors typically precedes neurologic findings and usually fluctuates in severity, with the worst symptoms occurring at night or when lying down due to dural distension [2]. The presence of dermatomal pain, either from root distension or infiltration by tumor, may also be the initial symptom [3]. Motor dysfunction can occur early in the disease process and manifest with developmental delay (crawling, standing), motor regression, or frequent falls. Weakness is often asymmetric as most lesions are eccentrically located. Kyphoscoliosis and torticollis may develop in patients with thoracic and cervical tumors, respectively, and may also indicate a specific pathology [4].

Torticollis is present when the patient's chin is rotated toward one shoulder, and the head is tilted toward the contralateral side. The most frequent cause in an infant is congenital muscular torticollis, due to a contracted sternocleidomastoid muscle. The acute condition in the older pediatric patient may be related to otitis media, ocular torticollis, trauma, or cervical spine subluxation [5]. Torticollis related to atlantoaxial rotatory instability is characterized by asymmetry of the odontoid process of C2 in relation to the lateral masses of C1, but diagnosis can be difficult by plain radiographs. Dynamic CT with the head rotated to the left and right provides more accurate information. Most cases will resolve spontaneously and those with symptoms less than 1 week are managed with immobilization, rest, muscle relaxants, and analgesics. Failure to improve after 1 week requires referral, imaging, and treatment [6].

A progressive spinal deformity can be due to a pathologic process. Tumors or syringomyelia in the thoracic spine can lead to progressive kyphoscoliosis, as seen in this patient. Idiopathic scoliosis is a three-dimensional spinal deformity associated with lateral curvature, apical lordosis, and rotation. Most (>95%) thoracic curves due to idiopathic scoliosis go to the right, due to preexisting deviation and rotation from the mediastinal structures; and therefore, left-sided curves should be suspect for an underlying pathologic process [7].

The decision to order advanced imaging should follow a systematic approach in the workup of pediatric neck pain to minimize radiation exposure, cost, and patient/parent anxiety [8]. Following a careful history and physical examination, the next study is plain radiographs to include posterior-anterior (PA) and lateral views of the specific area of concern. However, in spinal deformity, long films of the entire spine should be obtained. In a child with night pain or an abnormal examination (i.e., motor weakness, painful/persistent torticollis, spinal deformity, abnormal reflexes) and normal radiographs, a magnetic resonance imaging (MRI) is still indicated. Up to 75% of patients with pathology identified on MRI will have normal radiographs. The use of MRI in the evaluation of atypical pain or abnormal physical examination findings is validated [9]. In addition, advanced imaging with an MRI is recommended when soft-tissue pathology is suspected such as infection or malignancy. However, the sensitivity of MRI and the absence of radiation exposure must be weighed against the need for sedation in younger children [10]. If an MRI is indicated, the study can be ordered in consultation with the treating spinal surgeon after the referral is made.

Referral to a pediatric orthopedic spine specialist or neurosurgeon is indicated for atypical presentation of back or neck pain or pain-associated spinal deformity, torticollis, and neurologic deficits. Advanced imaging studies provide both diagnostic value and information important for surgical management. The finding of a spinal cord tumor often requires resection by a spine surgeon and adjunctive medical treatment. The most important prognostic factors are the patient's preoperative neurological state and the histological grade of the tumor [11], further emphasizing the need for prompt workup and referral to the appropriate specialist.

In this case example, an MRI indicated that the patient had a thoracic intramedullary spinal cord tumor with associated syrinx. He underwent staged right-sided T1-T11 hemilaminectomies with intraspinal tumor microdissection and shunt placement. Gross total resection of the tumor was achieved, and the patient did not require adjuvant therapy. He underwent an aggressive rehabilitation program and is doing well despite persistent motor deficits.

How to Approach the Case

If the presentation is atypical, the quality and timing of pain should raise suspicion and lead to immediate workup. Night pain, pain in a dermatomal pattern, motor weakness, abnormal reflexes, and bowel/bladder symptoms are some of the "red flags" in spinal pathology. A careful history and physical exam should evaluate for the presence of new or worsening spinal deformity. Imaging typically begins with plain radiographs, but pain associated with torticollis may limit the head positioning necessary for an accurate diagnosis on an x-ray. If a soft tissue pathology is suspected, an MRI should be obtained. Tumors that originate from bone are typically better visualized with CT. In some cases, blood tests and tissue biopsy may also be necessary, but this should be determined in conjunction with the treating surgeon.

 **Red Flags for Neck Pain and Acute Torticollis**
- Night pain
- Acute or worsening kyphoscoliosis
- Neural symptoms
- Changes in gait or coordination
- Focal weakness or other neurologic findings

Short Differential Diagnosis
- Infection – Meningitis or an epidural abscess must be ruled out in the initial evaluation of a patient with neck pain and torticollis.
- Primary tumors of bone – Osteoid osteomas and osteoblastomas can present with night pain and worsening spinal deformity. Neurologic deficits are less common than in tumors derived from neural elements.
- Congenital anomalies – Atlantoaxial rotatory instability can present with neck pain and torticollis. Neurologic symptoms may also be present.

Final Diagnosis

WHO Grade II Pilomyxoid astrocytoma from T3-T11 with associated syringomyelia due to CSF obstruction

Natural History and Treatment Considerations

The most common pediatric spinal cord tumors include astrocytomas, ependymomas, neuroblastomas, and primitive neuroectodermal tumors. As in this case example, patients typically present with pain or neurologic deficits. Motor or sensory sequelae can progress rapidly and are often irreversible. A progressive spinal deformity may also be present. Malignant spinal cord tumors ultimately require surgical resection and stabilization with adjuvant treatment in the form of chemotherapy and/or radiation.

Referral – When and to Whom?

A child presenting with back or neck pain at night, pain in a dermatomal pattern, weakness, abnormal reflexes, or bowel/bladder symptoms should be referred to a pediatric orthopedist or neurosurgeon with expertise in spinal pathology. If advanced imaging demonstrates the lesion involves the spinal cord rather than the bone, the tumor should be surgically managed by a neurosurgeon

The patient was found to have a thoracic intramedullary spinal cord tumor on MRI and underwent staged right-sided T1-T11 hemilaminectomies with intraspinal tumor microdissection and cardio-cervical decompression for a syrinx shunt. Gross total resection of the tumor was achieved, and the patient did not require any adjuvant chemotherapy or radiation.

> **Key Features and Pearls**
> - Torticollis has many benign causes, but patients presenting with worsening spinal deformity, night pain, or associated neural signs require a comprehensive workup to exclude infection and malignancy.
> - A timely diagnosis and appropriate treatment is critical to avoid neurologic deficits that are often permanent or do not fully recover.

Editor Discussion

The onset of torticollis, kyphoscoliosis, neck pain, and weakness in right-sided grip strength with changes in hand sensation in a previously healthy 10-year-old boy warrants immediate spine radiographs and referral to your closest neurosurgeon and/or pediatric orthopedic surgeon. This case jumps off the page with "badness." An astrocytoma is a cancer that can form in the brain or spinal cord. Astrocytomas begin in cells called astrocytes that support nerve cells. The signs and symptoms depend on the location of the tumor. Astrocytomas that occur in the brain can cause seizures, headaches, and nausea. As in this case, an astrocytoma in the spinal cord can cause weakness and sensory changes.

W.L. Hennrikus

Spinal cord tumors may present at any age and have a variety of signs and symptoms. Key symptoms are pain, sensory changes, and motor weakness. Pain can range from mild to so severe that the child is unapproachable. Sensory changes can be over dermatomes with very specific and unusual symptoms such as not wanting to keep a shirt on or asking for hot showers over that body part. Weakness can be subtle, such as new onset of clumsiness or a change in the gait. Parents are very observant of changes in their child's function, so should be taken seriously. The ASIA (American Spinal Injury Association) Classification is a good guide to approach the neurological examination. It consists of two sensory examinations (light touch and pin prick), motor testing of 11 muscle groups, and an impairment scale. Although you do not need to do the entire examination, it provides a useful framework.

R.M. Schwend

References

1. Wilne SH, Dineen RA, Dommett RM, Chu TPC, Walker DA. Identifying brain tumours in children and young adults. BMJ. 2013;347:f5844.
2. Wilne S, Walker D. Spine and spinal cord tumours in children: a diagnostic and therapeutic challenge to healthcare systems. Arch Dis Child Educ Pract Ed. 2010;95(2):47–54.
3. Binning M, Klimo P, Gluf W, Goumnerova L. Spinal tumors in children. Neurosurg Clin N Am. 2007;18(4):631–58.
4. Reimer R, Onofrio BM. Astrocytomas of the spinal cord in children and adolescents. J Neurosurg. 1985;63(5):669–75.
5. Korngold HW. Acute torticollis in pediatric practice. AMA J Dis Child. 1959;98:756–64.
6. Muñiz AE, Belfer RA. Atlantoaxial rotary subluxation in children. Pediatr Emerg Care. 1999;15(1):25–9.
7. Houten JK, Weiner HL. Pediatric intramedullary spinal cord tumors: special considerations. J Neuro-Oncol. 2000;47(3):225–30.
8. Feldman DS, Straight JJ, Badra MI, Mohaideen A, Madan SS. Evaluation of an algorithmic approach to pediatric back pain. J Pediatr Orthop. 2006;26(3):353–7.
9. Ramirez N, Flynn JM, Hill BW, et al. Evaluation of a systematic approach to pediatric back pain: the utility of magnetic resonance imaging. J Pediatr Orthop. 2015;35(1):28–32.
10. Shah SA, Saller J. Evaluation and diagnosis of Back pain in children and adolescents. J Am Acad Orthop Surg. 2016;24(1):37–45.
11. Nadkarni TD, Rekate HL. Pediatric intramedullary spinal cord tumors. Critical review of the literature. Childs Nerv Syst. 1999;15(1):17–28.

Chapter 27
Scoliosis Is Not Always Idiopathic: A Case of a Boy with Back Pain and Scoliosis

Arun R. Hariharan and Suken A. Shah

Brief Case Presentation

Chief Complaint

An 11-year-old boy presents with persistent low back pain after a twisting move while dancing.

History

The pain has been dull and constant with radiation down his left leg to the foot. The pain has been present during the day and night. His mother also notes that his posture has recently deteriorated. The pain had been limiting him from participating in sports and physical activities, such as basketball and surfing. He had been taking NSAIDs every 6 hours with only minimal relief. He had no fevers, chills, night sweats, weight loss, weakness, numbness, or bowel and bladder symptoms. He takes no other medications, his developmental history had been unremarkable, his past medical history is negative, and family history is negative for scoliosis.

A. R. Hariharan
Department of Orthopaedics, Nemours/Alfred I. duPont Hospital for Children, Wilmington, DE, USA

S. A. Shah (✉)
Division of Spine and Scoliosis, Department of Orthopaedics, Nemours/Alfred I. duPont Hospital for Children, Wilmington, DE, USA
e-mail: Suken.Shah@nemours.org

© Springer Nature Switzerland AG 2021
R. M. Schwend, W. L. Hennrikus (eds.), *Back Pain in the Young Child and Adolescent*, https://doi.org/10.1007/978-3-030-50758-9_27

Physical Examination

He is afebrile and his vital signs are within normal limits, and his BMI is in the ideal range. He is otherwise healthy, developmentally normal, and cooperative. His head and neck exams are normal. His breathing is non-labored and his abdomen is non-tender. His extremities are warm and well perfused.

On his musculoskeletal examination, he has a listing posture to the left, with a trunk shift both standing and walking. No rotational scoliosis is noted, and there are no overlying skin lesions or rashes on his back. He also demonstrates left-sided paraspinal muscle tenderness and spine stiffness with decreased spine flexion, extension, and lateral bending. He also demonstrates a positive straight leg raise test and difficulty with heel walking. His sensation is intact to light touch in all dermatomal distributions, and his reflexes are normal.

Questions About the Case the Reader Should Consider
1. Mechanical back pain is often responsive to non-steroidal anti-inflammatory drugs (NSAID) and self-limited. Why does this patient have persistent back pain refractory to NSAIDs?
2. Scoliosis is typically not painful or associated with mechanical pain with normal activity. What is the reason for the pain at night?
3. What is a possible explanation for his radicular symptoms?
4. What is the next diagnostic test that should be considered?
5. What is appropriate referral and treatment in this case?

Discussion

Back pain from a myriad of reasons is quite prevalent in children and adolescents. Most commonly, back pain is due to nonspecific pain or muscle strain. At times, back pain can result from other causes such as disk herniations, spondylolysis, infection, or tumor [1, 2]. Scoliosis, however, is typically not painful in children. Often, the back pain is self-limited, and most children do not seek medical attention. The American Academy of Family Physicians has recommended that children and adolescents with back pain who have no significant physical findings, a short duration of pain, and a history of minor injury can be treated conservatively without radiographic or laboratory studies. However, they also have a consensus level recommendation that children and adolescents with back pain, abnormal physical findings, constant pain, nighttime pain, or radicular pain should receive further evaluation. In patients with night time pain, pain that is persistent, pain that does not respond to NSAIDs, and pain with recent onset scoliosis, tumor and infection must be on the top of the differential diagnosis [2]. Additionally, the presence of radicular symptoms indicates a compressive process from a disk herniation, a spondylolisthesis, or a tumor [3–5].

Osteoblastomas, osteoid osteomas, and aneurysmal bone cysts (ABCs) are benign tumors that are commonly found on the posterior elements of the spine, including the spinous process, lamina. pars, and the pedicle. Osteoid osteomas are often less than 1 cm in size compared to osteoblastomas and ABCs which are greater than 2 cm in size. All of these benign tumors can cause night pain and pain at rest. However, since osteoid osteomas are relatively small in size, they infrequently cause neurological symptoms [6–8].

However, osteoblastoma is a bone-forming tumor greater than 2 cm that can expand the bone of the posterior elements and create nerve compression or inflammation. Forty percent of osteoblastomas involve the spine, especially the cervical and lumbar regions. This bone lesion, although benign, can be aggressive, destructive, and expansile and can compress or irritate the spinal cord or nerve roots [1, 6]. In addition to the spine, other sites of osteoblastomas include the diaphysis or metaphysis of long bones and the pelvis. Symptoms can include scoliosis, weakness, radicular pain, sensory changes, bladder dysfunction, and incontinence. Due to the nonmalignant nature of these tumors, patients do not usually display constitutional symptoms such as fever, anorexia, malaise, night sweats, and weight loss [1, 3, 9].

On examination, patients may display tenderness to the paraspinal muscles and decreased spine range of motion. The posterior elements of the spine are affected by extension of the spine, and thereby patients will be limited and report pain with spine extension. Of note, spondylolysis and spondylolisthesis also demonstrate increased back pain with extension. The exam may also reveal a spinal curvature, but the scoliosis is olisthetic, not similar to an idiopathic curve, which usually has a rotational component and compensatory curves above and below. In contrast, adolescent idiopathic scoliosis is usually not painful. The skin should also be examined for café-au-lait spots which indicate McCune Albright syndrome or neurofibromatosis. A thorough motor, sensory, and reflex examination is critical [1, 2, 9].

As previously stated, based on the AAFP recommendations, if a patient has back pain with abnormal physical findings, pain at night, constant pain, or radicular pain, additional evaluation should take place [2]. A plain radiograph focused on the affected area of the spine with orthogonal, posterior-anterior (PA), and lateral views should be obtained. A systematic approach when reading plain radiographs is helpful. In addition, a direct discussion with the radiologist may also be beneficial in some cases [10–12].

If, based on the history, physical examination, and plain radiographs, a tumor is suspected, referral to a pediatric orthopedic spine specialist is recommended. The orthopedic surgeon can then further workup the child with advanced imaging. In most cases of suspected tumors, a computed tomography (CT) scan and magnetic resonance imaging (MRI) are indicated. The CT scan better demonstrates bony involvement and can provide imaging in the axial plane which can be useful for surgical planning. MRI provides better visualization of the soft tissues, such as the surrounding ligaments and neural structures [10, 11, 13]. MRI can also provide information about the tumor itself such as fluid-fluid levels suggestive of an ABC [14].

Returning to the case of our 11-year-old boy – he was referred to our orthopedic spine service for scoliosis, but after his exam and X-rays demonstrated a possible tumor based on the blurring of a pedicle on the left side of L5 with a right-sided lumbar curvature (Fig. 27.1). MRI and CT scans were ordered. MRI scan demonstrated a heterogenous and expansile process about the left L5 posterior elements with near obliteration of the pedicle (Figs. 27.2 and 27.3). The T2-weighted images also show the aforementioned fluid-fluid levels in the axial and sagittal planes (Fig. 27.4). The CT scan in the axial images demonstrated an expansile and destructive lesion within the pedicle and transverse process extending anteriorly to the vertebral body (Fig. 27.5). The 3D CT reconstructions further illustrate the presence of this lytic mass on the posterolateral aspect of L5 on the left side (Fig. 27.6).

Differential Diagnosis

Based on the history of persistent back pain associated with scoliosis, radicular symptoms, and night-time pain combined with the clinical and imaging findings, the differential diagnosis for this 11-year-old boy included the following:

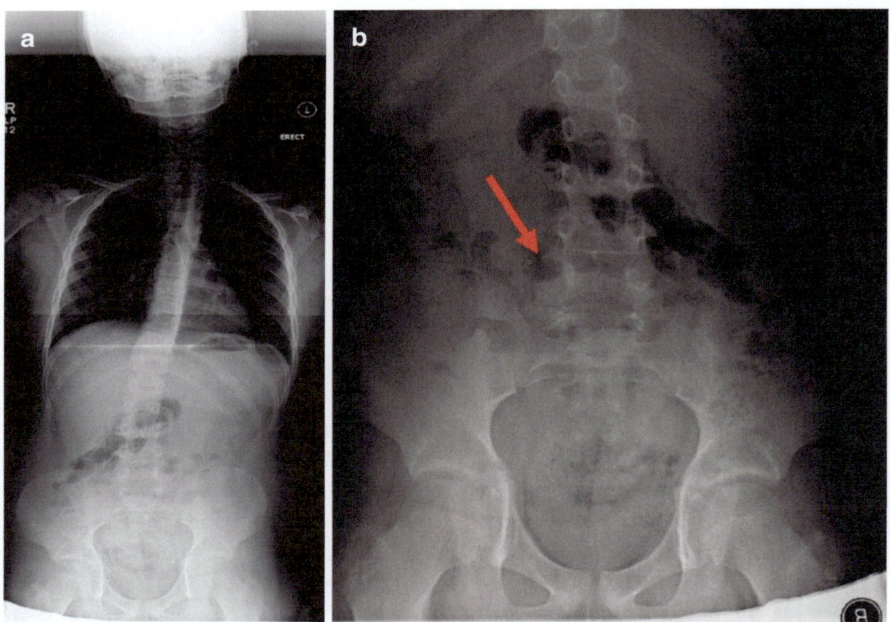

Fig. 27.1 (**a**) Posterior-anterior radiographs of the entire spine. A subtle right-sided lumbar curvature is seen. Otherwise no apparent abnormalities are evident. (**b**) A coned view of the lumbar spine X-ray. This shows an expansile lesion within the left pedicle of L5 with obliteration of clear pedicle margins (*arrow*)

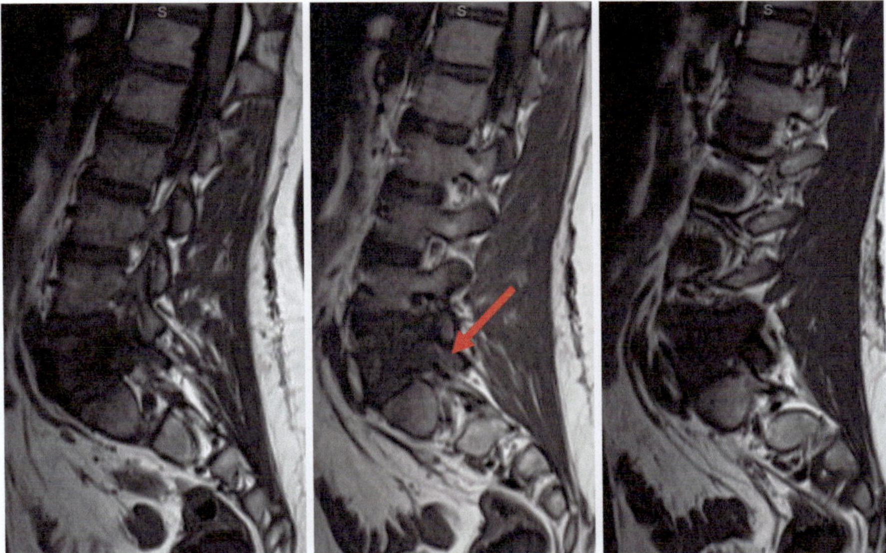

Fig. 27.2 Sagittal cuts of the T1 MRI. This demonstrates a heterogenous lesion within the L5 posterior elements involving the pars and the pedicle with anterior extension into the L5 vertebral body. Foraminal root compression of the L5 nerve root is also seen (*arrow*)

Benign Lesions
- Osteoblastoma
- ABC
- Giant cell tumor (less likely because these lesions are found in vertebral body rather than in posterior elements)
- Osteoid osteomas (less likely given the large size of this lesion and because osteoid osteomas are classically very responsive to NSAIDs)

Malignant Lesions
- Ewing's sarcoma
- Osteosarcoma
- Chondrosarcoma

Procedure

He was taken to the operating room for surgical treatment. Intraoperatively, a fleshy, reddish mass was encountered on the posterolateral aspect of the left side of the L5 vertebral body within the pedicle, transverse process, and extending into the lateral aspect of the vertebral body. The medial aspect of the vertebral body was noted to be well corticated and intact – the tumor did not involve the spinal canal. An intraoperative frozen section was suggestive of a benign bone lesion without giant cells.

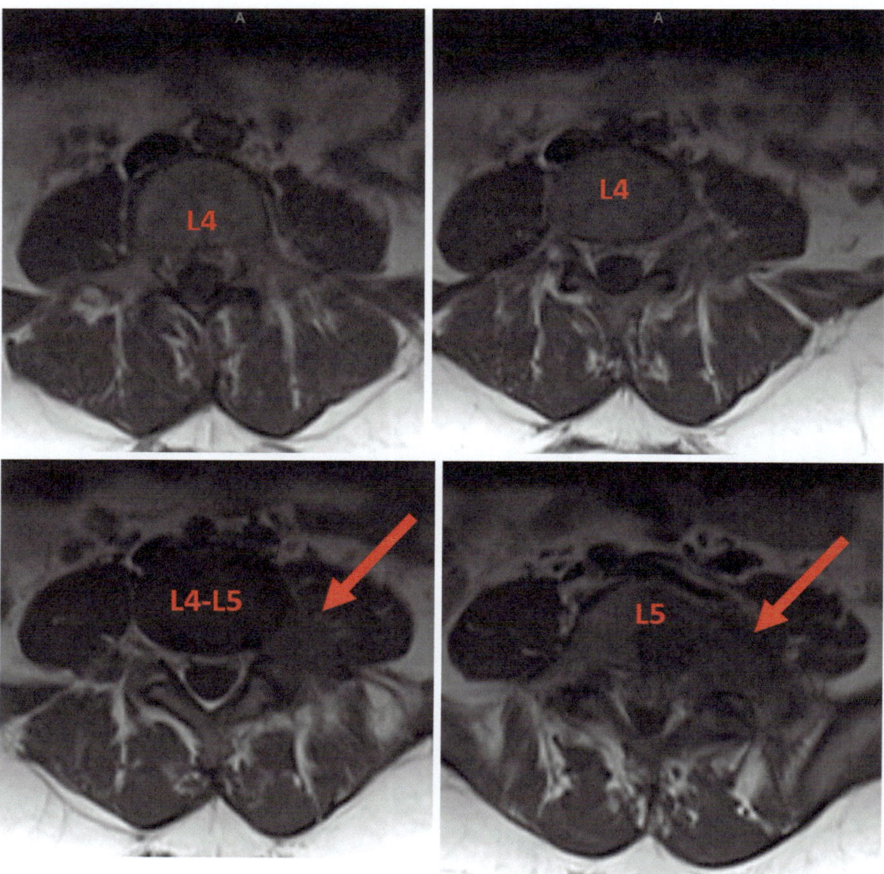

Fig. 27.3 Sequential axial MR cuts of the lower lumbar spine show the heterogenous, destructive, and expansile, although well contained, mass within the left-sided posterior elements of L5 (*arrows*)

Therefore, a marginal excision was performed, and the spine was stabilized with unilateral pedicle screws and a transforaminal interbody lumbar fusion (TLIF) from L4 to L5. Final pathology results demonstrated bony trabeculae lined by osteoblasts with uneven mineralization consistent with osteoblastoma (Fig. 27.7). Interestingly, the final histology also had evidence of giant cells surrounded by spindle cell proliferation without any cellular atypia (Fig. 27.7). These findings were interpreted as a case of a secondary ABC within an osteoblastoma, which can occur in up to 40% of cases. Both are benign lesions and the treatment protocol remains the same [15]. The patient tolerated the procedure well with complete resolution of all symptoms. Follow-up plain radiographs and surveillance CT images at 10 weeks postoperatively showed excellent fusion and resolution of the scoliosis (Fig. 27.8). Longer-term follow-up showed no recurrence and he resumed all sports.

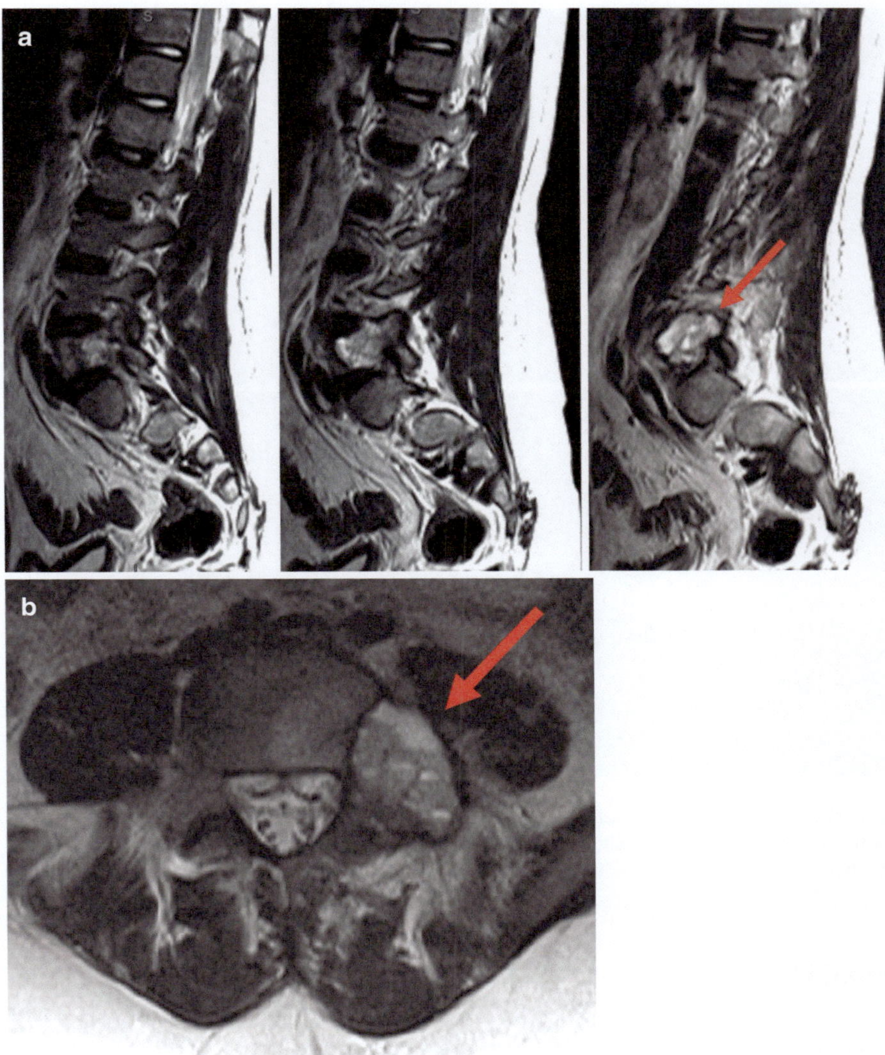

Fig. 27.4 (**a**) Sagittal cuts of the T2 MRI. This better demonstrates a heterogenous lesion within the L5 posterior elements. The fluid-fluid levels (*arrow*) and the well-circumscribed nature of the lesion are also seen here. (**b**) Axial cut of a T2 MRI at the L5 level which clearly shows the well-circumscribed nature of the growth as well as the fluid-fluid levels (*arrow*) which are indicative of a layering of blood and serous fluid when the patient is in the supine position in the MRI scanner

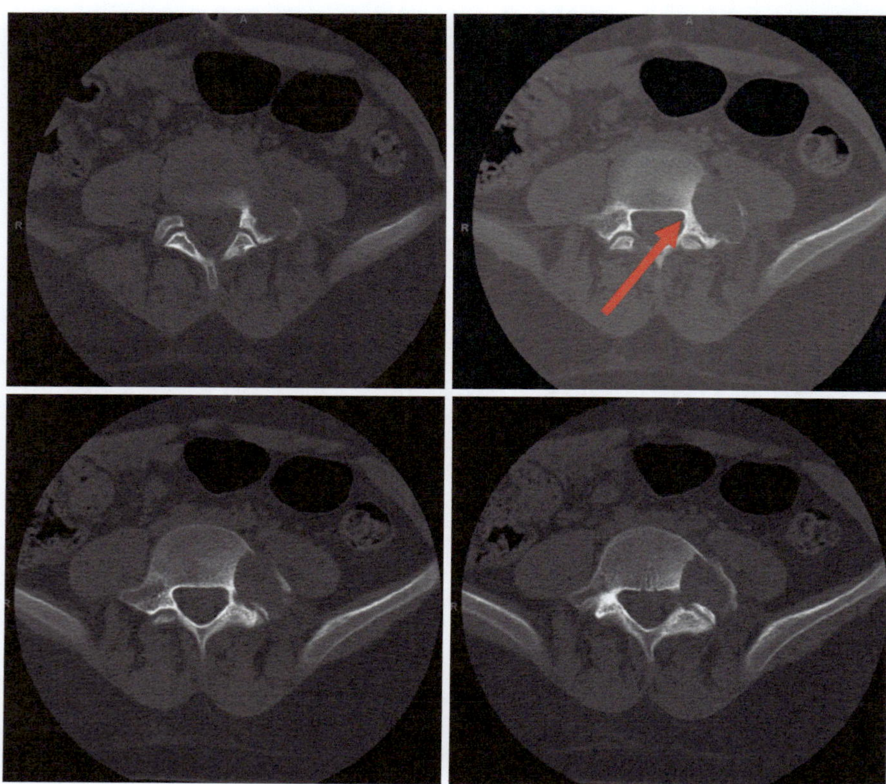

Fig. 27.5 Axial CT scan cuts of the L5 vertebral body demonstrate the lytic and expansile nature of the tumor. This also again shows that the growth is well contained and that the majority of the medial wall of the pedicle is uninterrupted (*arrow*), but not suitable for screw fixation after resection

Final Diagnosis

Osteoblastoma and ABC of L5 posterior elements on the left

How to Approach the Case (Fig. 27.9)

In a child or adolescent with persistent back pain refractory to NSAIDs, night time pain, and pain associated with development of new scoliosis, always be suspicious of infection or tumor. Spinal stiffness is also an abnormal finding, as are atypical features of the curve itself (no rotational component and a large trunk shift). Careful

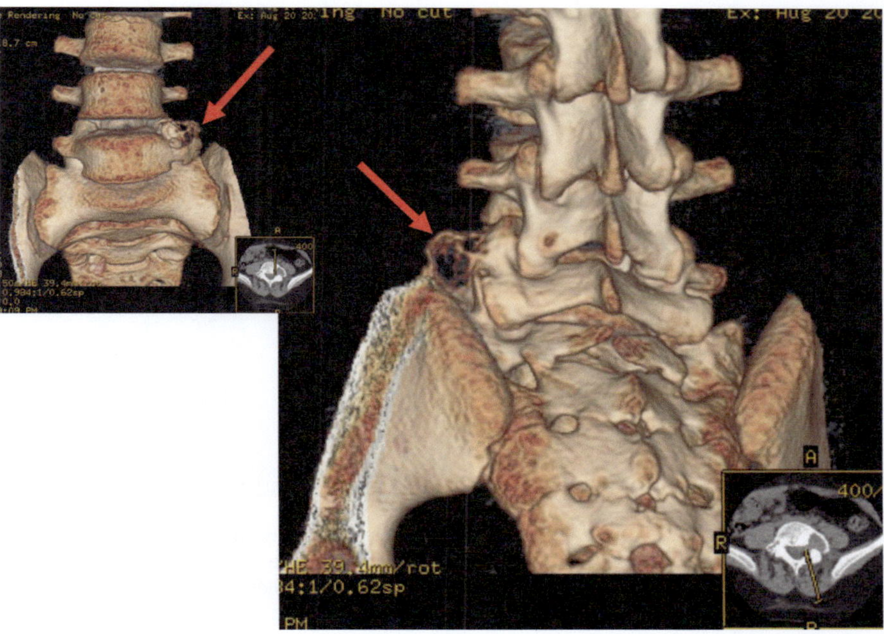

Fig. 27.6 3D reconstructions from the CT scan which again shows the lytic, lobulated mass within the posterolateral aspect of L5 on the left side (*arrows*)

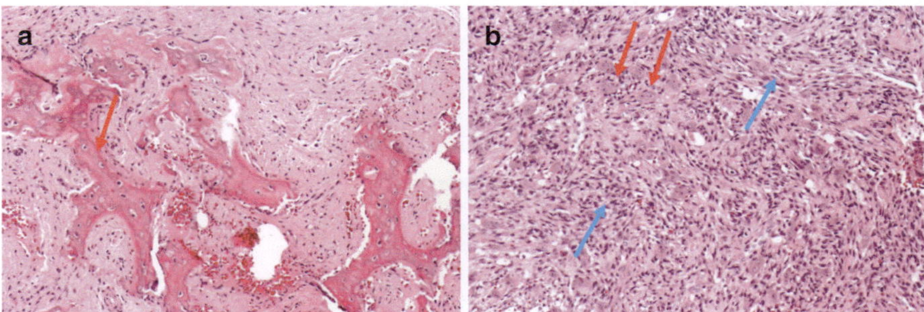

Fig. 27.7 Histologic images from intraoperative specimen of the tumor. (**a**) Areas of bony trabeculae (*red arrow*) lined by osteoblasts with uneven mineralization suggestive of an osteoblastoma. (**b**) Giant cells (*red arrows*) surrounded by florid spindle cell proliferation (*blue arrows*) without cellular atypia, suggestive of an ABC type tumor

history, physical examination, and review of X-rays are the essential three aspects of making an accurate diagnosis or for appropriate referral to a pediatric orthopedic surgeon. Advanced imaging studies such as MRI or CT scan can be instrumental in making the diagnosis and planning surgery.

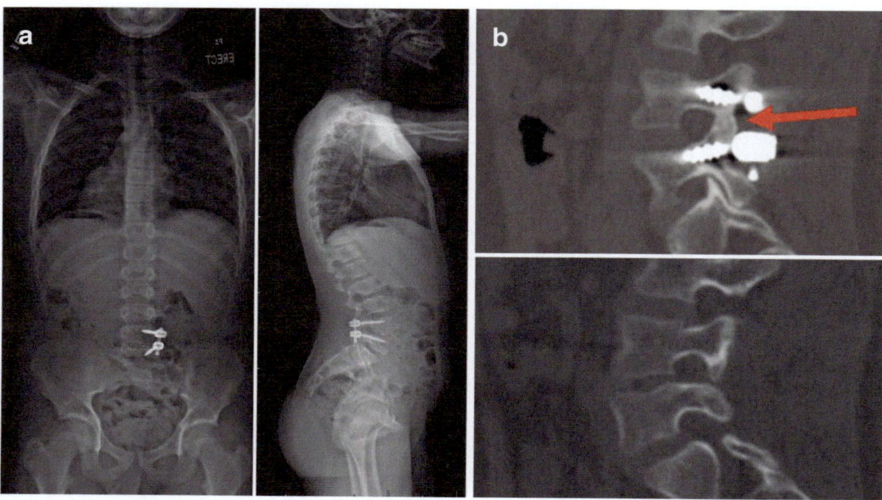

Fig. 27.8 X-rays and CT scan images, respectively, at approximately 10 weeks post-op (resection, fusion with interbody cage, and stabilization with unilateral pedicle screws). (**a**) Shows complete resolution of scoliosis and (**b**) shows that the implants are in excellent position with evidence of fusion posterolaterally (*arrow*) and in the interbody space

Fig. 27.9 How to approach the case

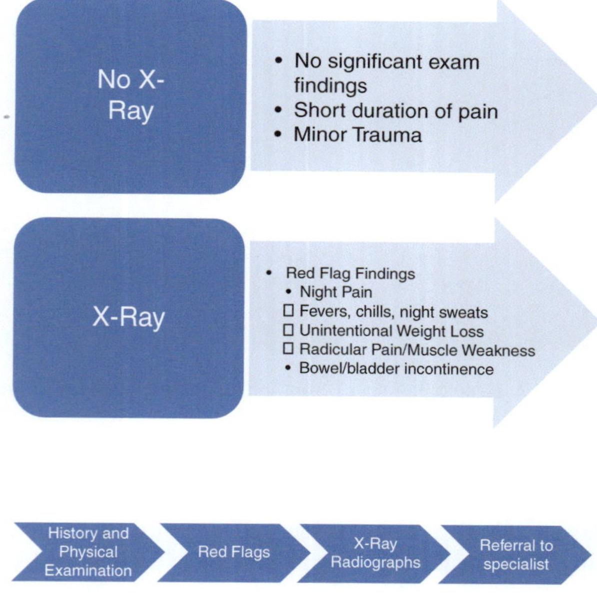

Natural History and Treatment Considerations

Although benign in nature, osteoblastomas and ABCs must be thoroughly excised in order to prevent recurrence. Recurrence rates of up to 20% for osteoblastomas and 25% for ABCs have been reported. Moreover, osteoblastomas have a small chance for metastases and for malignant transformation. In the process of appropriate and adequate removal, much of the structural elements of the spine, including the ligaments and bone, may be compromised. Therefore, treatment consists of not only removal of the tumor but also fusion and stabilization of the spine [1, 15, 16], if facets are violated or instability created.

Referral: When and to Whom?

Scoliosis that has atypical features such as significant pain, night pain, neurological symptoms or that has progressed to more than 20 degrees in a growing child should be referred to an orthopedic surgeon who has training, expertise, and experience in treating spinal deformities and spine tumors. In some instances, the tumor may be intradural or involve regions of the cervical spine where an orthopedic surgeon may not be comfortable operating. In these cases, the orthopedic surgeon may enlist the assistance of a neurosurgeon [1, 2, 5].

Discussion by Editors

Dr. Bob Hensinger of the University of Michigan, many years ago, taught us that back pain in children can be a symptom of infection or tumor. Additional red flags include night pain, pain associated with scoliosis, spine stiffness, neural symptoms, and neurologic findings. As illustrated by this case, an osteoblastoma is a benign (noncancerous) bone tumor. Adolescents are most often affected. The tumor is twice as common in males that in females. Because of the large size and destruction of normal bone by the osteoblastoma, surgery is necessary. This case is even more interesting because the pathology demonstrated additional findings consistent with an ABC. The causes of osteoblastomas and ABCs are unknown. Surgical excision may result in instability necessitating bone grafting, fusion, and instrumentation.

W.L. Hennrikus

It is very possible for a radiologist or a clinician to miss noticing a lesion on a plain radiograph. It is especially possible if the radiologist has given the image a "normal read" that the clinician will be influenced by the radiologist's report and either not directly examine the images or accept the normal report as accurate. When the clinical findings do not seem straightforward, or there are sufficient atypical findings, go back over the history, physical, and plain imaging studies, preferably with a wise colleague, and reexamine the actual X-ray, not just the report.

R.M. Schwend

A. R. Hariharan and S. A. Shah

References

1. Shah SA, Saller J. Evaluation and diagnosis of back pain in children and adolescents. J Am Acad Orthop Surg. 2016;24(1):37–45.
2. Bernstein RM, Cozen H. Evaluation of back pain in children and adolescents. Am Fam Physician. 2007;76(11):1669–76.
3. Payne WK, Ogilvie JW. Back pain in children and adolescents. Pediatr Clin N Am. 1996;43(4):899–917.
4. Hensinger RN. Acute back pain in children. Instr Course Lect. 1995;44:111–26.
5. Kordi R, Rostami M. Low back pain in children and adolescents: an algorithmic clinical approach. Iran J Pediatr. 2011;21(3):259–70.
6. Raskas DS, Graziano GP, Herzenberg JE, Heidelberger KP, Hensinger RN. Osteoid osteoma and osteoblastoma of the spine. J Spinal Disord. 1992;5(2):204–11.
7. Arkader A, Dormans JP. Osteoblastoma in the skeletally immature. J Pediatr Orthop. 2008;28(5):555–60.
8. Pettine KA, Klassen RA. Osteoid-osteoma and osteoblastoma of the spine. J Bone Joint Surg Am. 1986;68(3):354–61.
9. Herring J. The orthopaedic examination: a comprehensive overview. In: Tachdjian's pediatric orthopaedics from the Texas Scottish Rite Hospital for Children. 5th ed: Philadelphia: Saunders; 2013.
10. Riahi H, Mechri M, Barsaoui M, Bouaziz M, Vanhoenacker F, Ladeb M. Imaging of benign tumors of the osseous spine. J Belg Soc Radiol. 2018;102(1):13.
11. Canavese F, Dimeglio A. Normal and abnormal spine and thoracic cage development. World J Orthop. 2013;4(4):167–74.
12. Calloni SF, Huisman TA, Poretti A, Soares BP. Back pain and scoliosis in children: when to image, what to consider. Neuroradiol J. 2017;30(5):393–404.
13. Herring J. Imaging. In: Tachdjian's pediatric orthopaedics from the Texas Scottish Rite Hospital for Children. 5th ed. Philadelphia: Saunders; 2013.
14. Rapp TB, Ward JP, Alaia MJ. Aneurysmal bone cyst. J Am Acad Orthop Surg. 2012;20(4):233–41.
15. Harrop JS, Schmidt MH, Boriani S, Shaffrey CI. Aggressive "benign" primary spine neoplasms: osteoblastoma, aneurysmal bone cyst, and giant cell tumor. Spine. 2009;34(22 Suppl):S39–47.
16. Liu JK, Brockmeyer DL, Dailey AT, Schmidt MH. Surgical management of aneurysmal bone cysts of the spine. Neurosurg Focus. 2003;15(5):E4.

Chapter 28
A Middle School Student with Back Pain Due to a Heavy Backpack

Jessica M. Smith and Greg S. Canty

Brief Case Presentation

Chief Complaint

2-month history of low back pain

History

A 13-year-old girl presents with a 2-month history of intermittent low back pain. Pain is described as achy in her low back that does not radiate, is made worse by carrying her school backpack for long periods of time, and is alleviated with rest. The pain does not limit her from participating in school physical education activities nor does it wake her up at night. She does not participate in any organized sports. There are no bowel or bladder problems, recent illnesses, fevers, weight loss, morning stiffness, or lower extremity symptoms. Her parents are concerned that her backpack may be causing her pain. Her past medical history is unremarkable. Family history is negative for scoliosis, autoimmune disorders, or recent travel. Menarche was 2 months ago.

J. M. Smith (✉)
Pediatric Sports Medicine, Children's Mercy Kansas City, Kansas City, MO, USA

G. S. Canty
Sports Medicine Center, Pediatric Orthopaedic Surgery, Children's Mercy Kansas City, Kansas City, MO, USA

Department of Orthopaedic Surgery, University of Missouri-Kansas City School of Medicine, Kansas City, MO, USA

Department of Orthopaedic Surgery, University of Kansas School of Medicine, Kansas City, MO, USA

© Springer Nature Switzerland AG 2021
R. M. Schwend, W. L. Hennrikus (eds.), *Back Pain in the Young Child and Adolescent*, https://dci.org/10.1007/978-3-030-50758-9_28

"

Physical Examination

Weight 58.9 kg, height 160 cm, BMI 23 kg/m². She is healthy appearing, developmentally normal, and Tanner stage 4. Her back has no obvious curvature, erythema, or signs of trauma. There is no scoliosis or thoracic kyphosis on forward bend. A full active range of motion in flexion, extension, rotation, and side-bending is presented. Mild pain is reported with rotation and bending forward. There is no pain with extension-based maneuvers including the stork test. There is no paraspinal muscle pain or spinous process pain on palpation. Straight leg testing does not induce radicular pain. There is decreased core strength and control with single leg squats and unilateral gluteal bridge testing. Screening neurologic examination including sensory, motor, reflexes, and gait is normal.

Imaging and Radiographic Studies (Fig. 28.1)

Questions About the Case the Reader Should Consider
1. What is known about backpack use and adolescent back pain?
2. Why is it important to assess core strength and hamstring tightness when assessing a patient with back pain?

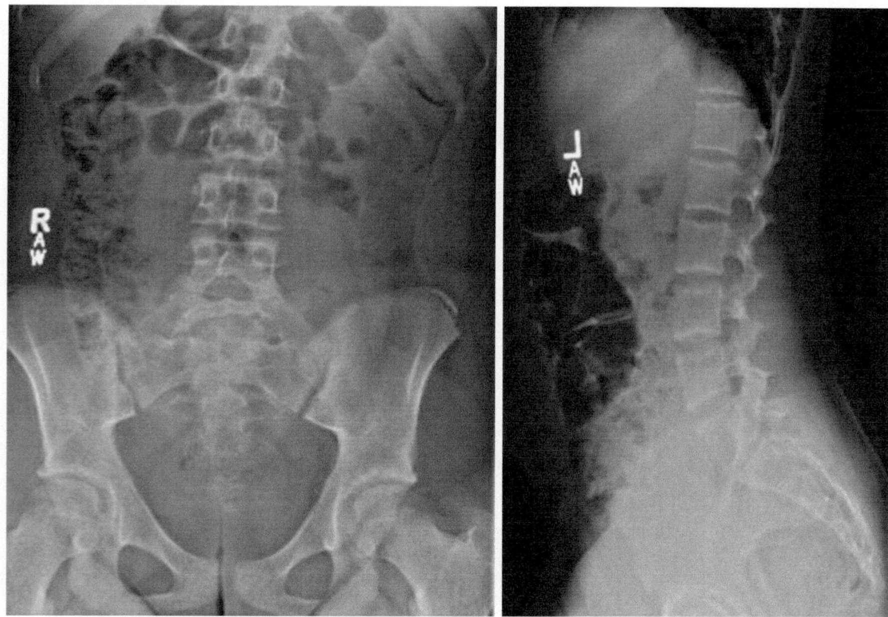

Fig. 28.1 Normal AP (left) and lateral (right) lumbar spine radiographs

3. What differential diagnosis should be considered with a complaint of low back pain?
4. Are there any other diagnostic tests that should be considered?

Discussion

Back pain is frequently reported by children and adolescents, with its prevalence increasing dramatically throughout adolescence from less than 10% in the pre-teenage years to 50% by middle adolescence [1]. The exact etiology of adolescent back pain is unknown; however, there has been recent and ongoing emphasis and concern regarding school backpacks as a potential cause [2, 3]. In studies looking at backpack use and back pain, several factors have been suggested as possible causes of back pain in adolescents including weight, type, and method of carrying (single strap, low on the back, cross-body single strap). However, a recent systematic review of research in this area has found no clear association between schoolbag characteristics and back pain in children and adolescents [2]. Heavy backpack loads or poorly distributed weight can put pressure on the lower back, shoulders, and neck. If the adolescent lacks the appropriate core muscle strength to maintain trunk stabilization, the back will compensate for an extended period of time, ultimately fatiguing, and lead to muscle imbalance. This muscle imbalance can cause an acute muscle strain, spasm, and back discomfort. To help decrease the burden of backpack use on the developing spine, The American Academy of Pediatrics has guidelines regarding safe backpack use (see below).

Examination of the pediatric back includes inspection of overall posture, spinal curvatures, and chest wall abnormalities; range of motion testing in flexion, extension, rotation, and lateral side bending and noting any pain; palpation of the spinous processes, paraspinal musculature, sacroiliac joints, and the hip/pelvic girdle; strength testing of the lower extremities and core musculature (trunk, pelvis, hips); and lastly a thorough neurological examination. Specifically testing patient's core muscle strength and hamstring flexibility are important, as poor core stability and tight hamstrings have been identified as risk factors for low back pain [4] (Figs. 28.2, 28.3, and 28.4). There are several clinical tests to assess core stability; however, an easy one for the busy pediatric office is the unilateral hip bridge test and single-legged squats [4, 5].

When presented with an adolescent patient having low back pain, the physicians should start with a broad differential diagnosis and narrow it following a thorough history and back examination. Factors to consider include duration of pain, location, aggravating and alleviating factors, participation in athletic activities/sports, and volume of repetitive motions.

If the history and physical examination are negative for red flags (see below) [6] and there is a high suspicion of mechanical low back pain, then lumbar radiographs are not required for diagnosis. However, if there is concern about other potential etiologies, it is reasonable for the physician to obtain an AP and lateral lumbar spine radiograph.

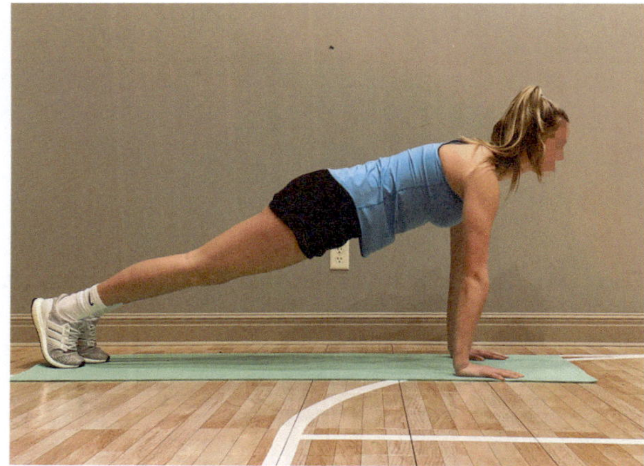

Fig. 28.2 Plank position with elbows extended. Have patient maintain a straight body posture as possible for 10 seconds

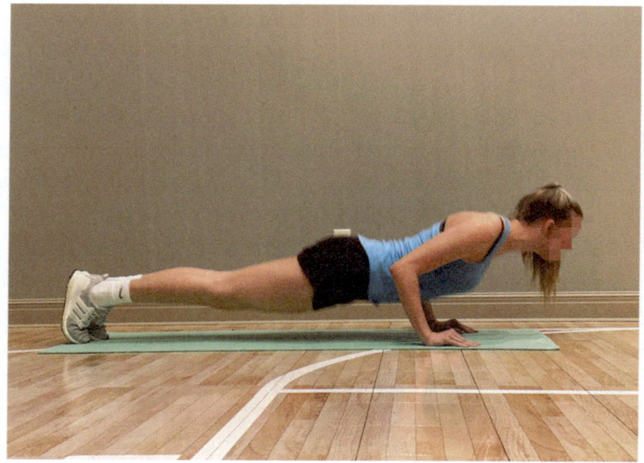

Fig. 28.3 Plank position with elbows bent. Maintain straight posture for 10 seconds, hands close to sides, body close to the floor but not touching. These positions test the strength of the trunk core muscles including the shoulder girdle

How to Approach the Case

Nonspecific low back pain is a common chief complaint in the primary care office. Features suggesting a diagnosis of mechanical low back pain include vague symptoms, worsening symptoms after exercise/activity that improve with rest and/ or stretching, and a normal physical examination with or without rotational pain if present. Always consider poor core muscle strength and tight lower extremity muscle groups as potential contributors to low back pain. Be mindful of atypical history and examination findings that may suggest more concerning pathology such as extension-based back pain (spondylolysis, especially in adolescent athletes), nocturnal symptoms (neoplasm, infection, trauma), neurological symptoms

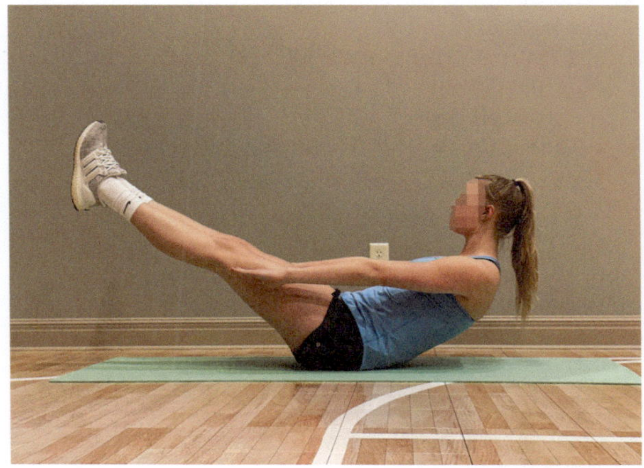

Fig. 28.4 Supine "V" position. Ask patient to first lift the lower extremities 30–40 degrees flexed at the hips with knees straight, then raise trunk 30–40 degrees and maintain this "V" position for 10 seconds. This tests strength and control of the anterior core muscles

(spondylolisthesis, intervertebral disc pathology), bowel and bladder dysfunction (spinal cord compression), or systemic symptoms (infection, neoplasm).

Although heavy backpacks and increased backpack weight to body weight ratios have been attributed to low back pain in adolescents in the past, it is likely not the backpack itself causing this patient's pain. The root cause is more likely attributed to poor core muscle strength and overall trunk stability which is aggravated by prolonged heavy backpack use.

Management of mechanical back pain includes relative rest from activities that exacerbate symptoms, physical therapy exercises to increase core muscle strength, and advocating for an active lifestyle. Educate patients and parents on current AAP recommendations including proper backpack wear, limiting backpack weight to 10–20% of the child's body weight, and trying to limit use and time wearing a backpack [7]. If pain persists despite an initial conservative approach, then routine referral to a specialist with expertise in adolescent back pain is warranted.

Red Flags for Low Back Pain with Backpack Use
- Younger child (age < 10)
- Nocturnal pain
- Bowel or bladder symptoms
- Neurological findings
- Pain not associated with activities or severe pain
- Pain with extension-based movements
- Systemic symptoms

> **Short Differential Diagnosis for Low Back Pain**
> - Musculoskeletal: mechanical back pain, paraspinal muscle spasm, spondylolysis
> - Inflammatory: ankylosing spondylitis
> - Neoplastic: leukemia, lymphoma
> - Infectious: discitis, osteomyelitis

Final Diagnosis

Mechanical low back pain with weak core muscles

Natural History and Treatment Considerations

Nonspecific musculoskeletal low back pain accounts for up to 50 percent of case presentations for back pain in the primary care office [8]. Mechanical back pain, synonymous with musculoskeletal back pain, refers to pain derived from the musculature and bony articulations of the spine. Typical presentation includes vague low back pain that is associated with physical activity, which gets better with rest. Physical examination will most likely be normal; however, there may be some tenderness to palpation of paraspinal musculature or pain with rotational movement.

Although the exact etiology of what causes mechanical adolescent back pain is unknown, poor core and trunk stabilizing muscle strength are a likely contributor. Several aspects of heavy backpack use have been proposed to contribute to mechanical back pain in adolescents, including improper use, increased backpack weight to body weight ratio, sedentary lifestyle, and female sex [2]; however, current systematic literature reviews suggest poor research evidence that weight of the backpack is the root cause of back pain.

Treatment considerations include rehabilitation with an emphasis on core strengthening, trunk stabilization, and stretching of the hamstring muscles [9].

Referral – Emergency, Urgent, or Routine: And to Whom?

Mechanical low back pain without atypical features or red flags can be managed by the primary care physician and does not need referral to a specialist. If pain persists despite conservative management, then consider a *routine* referral to specialists such as a pediatric sports medicine physician or a pediatric orthopedic surgeon.

AAP Guidelines for Backpack Safety [7]
- Backpack characteristics:

  - Wide padded shoulder straps
  - Two shoulder straps to evenly distribute the weight
  - Padded back
  - Waist strap
  - Lightweight backpack
  - Rolling backpack

- Guideline for safety while wearing backpack

  - Always wear both shoulder straps
  - Tighten the straps so that the backpack is close to the body and 2 inches above the waist
  - Backpack should weigh less than 10–20 percent of the student's body weight
  - Stop and unload unneeded items in school lockers when able or available

Brief Summary

Backpack use and weight have been suggested as possible causes of back pain in adolescents. Current literature reviews show that evidence is lacking to link backpack use and backpack characteristics with the increasing rates of adolescent back pain [2]. Any association is more likely related to fatigue and loss of core/trunk stabilization strength when carrying a backpack for extended periods of time. The American Academy of Pediatrics offers recommendations on the proper use, fit, and weight of backpacks as a means to decrease strain on the adolescent spine.

Key Features and Pearls
- Adolescent back pain is a common chief complaint in the primary care office, and the exact etiology of mechanical back pain is unknown.
- Mechanical back pain refers to pain due to the paraspinal muscles and bony structures of the spine and is typically worse with rotational movements.
- Mainstay of treatment includes increasing physical activity and trunk/core muscle development in adolescents and may require guided physical therapy to achieve this.

- Current evidence is lacking linking heavy backpack use as the cause of adolescent mechanical back pain; however, heavy backpack use may exacerbate mechanical low back pain symptoms in patients with weak core and trunk stabilizing musculature.
- Most importantly, low back pain that is associated with red flag symptoms should be investigated further to assess for more severe diagnoses.

Editor Discussion

Pediatric back pain due to backpacks is a "hot topic." The cause and effect is not completely clear. Confounding the situation is the fact that many middle school and high school student athletes are carrying not only a backpack to school but a laptop and a gym bag. The combined weight of these three objects often exceeds 20% of the patient's body weight. In addition, some schools have eliminated lockers due to vandalism, gang-related issues, and space constraints. No lockers compounds the problem because the student athlete then needs to carry the backpack, laptop, and gym bag from class to class during the day.

W.L. Hennrikus

For evaluating core trunk stability, I prefer to ask the child to do two simple tests:

1. Ten well-executed pushups (plank position) to test trunk and upper extremity strength. The child should have straight body alignment in up position (Fig. 28.2) and straight body position near the floor with hands positioned close to the sides (Fig. 28.3).
2. Holding a supine V position for 10 second with the shoulders and chest elevated from the table, hips flexed 30 degrees with the knees extended (Fig. 28.4).

   If the child cannot do these two tests, then they and their parents will readily see for themselves that they need to work on their core muscle strength.

R.M. Schwend

References

1. Sheir-Neiss GI, et al. The association of backpack use and back pain in adolescents. Spine (Phila Pa 1976). 2003;28(9):922–30.
2. Yamato TP, et al. Do schoolbags cause back pain in children and adolescents? A systematic review. Br J Sports Med. 2018;52(19):1241–5.
3. Skaggs DL, et al. Back pain and backpacks in school children. J Pediatr Orthop. 2006;26(3):358–63.
4. Butowicz CM, Ebaugh DD, Noehren B, Silfies SP. Validation of two clinical measures of Core stability. Sports Phys Ther. 2016;11(1):15–23.
5. Miller MM, Grooms D, Schussler E, et al. Single leg Glute bridge: a clinical test for gluteal muscle endurance. Med Sci Sports Exerc. 2013;45(5):430.
6. Premkumar A, Godfrey W, Gottschalk MB, Boden SD. Red flags for low back pain are not always really red: a prospective evaluation of the clinical utility of commonly used screening questions for low back pain. J Bone Joint Surg Am. 2018;100(5):368–74.

7. Back to School Tips on Getting the Year Off to a Good Start – from the American Academy of Pediatrics. AAP.org. https://www.aap.org/en-us/about-the-aap/aap-press-room/news-features-and-safety-tips/Pages/Back-to-School-Tips-Getting-the-Year-Off-to-a-Good-Start-from-the-AAP.aspx. Published 2018. Accessed 15 Mar 2019.
8. Nigrovic, P. Evaluation of the child with back pain. In: Drutz J, et al. UpToDate. Waltham: UpToDate; 2019. www.uptodate.com. Accessed 13 Mar 2019.
9. Anderson, Steven J., and Sally S. Harris. Care of the Young Athlete. 2nd ed., Am Acad Pediatr, 2010, pp. 341–342.

Additional AAP Resources

HealthyChildrenOrg – Back Pain in Children & Teens. Available online at: https://www.healthychildren.org/English/health-issues/conditions/orthopedic/Pages/Back-Pain-in-Children-Teens.aspx. Accessed 2/26/2020.
HealthyChildrenOrg – Backpack Safety. Available online at: https://www.healthychildren.org/English/safety-prevention/at-play/Pages/Backpack-Safety.aspx. Accessed 2/26/2020.
Pediatric patient education. Patient education Handouts - Core exercises (Care of the Young Athlete). Available online at: https://patiented.solutions.aap.org/handout.aspx?gbosid=156779. Accessed 2/26/2020.

Chapter 29
Case of an Obese Adolescent with Back Pain: Studies Normal

Natalie Ronshaugen and Kody Moffatt

Brief Case Presentation

This 12-year-old girl had been having frequent complaints of back pain after sliding into home plate while playing softball. She continued to have pain with physical activity particularly softball and seemed to be having more pain and difficulty than the other girls. Her mother and coach commented that she "looked like an old lady walking out onto the field." Her past medical history is negative for any significant musculoskeletal pathology. Her family history is negative for Charcot-Marie-Tooth (CMT) disease or other peripheral neuropathies. Her father and multiple fraternal family members have feet with "high arches" similar to our patient.

Physical Examination

Weight 83 kg, height 163 cm, BMI 31 (>95% for age and sex). She is otherwise healthy and developmentally normal. Her exam demonstrated bilateral lumbar paraspinous muscular pain and tenderness at the L1 to L3 levels with minimal midline symptoms which mildly increased with left-sided side bending. She had normal active range of motion in all planes, no point tenderness, no midline defects, negative Stork sign bilaterally, equal leg lengths, equal shoulder height, no trapezial fullness, balanced trunk shift, and normal waistline symmetry; her neurologic exam was normal. She was also noted to have forefoot pronation with a significantly elevated medial arch and calcaneal supination consistent with cavovarus feet.

N. Ronshaugen (✉) · K. Moffatt
Sports Medicine, Orthopedics, Children's Hospital & Medical Center Omaha, Omaha, NE, USA
e-mail: nronshaugen@childrensomaha.org

© Springer Nature Switzerland AG 2021
R. M. Schwend, W. L. Hennrikus (eds.), *Back Pain in the Young Child and Adolescent*, https://doi.org/10.1007/978-3-030-50758-9_29

Radiographs of her spine were normal (negative for bony pathology). Non-contrasted magnetic resonance imaging (MRI) of her spine was performed due to her physical finding of bilateral cavovarus feet (not her back pain). This demonstrated bone marrow edema in the pedicles and possibly the pars interarticularis of the fifth lumbar vertebra without evidence of spondylolisthesis, potentially indicating a stress injury or stress fracture. This radiographic finding did not correlate with the location of pain.

Imaging and Radiographic Studies *(Figs. 29.1, 29.2, 29.3, and 29.4)*

Questions About the Case the Reader Should Consider

1. What is the epidemiology of obesity in children and adolescents in the United States?
2. What is the association between obesity and musculoskeletal pain?

Fig. 29.1 Standing lateral radiograph of the entire spine demonstrating no bony pathology, specifically no evidence of spondylolysis or spondylolisthesis

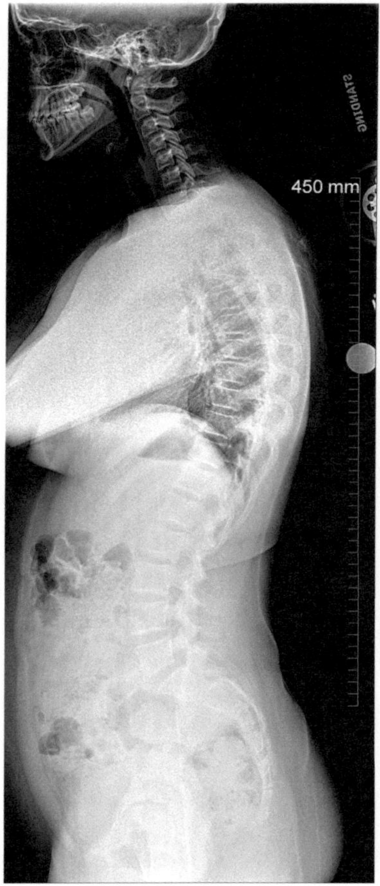

Fig. 29.2 Standing lateral radiograph of the lumbar spine demonstrating no bony pathology, specifically no evidence of spondylolysis or spondylolisthesis

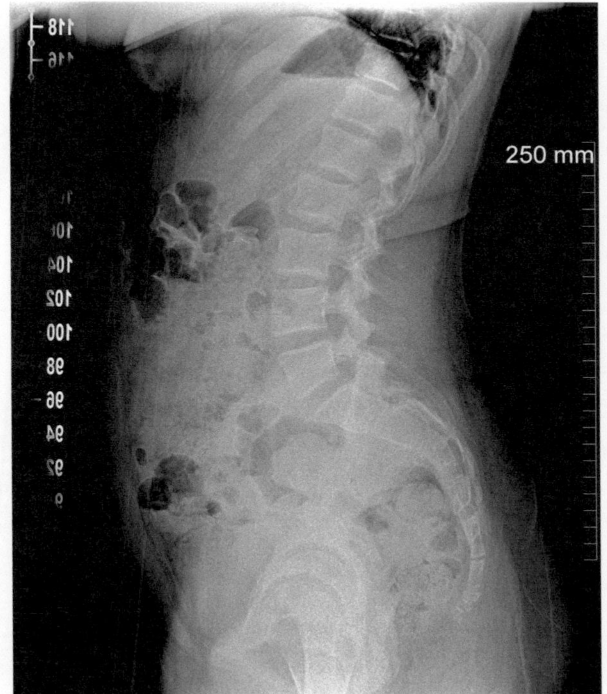

3. What is the most likely diagnosis for the patient's back pain?
4. When is imaging indicated for a complaint of low back pain?
5. If she had presented for back pain only, would imaging be indicated?
6. What is the natural history of a spondylolysis injury, including mechanism of injury, pain pattern, and physical exam?
7. Why is imaging of the back important for the evaluation of cavovarus feet?
8. What is the most appropriate way to treat her back pain?

Discussion

The differential diagnosis of this 12-year-old female with low back pain, obesity, and cavovarus feet includes muscular strain, bony pathology (e.g., spondylolysis, spondylolisthesis, etc.), neuropathic pain (e.g., CMT, genetic sensory or autonomic neuropathy), degenerative disk disease, rheumatologic disease (e.g., ankylosing spondylitis), infection (e.g., osteomyelitis), pancreatitis, renal disease (e.g., pyelonephritis), and gastrointestinal etiology (e.g., constipation). Like any other condition, the diagnostic workup should flow from the history and physical examination.

The worldwide prevalence of pediatric obesity has increased severalfold in recent years. Obese children can develop serious health, medical, and psychosocial complications. They are at increased risk for breathing disorders such as sleep

Fig. 29.3 T2-weighted magnetic resonance imaging sagittal view of the entire spine demonstrating no bony pathology, tethered spinal cord, or syrinx

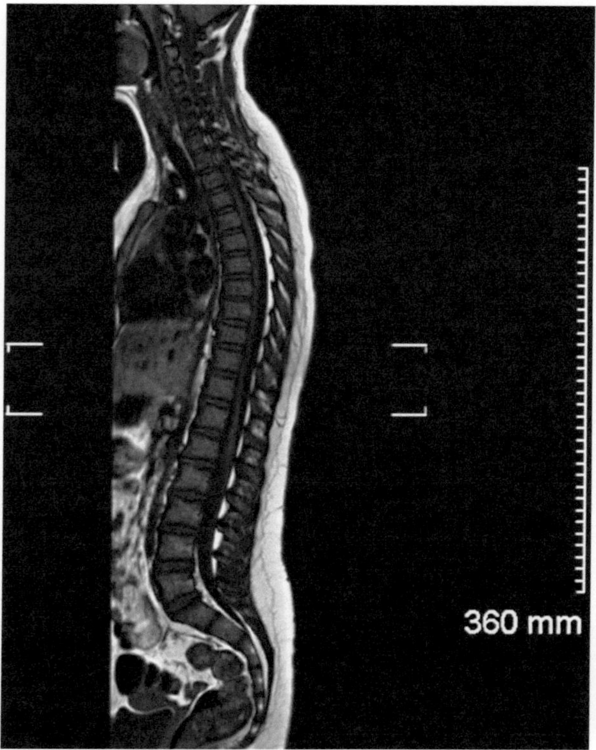

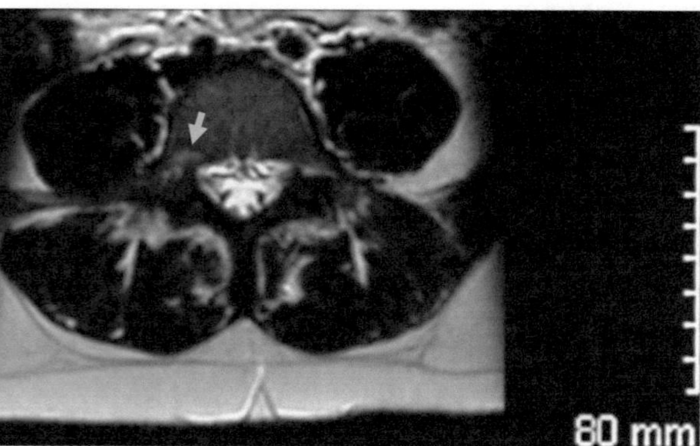

Fig. 29.4 T2-weighted magnetic resonance imaging axial view of the fifth lumbar vertebrae demonstrating bone marrow edema in the pedicles and possibly the pars interarticularis without evidence of spondylolisthesis, potentially indicating a stress injury or stress fracture. This radiographic finding did not correlate with the location of pain

apnea, metabolic syndrome, type 2 diabetes, depression, liver and gall bladder pathology, gastroesophageal reflux, hypertension, elevated cholesterol, and musculoskeletal pain [1]. These short- and long-term health problems may continue into adult life [1, 2]. Obesity specifically has been associated with an increased incidence of low back pain in the past 12 months [3].

While the association between obesity and low back pain is commonly reported, there may not be a direct causal relationship between the two. With regard to sedentary lifestyle, both extremes have been associated with back pain, very sedentary and highly active [4]. Overweight and obese children report musculoskeletal pain primarily due to changes causing muscular pain and additional pain with articulating joints and as a result of fractures. However, while parents often attribute their decreased activity level to their weight, children are more likely to report that pain is in fact limiting them [2, 5].

Low back pain in youth has been linked to obesity, early degeneration of intervertebral discs, rapid growth spurts, female sex, smoking, and psychosocial risk factors [3, 6]. The relationship between increase in BMI, weight, and pain demonstrates a risk factor for damage to the musculoskeletal structure, and this damage is often expressed by the child as pain [5]. Evidence is emerging to suggest that a reduction in physical functioning of obese and overweight children may occur and be evident through the child's expression of pain, further impacting on their self-esteem resulting in a poorer quality of life [2, 5].

Changes to the musculoskeletal system in overweight and obese children have been shown to negatively influence motor performance, including muscle strength, balance, and walking. The reporting of musculoskeletal pain by overweight children may reflect a significant marker of a reduction in osteoarticular health and changes to skeletal structure. In children, there appear to be links between bone health, pain, physical activity, and quality of life [2].

The relationship between being overweight and musculoskeletal pain might induce a vicious circle in which being overweight, having musculoskeletal pain, and low fitness level reinforce each other. After an episode of back pain, body mass index (BMI) also has been found to continue to increase in children and adolescents [6].

Muscle strain is a very common cause of back injury. Back pain, in the absence of any of focal bony or neurologic findings, and with tenderness over the paraspinal muscles, particularly in the setting of an acute injury, is consistent with muscle strain. In such cases, imaging is not helpful [4, 7]. Treatment for back strain consists of physical rehabilitation, focused on pain management, movement control, flexion, strength training, and functional optimization.

Spondylolysis is a stress injury of the pars interarticularis which our patient did not have but is in the differential diagnosis. Most commonly, the injury occurs at L5 (85–95%) followed by L4 (5–15%). Studies have shown an incidence of pars defect to be 3–5% in the general population and 11–15% of adolescent athletes; however, most of these are asymptomatic [8]. Symptomatic spondylolysis is most frequently seen in adolescent athletes who repetitively arch their backs for their sport (e.g., gymnasts, divers, football linemen, weight lifters, and wrestlers) [8]. The repetitive extension of the lumbar spine stresses the pars and puts it at risk of stress injury. Patients with spondylolysis classically present with focal low back pain that worsens over time. Presenting after an acute injury is less common. The pain will occasionally be reported as radiating into the buttocks or upper thigh [8]. Patients generally have a hyperlordotic posture with tight hamstrings [8]. Pain with extension, while standing on one leg (Stork sign), is thought by many to be pathognomonic [8].

In the case of this patient, imaging was obtained, not because of her back pain but because of a clinical finding of cavovarus feet. Cavovarus foot deformity is characterized by abnormally elevated medial arch and supination of the calcaneus and is associated with neurologic abnormalities, both progressive, such as CMT, spinal cord tumors, and an early sign of Freidreich's ataxia, as well as nonprogressive causes like poliomyelitis, cerebral palsy, tethered spinal cord, and syrinx [9]. A complete neurologic evaluation should be completed at the time a cavovarus foot is identified. Evaluation for spinal dysraphism or tumor would include spine radiographs and/or MRI.

Again, this patient had no abnormal neurologic findings on exam, but because cavovarus foot deformity can be caused by neurologic pathology, a full evaluation was pursued, including MRI of the spine. In ordering an imaging study directed at evaluating her cavovarus foot deformity, a positive result would be primarily due to pathology affecting the nerve roots and spinal cord [9]. While no cause of her foot deformity was found on her imaging, she did have subtle edema noted in the pedicle and/or pars interarticularis at the L5 level. Spondylolysis in an early stage, without significant spondylolisthesis, is not associated with cavovarus foot deformity.

There is a temptation to image all adolescents with back pain in order to not miss a specific anatomic cause of their back pain such as spondylolysis. However, unnecessary imaging is expensive and can result in unrelated incidental findings [4]. Without specific concern for spondylolysis on history and clinical exam, one may find an asymptomatic spondylolysis and not actually find the source of the patient's pain. There is no difference in outcomes between patients with nonspecific back pain who received imaging immediately versus those who were treated conservatively for 3 months and then received imaging. In fact, in most cases of nonspecific back pain, a cause cannot be identified on imaging [7]. Increased imaging in nonspecific low back pain has been linked to increased injections and surgeries [4].

Imaging should be considered when a diagnosis of tumor, disc herniation, fracture, or spondylolysis is consistent with history and physical exam. History of unintentional weight loss, night sweats, or pain that keeps them up at night is concerning for tumor. History of radicular pain, positive straight leg raise, or cross straight leg raise is consistent with disc herniation. Saddle anesthesia, bowel or bladder dysfunctions, and lower extremity weakness are associated with cauda equina syndrome. Athletes with midline point tenderness or extension causing back pain raise concern for spondylolysis. History of trauma, midline point tenderness, step-offs, or crepitus is consistent with spine fracture [4].

Since spondylolysis on imaging is found in 11–15% of adolescent athletes, with or without symptoms, it is important to evaluate if her back pain seems to be secondary to the spondylolysis [8]. Edema in the pars, in the setting of slowly progressive back pain with extension, would cause concern that her back pain was secondary to spondylolysis. However, our patient's back pain was acute and primarily in her paraspinal muscles. Her presentation was therefore unlikely secondary to the spondylolysis and more likely from a muscle strain.

Once made aware of an incidental finding, even if not felt to be causing symptoms, the question becomes: Should it be treated? Some incidental findings warrant treatment, as is the case of an incidental finding of malignancy. In the case of true and symptomatic spondylolysis, 62–75% of early stage spondylolysis cases undergo bone healing. Bony healing can be obtained with or without bracing but does require relative rest and may benefit from physical rehabilitation. Even without radiographic healing, excellent clinical outcomes can be achieved [8]. Meaning that successful treatment is resolution of symptoms and not necessarily bone healing.

Our patient was treated with physical rehabilitation with a presumed muscular source of her back pain and responded well to her treatment. She returned to activities of daily living including competitive sports without pain.

Low back pain can also be treated with analgesic medications. Primarily nonsteroidal anti-inflammatory drugs (NSAIDs) and muscle relaxants have been found to be clinically helpful. Paracetamol is ineffective in treating back pain. Opioids have not fully been evaluated for benefit. With any analgesic medication, risks of side effects should be weighed against the benefits of pain relief [4].

In order to comprehensively treat nonspecific back pain in an adolescent or child with obesity, the obesity itself should be addressed as well. Treatment for obesity should include lifestyle changes which incorporate the whole family. Children and adolescents should be encouraged to engage in moderate to vigorous exercise at least 20 minutes but ideally 60 minutes daily, and nonacademic screen time should be limited to no more than 1–2 hours. They should also be counseled on decreasing fast foods, high-fat, high-sodium, or processed foods, added sugars including eliminating sugar-sweetened beverages. Increasing dietary fiber, fruits, and vegetables should be encouraged. A complete look at daily stressors and family dynamics should also be completed as this often significantly contributes to weight loss outcomes. Many institutions have comprehensive weight loss programs for children and adolescents, and these should be considered for obese and very obese patients when they are available [10].

How to Approach This Case

The history of an acute event (such as sliding into home plate) followed by low back pain with activity without radicular symptoms is most consistent with a muscular etiology such as a paraspinous muscle strain. Bony injuries such as spondylolysis or spondylolisthesis are also possible. Midline back pain which does not resolve within 3 months, or back pain with extension should prompt an evaluation with x-rays [7, 11]. It is important to note the advanced imaging in our case was performed to evaluate for findings associated with cavovarus feet and shuffling gait such as a tethered spinal cord, CMT, or syrinx [9]. These were not found in our case, but our patient did have subtle suggestions of edema in the L5 pars interarticularis or more specifically the pedicle. The location of pain by history and physical exam findings did not correlate with pathology at this location, and her neurologic examination was normal. Advanced imaging studies such as computerized tomography (CT) or MRI can produce findings which may or may not be related to the actual cause of the pain and should not be used to search for a diagnosis, but to confirm an already suspected diagnosis or to evaluate for specific known associated findings. The patient became pain free and returned to normal activity after a brief course of physical rehabilitation which has been demonstrated to be an effective treatment for muscular back pain [4]. Physical exercise is an important nonpharmacological treatment for low back pain and obesity.

> **Red Flags Requiring Imaging in Low Back Pain of the Child or Adolescent Athlete**
> - Midline point tenderness
> - Positive stork sign or extension back pain
> - Positive straight leg raise, slump test, or cross straight leg raise
> - Numbness or weakness of the lower extremities
> - Step offs or crepitus along the spine
> - Visible deformity
> - Saddle anesthesia
> - Bowel or bladder dysfunction
> - Fever or Night sweats
> - Unintentional weight loss

> **Short Differential Diagnosis**
> - Muscle strain – Common in athletes. Her acute onset of pain and location of tenderness is most consistent with this diagnosis.
> - Symptomatic spondylolysis – A thorough exam that includes evaluation for extension pain should be done in the setting of incidental finding on MRI when back pain is noted in history.
> - Nonspecific low back pain – While athletes tend to have a cause for their back pain, nonspecific low back pain is common in the general population and is more common in adolescents with obesity.

Final Diagnosis

Lumbar strain

Natural History and Treatment Considerations

Low back pain is the most common type of back pain, often begins in childhood, has high recurrence, and can return more intensely than previously experienced [11]. The majority of children with low back pain presenting to the sports medicine clinic have an underlying musculoskeletal or biomechanical cause [11]. Fortunately, muscular back pain/muscular strain often responds well to conservative treatment such as physical rehabilitation and/or a brief course of pharmacological therapy.

Pediatric or childhood obesity is a growing global epidemic that requires attention due to the burden placed on the healthcare system for children and adults [1]. Obesity affects 34% of children in the United States and is considered a top public health concern due to the high level of morbidity and mortality [1].

The link between being overweight and musculoskeletal pain might induce a vicious cycle in which being overweight, musculoskeletal problems, and low fitness level reinforce each other [12]. The importance of effective weight loss interventions for overweight children is evident if the cycle of being overweight and musculoskeletal pain is to be broken [12]. The use of imaging is guided by history and physical examination. The use of diagnostic radiographs is controversial, and there is no universal imaging screening protocol [11]. Advanced imaging such as CT or MRI should be reserved to either confirm a diagnosis (if needed) or evaluate for other comorbid pathology [11].

In this case, radiographs and MRI failed to demonstrate definitive pathology. Bone marrow edema was noted in a location which did not correlate with her history or physical exam likely representing an incidental finding. She responded well to physical therapy, her pain resolved, and she returned to normal function. Obesity is an independent risk factor for back pain [6] and likely was a contributing factor in her course.

Referral – Emergency, Urgent, or Routine: And to Whom?

Low back pain is common and infrequently catastrophic, particularly in childhood and adolescence [4]. However, emergent referral is necessary in the case of potential permanent nerve damage, as would be the case for a confirmed cauda equina syndrome, spinal infection, or severe neurological deficits, which require emergent surgical intervention. Tumor identification requires urgent referral, unless it is associated with acute neurologic findings, in which case emergent referral may be necessary. Given that spondylolysis generally has a good prognosis, they can often be managed in a primary care setting, if the stress injury is in its early stages. Routine referral to orthopedics would be appropriate for lesions which are more advanced or symptomatic. Urgent referral would be more appropriate in the case of acute spondylolisthesis or shifting of the vertebrae. Symptomatic significant slipping is traditionally treated with fusion, and lower grade slips are treated nonoperatively with nonsteroidal anti-inflammatory drugs, activity restriction to avoid excessive lumbar extension, physical rehabilitation, and sometimes bracing.

Since obesity and lifestyle have been associated with low back pain, and because nonspecific low back pain has a propensity to recur, addressing these issues is an important part of treatment. Appropriate referrals to nutrition and comprehensive obesity programs and discussions about over training are important [6].

Brief Summary

Low back pain is a common problem among children and adolescents; however, permanent or catastrophic outcomes are rare. Radiologic, anatomic causes of back pain are infrequent, though incidental findings and false-positives are common. Treatment for nonspecific low back pain should be focused on physical rehabilitation and lifestyle changes. Imaging should be reserved for specific concerning findings, which might alter management.

Obesity is strongly associated with musculoskeletal pain, including low back pain. Treatment of children and adolescents with obesity and low back pain should include both addressing their current weight and working to prevent further weight gain in the setting of back pain.

Key Features and Pearls
- Back pain without red flag symptoms concerning for fracture, disc herniation, tumor, infection, or spondylolysis does not require imaging. Imaging should not be pursued unless specifically evaluating specific worrisome findings.
- Cavovarus foot formation requires a thorough neurologic exam and possible hip and back images to evaluate for a neurologic cause including Charcot-Marie-Tooth.
- Imaging findings should always be correlated with the history and physical exam before diagnosis can be made in order to avoid placing causation on an asymptomatic finding.

Editor Discussion

Lumbar sprain is a diagnosis of exclusion. A detailed history and careful physical exam are key. Plain films are indicated in most patients such as in this patient with a minor trauma from siding into home plate. If the patient with presumed lumbar sprain does not improve after 6 weeks of conservative treatment, then referral is indicated. Findings such as night pain, weight loss, fever, neurologic deficits, or a history of a significant trauma should prompt an urgent referral.

W.L. Hennrikus

Back pain related to general musculoskeletal strain, weak core muscles, and general deconditioning is common. Spondylolysis and stress reaction in the pars interarticularis, especially at L5 level is also common, seen in up to 15% of the adolescent population. Uncommon, but seen in this patient, was a presumed diagnosis of CMT, which should be confirmed by genetic testing. Hereditary motor and sensory neuropathies types 1 and III have associated enlarged peripheral nerves, and back pain has been described as the most common anatomic site for pain, more common than pain in the lower extremities or feet. Although very unlikely to be present at this young age, there have been reports of severe back pain due to cauda equina syndrome related to hypertrophied nerve roots that can be found in CMT or chronic inflammatory demyelinating polyneuropathy (CIDP). Once the diagnosis of CMT or other peripheral neuropathy is made, referral to a pediatric neurologist is necessary to confirm the diagnosis, which nowadays is performed by genetic testing. If genetic testing does not confirm CMT, electrophysiologic testing will confirm a peripheral neuropathy such as CIDP. With a normal MRI, this patient's back pain can be treated as typical musculoskeletal back pain.

R.M. Schwend

References

1. Xu S, Xue Y. Pediatric obesity: causes, symptoms, prevention and treatment. Exp Ther Med. 2016;11(1):15–20.
2. Smith SM, Sumar B, Dixon KA. Musculoskeletal pain in overweight and obese children. Int J Obes. 2014;38(1):11–5.
3. Mikkonen PH, Laitinen J, Remes J, Tammelin T, Taimela S, Kaikkonen K, et al. Association between overweight and low back pain: a population-based prospective cohort study of adolescents. Spine (Phila Pa 1976). 2013;38(12):1026–33.
4. Maher C, Underwood M, Buchbinder R. Non-specific low back pain. Lancet. 2017;389(10070):736–47.
5. Taylor ED, Theim KR, Mirch MC, Ghorbani S, Tanofsky-Kraff M, Adler-Wailes DC, et al. Orthopedic complications of overweight in children and adolescents. Pediatrics. 2006;117(6):2167–74.
6. Jones GT, Macfarlane GJ. Epidemiology of low back pain in children and adolescents. Arch Dis Child. 2005;90(3):312–6.
7. Chou R. In the clinic. Low back pain. Ann Intern Med. 2014;160(11):ITC6-1.
8. Standaert CJ, Herring SA. Spondylolysis: a critical review. Br J Sports Med. 2000;34(6):415–22.
9. Schwend RM, Drennan JC. Cavus foot deformity in children. J Am Acad Orthop Surg. 2003;11(3):201–11.

10. Styne DM, Arslanian SA, Connor EL, Farooqi IS, Murad MH, Silverstein JH, Yanovski JA. Pediatric obesity—assessment, treatment, and prevention: an endocrine society clinical practice guideline. J Clin Endocrinol Metab. 2017 Mar 1;102(3):709–57.
11. Taxter AJ, Chauvin NA, Weiss PF. Diagnosis and treatment of low back pain in the pediatric population. Phys Sportsmed. 2014;42(1):94–104.
12. Paulis WD, Silva S, Koes BW, van Middelkoop M. Overweight and obesity are associated with musculoskeletal complaints as early as childhood: a systematic review. Obes Rev. 2014;15(1):52–67.

Chapter 30
Case of an Immigrant Child with Back Pain Due to Tuberculosis

Krishn Khanna, Mathew Varghese, and Sanjeev Sabharwal

Case Presentation

Chief Complaint

Back pain after a fall

History

A 3-year-old child from Mumbai, India, presented after a fall from a height of 5 feet. He could get up after the fall. The parents took him to a local hospital where after examination they were told all was well and the child was sent home. A few weeks later, he complained of back pain, was seen as an outpatient, and prescribed over-the-counter analgesics.

Two months after initial presentation, he started having low-to-moderate grade fever, with the highest recorded temperature being 101 °F, without a definite pattern. He was taken to a local practitioner who prescribed antipyretics and also ordered a peripheral smear for malaria, a Widal test for enteric fever, and a routine urinalysis.

K. Khanna
Department of Orthopaedic Surgery, University of California – San Francisco, San Francisco, CA, USA

M. Varghese
Department of Orthopaedics, St. Stephen's Hospital, New Delhi, Delhi, India

S. Sabharwal (✉)
Department of Orthopaedic Surgery, University of California – San Francisco, Benioff Children's Hospital of Oakland, Oakland, CA, USA

© Springer Nature Switzerland AG 2021
R. M. Schwend, W. L. Hennrikus (eds.), *Back Pain in the Young Child and Adolescent*, https://doi.org/10.1007/978-3-030-50758-9_30

All were normal. The fever did not resolve over the course of the next week, and the patient was empirically started on Amoxicillin/Clavulanic acid for a presumed diagnosis of enteric fever.

Imaging and Radiographic Studies

Imaging was obtained 10 days later. Initial radiographs were all AP images (no Lateral views) and were normal (Fig. 30.1).

During the next 3 months, the patient underwent additional testing and symptomatic treatments, which did not provide a diagnosis nor pain relief. Testing including imaging (numerous chest and abdominal radiographs as well as an abdominal ultrasound) were all normal.

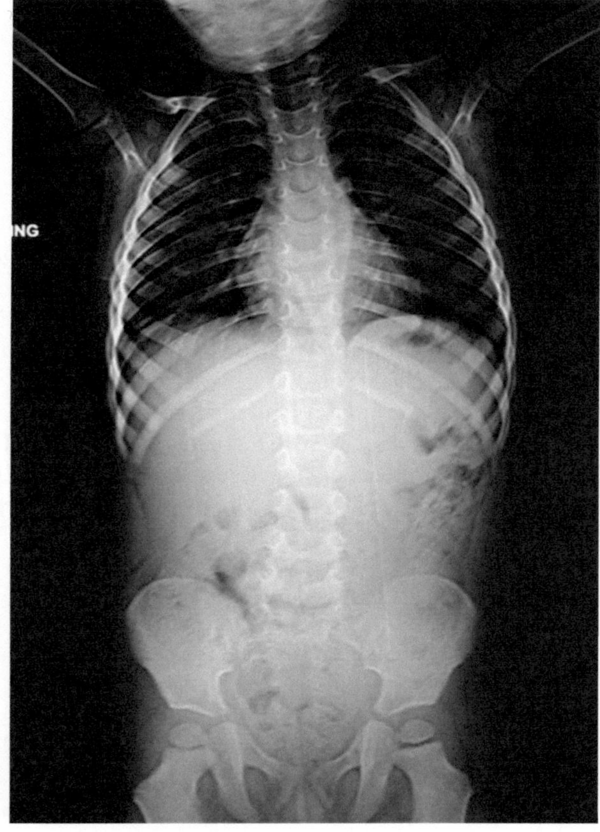

Fig. 30.1 Initial radiographs of the patient were all AP images and showed no obvious abnormality

Laboratory Testing

Laboratory tests including CBC, ESR and urinalysis. Tests for enteric fever and malaria were repeated. All were normal. Suspecting smear negative malaria, chloroquine was started. He was also placed on a second course of antibiotics for possible enteric fever. The patient continued to be febrile and began to lose weight – approximately 3 lbs. in the last 3 months. The parents also noticed that he had started to stoop forward while walking. He had no bowel or bladder symptoms.

Physical Examination

On examination, he was very apprehensive and would not let anyone touch him. He was afebrile and had normal height and weight for his age. He did not demonstrate pallor or lymphadenopathy. Exams of his heart, lungs, and abdomen were normal. Motor and reflex exams were normal. His back exam demonstrated a Gibbus (kyphotic deformity) in the mid thoracic spine, with a compensatory lordosis (Fig. 30.2). The posterior prominence was tender, but no swelling was noted.

Diagnostic Tests

AP and lateral radiographs of the spine were obtained (Fig. 30.3) which showed a very large paraspinal shadow at the lower thoracic spine extending from T5 to T10 with a slight coronal convexity to the left. There was no bone destruction. The sagittal plane did not suggest an abnormal shadow nor a bone lesion.

An MRI screening of the entire spine demonstrated destruction and collapse of the T8 vertebra, end plate destruction of the caudal end plate, intact intervertebral disc space, and decreased T9 vertebral height (Fig. 30.4). There were signal changes in both these vertebrae with a large prevertebral, epidural, and paraspinal fluid collection. The epidural collection indented the spinal cord. There was an intradural component of the abscess (Fig. 30.5). The child was admitted due to a possibility of impending neurological deficit. Laboratory investigations revealed a hemoglobin of 10.9, WBC count of 16,000/mm^3, and an ESR of 27.

Questions About the Case the Reader Should Consider
1. What clinical features about the case suggest spinal tuberculosis?
2. Why does the child not have neurological deficit despite impressive MRI?
3. What is the natural history of this thoracic spinal tuberculosis with kyphosis if left untreated?
4. For this child what are the best laboratory tests for confirming the diagnosis?
5. What is the importance of using many drugs at one time to treat tuberculosis?
6. What are the indications for surgical treatment? Bracing? Does the abscess need to be surgically drained? Does the spine need to be surgically stabilized?

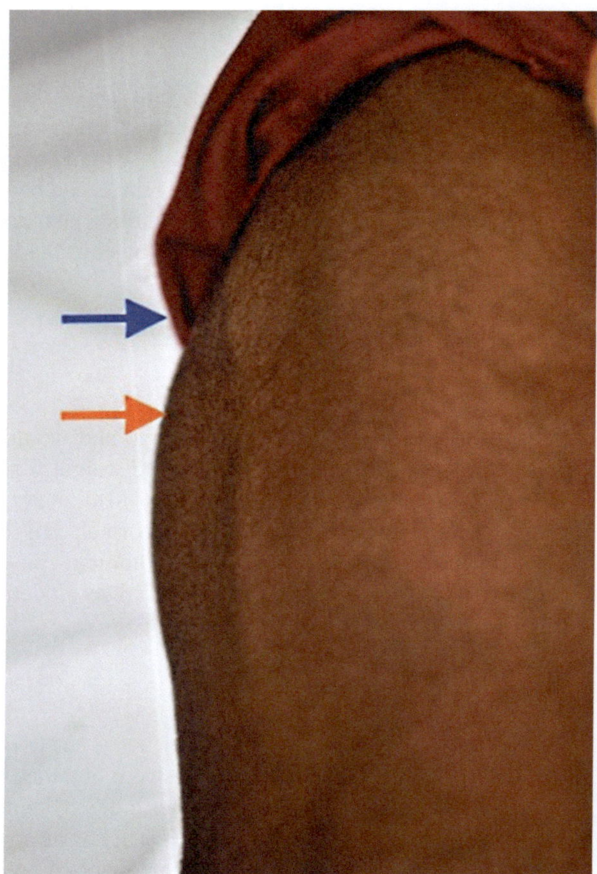

Fig. 30.2 A thorough examination of the back showed a Gibbus (kyphotic deformity) in the mid thoracic spine (*blue arrow*), with a concavity just caudal to the gibbus suggesting a compensatory lordosis (*orange arrow*)

Case Discussion

We have presented the case of a 3-year-old boy with nonspecific symptoms, including fever, weight loss, and a stooped posture. The symptoms persisted for months without a diagnosis, and he was treated inappropriately. Through this case, we will demonstrate the importance of a thorough history and physical exam, the characteristic imaging and laboratory findings, and the historic and current medical and surgical treatment protocols for this disease – spinal tuberculosis. Although uncommon in the developed world, with migration between people of all nationalities on the rise, we hope to inculcate an index of suspicion for tuberculosis when evaluating patients with such vague symptoms.

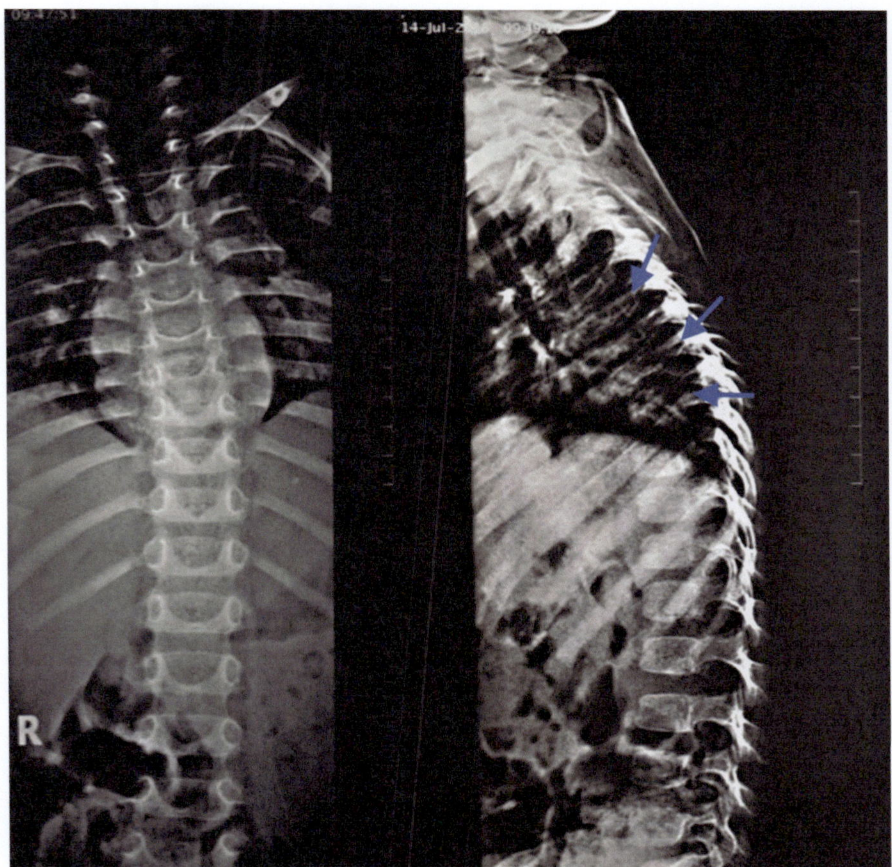

Fig. 30.3 AP (left) and lateral (right) X-rays of the spine showed a very large paraspinal shadow at the lower thoracic spine extending from T5 to T10, best seen on the lateral imaging (*blue arrows*), with a slight coronal convexity to the left seen on the coronal

Geography and Epidemiology

Tuberculosis is one of the oldest known infectious diseases of man – seen in mummies dating 9000 BC [1]. However, only in the last 60 years has an effective treatment for the disease been established [2].

Today, approximately 2 billion people worldwide are infected with tuberculosis. Only 5–15% are symptomatic. The remainder are carriers and have a latent infection [3]. Extrapulmonary tuberculosis is seen in 20% of infected individuals; however, the exact incidence of spinal tuberculosis is unclear [4]. Skeletal tuberculosis is seen in nearly 10% of patients with active pulmonary disease, and up to 50% of these cases involve the spine [5].

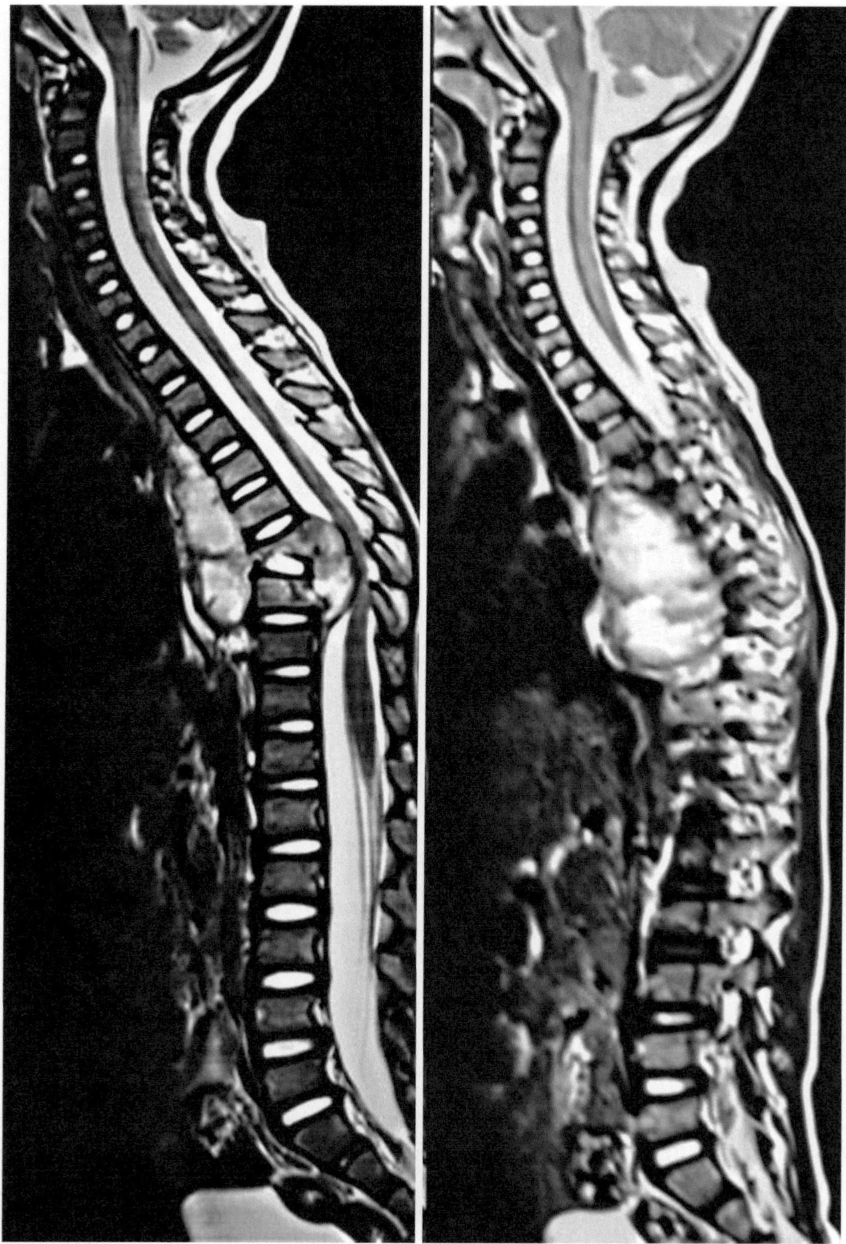

Fig. 30.4 The left image is the central sagittal cut and the right image in the para-central sagittal cut of the patient's full spine MRI. There is destruction and collapse of the T8 vertebra, with some end plate destruction of the caudal end plate, intact intervertebral disc space, and decreased T9 vertebral height. There is signal change in both of these vertebrae with a large prevertebral, epidural, and paraspinal collection. The epidural collection is indenting the cord

Tuberculosis disproportionately infects the poor regardless of the nation [6, 7]. Among the most important risk factors for tuberculosis infection is HIV [3]. Those with HIV are at a 21–30-fold increased risk of developing tuberculosis [5]. Other patients at increased risk for tuberculosis include immune-compromised patients [8], those at the extremes of age, diabetics, smokers, cancer patients, and alcoholics [3]. Overcrowded living conditions, such as prisons or shelters, are also a risk factor.

There are endemic regions in the world for tuberculosis (Fig. 30.6). For example, due to high HIV infection rates, sub-Saharan Africa is the most densely burdened

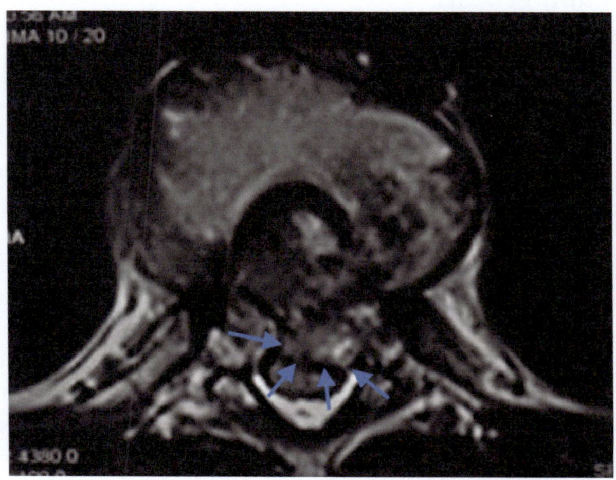

Fig. 30.5 This is a T2-weighted axial MRI image of the patient's T8 vertebral body showing intra-dural abscess (*blue arrows*)

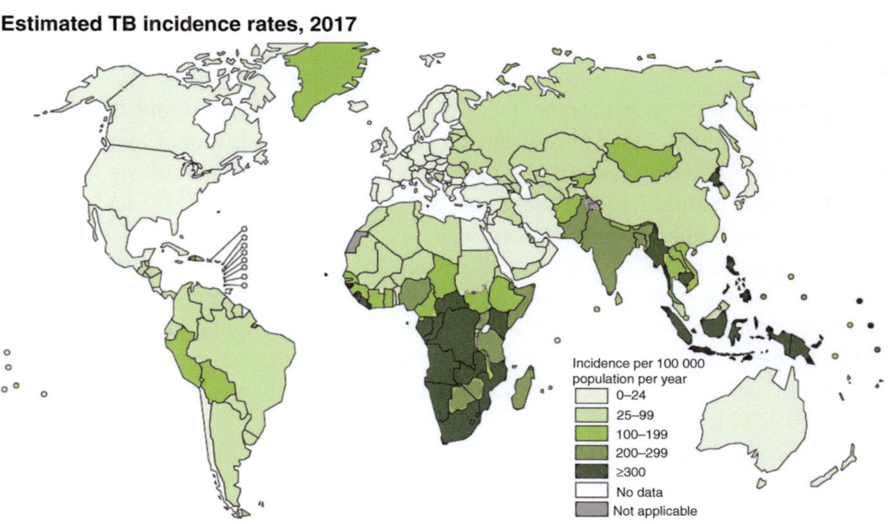

Fig. 30.6 This map from the World Health Organization's 2018 tuberculosis report shows the endemic regions of tuberculosis (Reprinted with permission from Global Tuberculosis Report 2018. Geneva: World Health Organization ©2018)

[3]. In addition, about 60% of new cases of tuberculosis come from 6 countries: India, Indonesia, China, Nigeria, Pakistan, and South Africa [3]. In the United States, the incidence of tuberculosis is 4 times higher in foreign-born persons [9], especially immigrants from sub-Saharan Africa and Southeast Asia [10]. This epidemiology is crucial to inculcate an index of suspicion when evaluating a patient who may be at risk for this disease.

Pathogenesis

Tuberculosis is caused by *mycobacterium tuberculosis complex bacillus* [5]. 50% of all tuberculosis patients have a primary lung foci or history of pulmonary tuberculosis [4]. Spinal tuberculosis is a secondary infection [11]. It is unclear whether spinal tuberculosis requires active disease elsewhere or whether spinal tuberculosis can be present in latent tuberculosis. It is also unclear whether spinal tuberculosis implies the patient is contagious [4].

Unlike most infections of the spine, spinal tuberculosis begins in the anterior vertebral body [11]. The infection spreads posteriorly. In adults, the vertebral body is nearly always involved, and the intervertebral disc is usually the last segment to be affected [5, 11]. However, children have a more vascular intervertebral disc, and the disk may be the focus of disease [12]. The bony involvement in spinal tuberculosis results in destruction of the anterior vertebral bodies, leading to kyphosis or a forward bend of the spine.

Natural History

Spinal tuberculosis is a chronic manifestation of the disease. Only 20–30% of patients with spinal TB demonstrate the traditional constitutional symptoms of tuberculosis – malaise, weight loss, and fever [11]. Spinal tuberculosis has three major clinical features: (1) cold abscesses, (2) neurologic deficit, (3) and, in long standing cases, kyphotic spine deformity.

Cold abscess refers to a collection of purulence originating from the infected vertebrae. However, unlike the typical abscesses in pyogenic infections, there is no surrounding inflammatory response [5, 11]. Seen in 70% of spinal tuberculosis [13], cold abscesses are slow growing and are often located in the paravertebral tissue [14]. Cold abscesses can cause a mass effect – variable depending on the location (Table 30.1) [11, 15].

Neurologic deficit can occur up to 40% of cases in low-income countries and up to 20% of cases in high-income countries [16]. Neurologic deficits are more

Table 30.1 Location of cold abscesses

Location	Incidence	Characteristics
Cervical and upper thoracic spine	10%	Retropharyngeal abscesses can result in dysphagia, hoarseness, and respiratory distress
Lower thoracic spine	40–50%	Fusiform paravertebral swellings
Lumbar spine	35–45%	Descends down beneath the inguinal ligament to appear in groin/ thigh. It can also track into the gluteal region as it follows the iliac vessels

likely to occur when the disease involves the cervical and thoracic spine due to the narrower spinal canal compared to the lumbar spine. Radicular pain, focal nerve root weakness, and sensory changes are the early neurologic signs. Myelopathy and paraplegia can result from untreated disease [11].

Neurologic changes are divided into early onset or late onset [17]. Early-onset deficits have multiple causes including cord compression secondary to a mass effect, mechanical spine instability due to vertebral bone destruction, cord infection, edema, and arteritis of the spinal artery [5, 11, 12, 16, 17].

Late-onset deficits occur years and decades after treatment and healing of the active tuberculosis. The most common cause of late neurologic changes is severe kyphotic deformity resulting from spinal tuberculosis [5, 16–18]. The spinal cord is compressed as it drapes over the kyphosed vertebral column [11]. The magnitude and location of vertebral body collapse impacts the degree of sagittal plane deformity and risk for neurologic deficits. For example, type A reconstitution results from minimal vertebral body destruction and an intact posterior column. Type B reconstitution occurs when the antero-inferior edge of superior body rests on the inferior vertebral body and causes a 40–60 degree kyphosis. Type C reconstitution occurs when the anterior edge of superior bodies rest on anterior edge of inferior body and typically causing a progressive kyphosis greater than 100 degrees (Fig. 30.7). Overall, kyphosis in spinal tuberculosis is extremely common [19–23]. The degree of kyphosis can reach over 100 degrees and is determined by whether the posterior structures of the spine remain intact or fail [13].

The initial degree of kyphosis is generally less than 30 degrees in adults diagnosed with spinal tuberculosis. The kyphotic deformity progresses an average of 15 degrees after medical treatment. However, if the initial kyphosis is greater than 60 degrees, the deformity will continue to progress despite medical treatment and healing [24]. In children, the continuation of growth of the spine can also cause the kyphosis to progress [19, 20]. Four radiographic signs predicting kyphotic collapse in children have been reported. These "spine-at-risk" signs include dislocation of the facets, posterior retropulsion of the diseased fragments, lateral translation of the vertebrae in the coronal plane, and toppling of the superior vertebra [23].

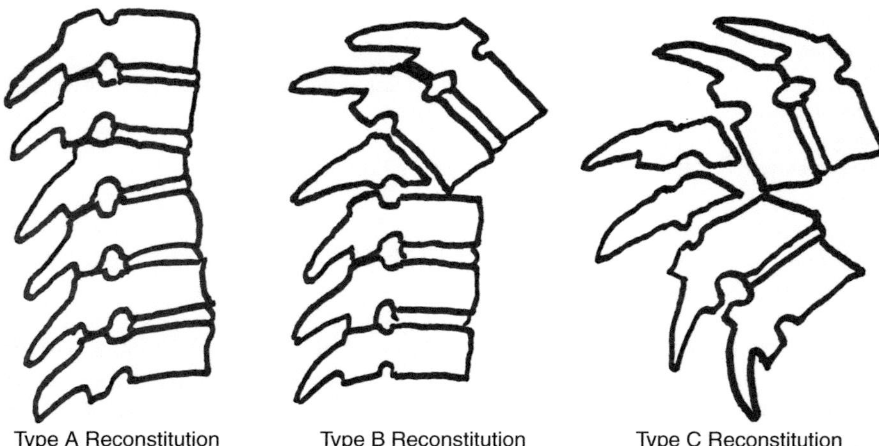

Fig. 30.7 Type A reconstitution results from minimal vertebral body destruction and an intact posterior column. Type B reconstitution is a result when the anteroinferior edge of superior body rests on the inferior vertebral body and causes a 40–60 degree kyphosis. Type C reconstitution occurs when the anterior edge of superior bodies rest on anterior edge of inferior body and typically causes a kyphosis greater than 100 degrees which grows

History and Physical Exam

Spinal tuberculosis is an insidious disease. The time from onset of symptoms to diagnosis is often delayed 3–6 months [13]. Therefore, a high index of suspicion is essential. Immigrants from sub-Saharan Africa and Southeast Asia, chronically ill individuals, the homeless, IV drug abusers, and patients on immunosuppressant medications presenting with spine symptoms are all at high risk. In urban regions, contact with a high risk patient is also a risk for disease transmission.

The constitutional symptoms such as weight loss, malaise, night sweats, low grade temperatures, body aches, and fatigue are associated with active pulmonary tuberculosis but only present in 20–38% of skeletal tuberculosis [11, 25].

As demonstrated in this case presentation, back pain is the most common complaint of spinal tuberculosis. Back pain is reported in 90–100% of all spinal tuberculosis and is the sole symptom in 61% of cases [5, 25]. Back pain can be a symptom of tissue destruction of the vertebral bodies, mass effect, or instability of the spine. Radicular pain is often secondary to nerve root compression by a cold abscess or vertebral body collapse. Neurologic deficit may be the presenting symptoms in 23–76% of patients [26].

Neurologic deficits require an astute clinical exam. Neurologic findings can be as subtle as a clumsy gait or worsening hand dexterity, or as severe as quadriparesis. Patients with myelopathy can present with bowel incontinence or urinary retention [13]. Upper motor neuron involvement can result in symptoms like hyperreflexia and clonus which are often noticed by a physician and not sensed by the patient [27].

Spinal deformity, such as the gibbus seen in the case presentation, is a late physical exam finding of spinal tuberculosis. The degree of deformity is dependent on the number of vertebrae involved [13]. A knuckle deformity implies involvement of a single vertebra. A gibbus is seen when 2–3 vertebrae are involved. A global kyphosis represents involvement of multiple vertebrae [13].

Diagnostic Work-Up

The diagnosis of spinal tuberculosis can be established using laboratory studies, imaging, and tissue diagnosis.

Laboratory Tests

A complete blood count (CBC), erythrocyte sedimentation rate (ESR), and C-reactive protein (CRP) are nonspecific markers of an infectious process [5, 11, 13, 18]. Peripheral leukocytosis may be noted in cases of active pulmonary disease and is present in 30–50% of patients with spinal tuberculosis [5]. Anemia of chronic disease is common. An ESR > 20 mm/h has been reported in over 60% of patients [13]. A CBC with cell differential should be obtained, as a lymphocyte-to-monocyte ratio can be used to monitor response to therapy [28].

The Mantoux test, the purified protein derivative (PPD) or tuberculosis skin test, can be used to screen for tuberculosis; however, the skin test does not differentiate active from latent disease. The skin test is positive in 63–90% of spinal tuberculosis [5]. In endemic regions, a negative test is more helpful than a positive test because many patients in endemic areas have received Bacille Calmette-Guerin vaccination resulting in a positive skin test. Interferon-γ release assay – QuantiFERON – is a serologic option, which tests for *M. tuberculosis* antigens and is not affected by prior Bacille Calmette-Guerin vaccination [29].

Imaging

Imaging of back pain in a patient suspected of having tuberculosis begins with a chest X-ray because concomitant pulmonary tuberculosis is present in nearly half of the patients with spinal disease [4]. Next, AP and lateral radiographs of the entire spine should be obtained. Spine radiographic findings are generally not present until later stages of the disease [30]. Radiographs of a patient with spinal tuberculosis can demonstrate a loss of bone density in the anterior spine and paradiscal regions [5]. Radiographs can also show soft tissue shadows in the paraspinal region indicative of cold abscesses. The presence of calcifications in these soft tissue shadows is pathognomonic for spinal tuberculosis [11]. Radiographs can also demonstrate kyphotic deformity of the spine [13].

Magnetic resonance imaging (MRI) is more sensitive than radiographs (93%) and more specific than CT (96%) [31]. Contrast-enhanced MRI increases the diagnostic accuracy and can be used when malignancy is suspected [5]. Tuberculosis in the bone appears hypointense on T1 sequences and hyperintense on T2 sequences. The discs are well preserved [5]. An MRI of the entire spine should be obtained to identify non-contiguous lesions [13]. Cold abscesses appear different than pyogenic bacterial abscesses on MRI. For example, cold abscesses have smooth thin walls as opposed to thick, irregular, contrast-enhancing walls in bacterial abscesses [14]. Myelopathy, myelomalacia, and cord edema visualized on MRI can help assess the prognosis of recovery in patients with neurological deficits [18]. Some centers are now recommending the use of full spine MRI as soon as spinal tuberculosis is suspected. This approach has two advantages. Firstly, it allows for earlier diagnosis. Secondly, MRI of the entire spine identifies skip lesions. If MRI is omitted and only repeat plain radiography performed, progression of initial less involved segments not noted on initial radiographs may be misinterpreted as a new lesions, leading to the misdiagnosis of multidrug-resistant tuberculosis.

Computed tomography (CT) of the spine can detect osteopenia and smaller lytic lesions earlier than plain radiographs [18]. Soft tissue calcifications and spinal canal encroachment are also more accurately depicted on CT scans [11, 13]. However, CT is rarely utilized in cases of spinal TB unless there is a contraindication to the use of MRI.

Other imaging modalities, such as positron emission tomography (PET) and bone scan, have had smaller, experimental roles in assessing spinal tuberculosis. However, recent reports on the use of PET/CT to assess disease activity and monitoring response to treatment are encouraging [32].

Tissue Diagnosis

The gold standard diagnostic test for spinal tuberculosis is tissue diagnosis [5, 11, 13, 14, 18]. All tissue samples should be sent for culture, histopathology, and a real-time polymerase chain reaction (PCR) [13]. Tissue samples can be obtained via image-guided needle biopsy or open surgical biopsy [11]. Histopathology is considered the gold standard diagnostic method, with 100% confirmation of diagnosis in one report [33]. The microscopic examination of the samples show epithelioid cell granulomas, caseous necrosis, lymphocytes, and Langerhans giant cells [34].

Real-time PCR is another helpful diagnostic method with a sensitivity of 90% in spinal tuberculosis samples [35, 36] and a specificity of 83–90% [37]. The diagnosis can be obtained within 24 hours [35] and can detect as few as 10–50 tubercle bacilli [5].

Unlike other bacterial infections, cultures and smears are not the gold standard diagnostic test in spinal tuberculosis. Tuberculosis is a paucibacilar disease [13], and only 52% of smears on Ziehl-Neelsen staining and 83% of cultures Lowenstein–Jensen media are positive [38]. Furthermore, the culture process can take 1–2 months [18]. Newer mediums such as BACTEC 12 B and GeneXpert MTB/RIF require only 1–2 weeks of incubation time and have sensitivities and specificities approaching 90% [5, 13]. The role for culture is now focused on obtaining antimicrobial sensitivities to identify and treat multidrug-resistant (MDR) tuberculosis [13].

Treatment Algorithm

The historic treatment of tuberculosis had been supportive for millennia. In the pre-antibiotic era, sanatoria formed the mainstay of treatment, with heliotherapy (use of natural sunlight) and nutrition the major interventions which treated only the constitutional symptoms rather than the underlying pathogen [18, 39].

The most dramatic change in the treatment of spinal tuberculosis was the advent of antimicrobial therapies in the 1940s [39]. In 1943, streptomycin was the first antimicrobial therapy used for tuberculosis. Additional antibiotics were produced in subsequent decades and compose the pillars of the current ambulatory multidrug chemotherapy regimens for tuberculosis [40–42]. The antimicrobial concentrations in and around the infected tissue exceeded minimum inhibitory concentrations [43, 44] resulting in resorption of abscesses and repair and filling in of new bone. In some cases, medical management alone enhanced neurologic recovery [41, 42]. During this similar time frame, surgical treatment of spinal tuberculosis advanced to include abscesses drainage, anterior surgical debridement, and fusion [45–47].

As a result of the advances in medical and surgical treatment of tuberculosis, the "middle path" approach was developed in the 1960s [39, 48]. Patients who presented as poor surgical candidates were initially treated with triple agent anti-tuberculosis chemotherapy, regardless of neurologic deficit. Patients who showed no improvement of neurologic symptoms 1 month after therapy underwent surgery. Using the "middle path approach," initial reports showed that surgery was necessary in only 6% of patients without neurologic deficits and 60% of patients with neurologic deficits. Subsequently, chemotherapy was considered the first line of treatment. Surgery was reserved for cases presenting with an evolving neurological deficits and cases that did not improve with medial management alone [11, 13, 16, 27, 49, 50]. The 2006 Cochrane review did not find sufficient evidence to conclusively recommend routine surgical treatment for the treatment of spinal tuberculosis [51]. Currently, there is no consensus on the surgical indication for patients presenting with neurologic deficits [16, 50, 52–54]. Some recommend surgical management only for complete paraplegia [54]. Others recommend surgical management of all neurologic deficits [53]. Overall, given the success of medical management of spinal tuberculosis [39, 43, 48, 52] in treating the disease and in resolving neurologic symptoms, surgery should be utilized judiciously.

Kyphotic deformity is a critical component of the natural history of spinal tuberculosis [19–23]. Surgery for deformity correction is recommended for patients with a kyphosis greater than 60 degrees and in pediatric patients with a risk for deformity progression due to remaining growth. Figure 30.8 shows a current treatment algorithm for spinal tuberculosis.

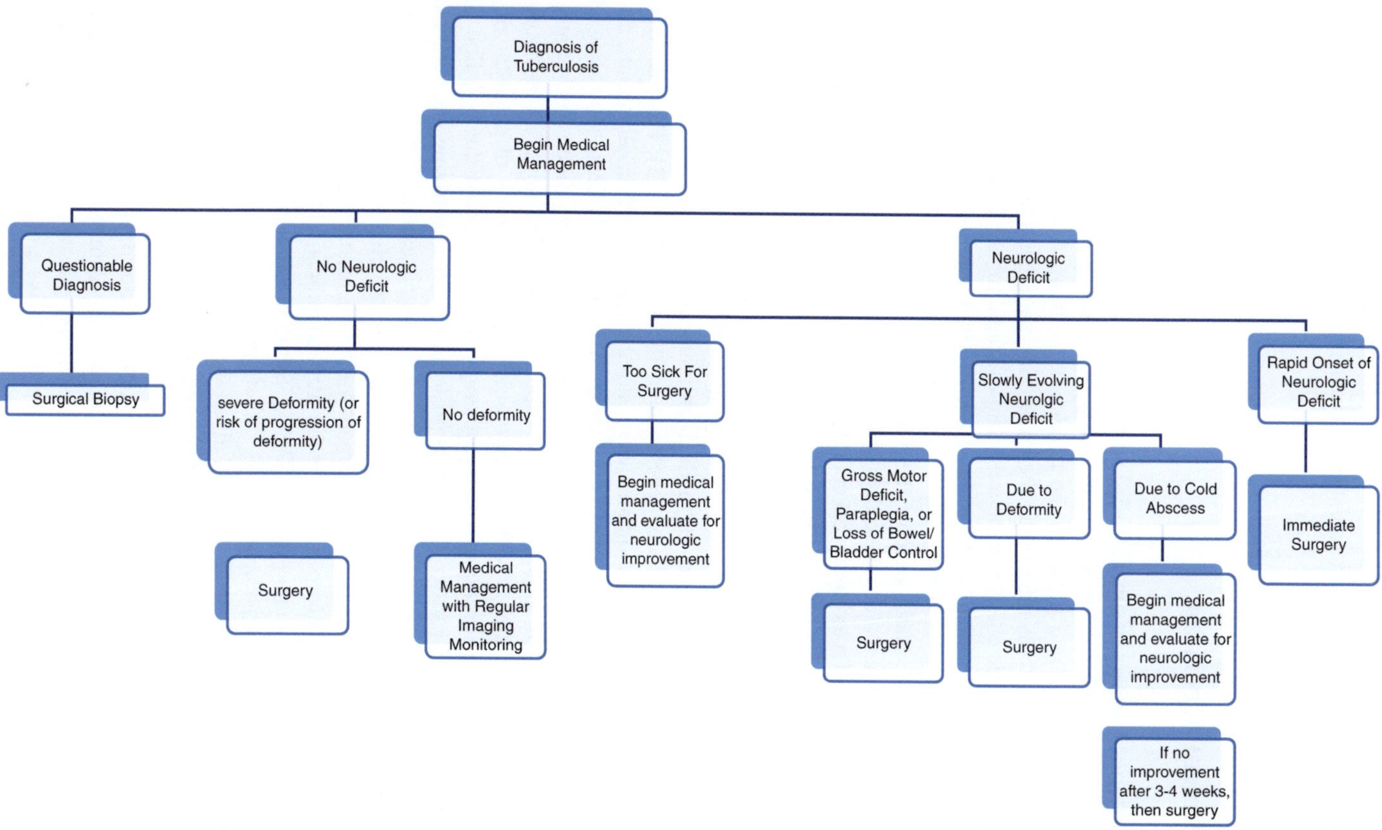

Fig. 30.8 Treatment algorithm for spinal tuberculosis

Medical Management

There are three primary objectives of medical management of spinal tuberculosis: (1) cure the patient of infection and associated sequelae, (2) prevent development of drug-resistant tuberculosis, and (3) prevent relapse of disease.

Numerous drugs have been used to treat spinal tuberculosis. The WHO has classified the medications as shown in Table 30.2 [55].

When choosing a regimen, it is crucial to consider the development of resistance. Drug-resistant strains occurred after single-agent therapy. However, the risk of developing resistance becomes negligible with the use of 3 or more agents [40]. All medical regimens share an intensive phase to eradicate rapidly multiplying bacilli, followed by a longer continuation phase to eradicate the slower intracellular bacilli. A recent study demonstrates a 0% relapse rates after 6 months of rifampin, isoniazid, and pyrazinamide [56].

The most commonly prescribed multidrug regimen for sensitive TB is 2 months of rifampin, isoniazide, pyrazinamide, and ethambutol followed by 4 months of Rifampin and Isoniazid. This recommendation is also supported by the WHO [55]. Daily multidrug administration is recommended; however, in the resource-limited environment, medicine can be administered every 2–3 days [57].

Incomplete drug regimens and noncompliance can lead to the development of drug resistance. This ranges from multidrug-resistant tuberculosis (MDR) to extensively drug-resistant tuberculosis (XDR) to total drug-resistant tuberculosis (TDR) [58]. In endemic regions, it is critical to obtain cultures to identify antimicrobial sensitivities and hopefully prevent resistant tuberculosis.

If medical treatment is not effective, a tissue diagnosis must be obtained. Adding a single agent to the current regimen (addition syndrome) is not recommended [59]. An infectious disease expert with an understanding of the regional resistance profiles should be consulted.

Table 30.2 WHO classification of anti-tuberculous drugs

Group	Drugs
Group 1: First line oral agents	Isoniazid, rifampin, ethambutol, pyrazinamide, rifabutin
Group 2: Injectable agents	Kanamycin, amikacin, capreomycin, and streptomycin
Group 3: Fluoroquinolones	Moxifloxacin, levofloxacin, gatifloxacin, ofloxacin
Group 4: Oral bacteriostatic second-line agents	Ethionamide, protionamide, cycloserine, terizidone, para-aminosalicylic acid
Group 5: Agents with unclear efficacy	Clofazimine, linezolid, amoxicillin-clavulanate, thiacetazone, clarithromycin, carbapenems

Reprinted with permission from World Health Organization. Companion Handbook to the WHO Guidelines for the Programmatic Management of Drug-Resistance Tuberculosis. The World Health Organization © 2014

Surgical Management

In cases of neurologic deficit due to cord compression, the decompression of the cold abscess is an important factor for recovery [11, 12, 16, 18, 39, 50]. Neurologic recovery can be observed after decompression of long-standing neurologic deficits because the cord compression in spinal tuberculosis is gradual. Both decompression and fusion are often necessary [45–47]. As initially reported by Percival Pott, bone healing and fusion are crucial to the success of treatment.

With the advent of modern spine instrumentation with pedicle screws, posterior approaches to correcting spinal deformity and achieving stable fusion have become more successful. Modern antitubercular medications can facilitate resorption of the anterior abscesses. Anterior access and debridement can also sometimes be achieved through the posterior approach [13].

Outcome

Following appropriate medical and surgical treatment, spinal tuberculosis has nearly 90% good outcomes for pain, neurologic recovery, and deformity [12, 13]. The cornerstone of treatment is multidrug anti-tubercular chemotherapy. Relapse rates have been shown to be ~2% with completion of anti-tubercular chemotherapy [60]. In addition, modern surgical spine techniques and instrumentation have resulted in improved deformity correction.

Neurologic recovery can be expected with appropriate treatment. 92% of patients demonstrate marked improvement and 74% of patients becoming ambulatory after presenting non-ambulatory [61]. Younger age, incomplete paraplegia, and surgery are associated with improved neurologic outcomes [62].

How to Approach the Case

As the patient was neurologically intact, the decision to start anti-tubercular treatment was made. A weight-based four drug regimen was started: Rifampicin, Isoniazid, Ethambutol, and Pyrazinamide. He was prescribed a thoracolumbar brace to protect the spine and was monitored closely for the development of any neurological deficit. Within 3 weeks of treatment, he was afebrile and became more active. At 6 months, repeat MRI (Fig. 30.9) and PET imaging (Fig. 30.10) were obtained which showed resolution of the intra-dural abscess, but persistent metabolic activity in the spine and lung. He is currently in his eighth month of the pharmaceutical regimen and remains neurologically intact. Surgical treatment was not necessary because he responded appropriately to medical management, did not have progressive kyphosis >60 degrees or at risk signs for instability, and had no myelopathy needing decompression and stabilization.

Fig. 30.9 This is a T2-weighted axial MRI image of the patient's T8 vertebral body 6 months after starting anti-tuberculous treatment, showing resolution of the intra-dural abscess but persistence of the extra-dural abscess (*orange arrows*)

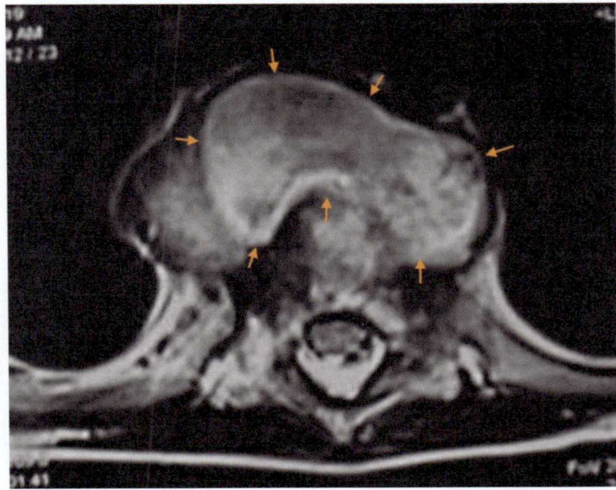

Fig. 30.10 This is an axial PET image 6 months after starting anti-tuberculous treatment showing persistence of FDG avid area not only in the spine (*blue arrow*) but also in the chest (*orange arrow*)

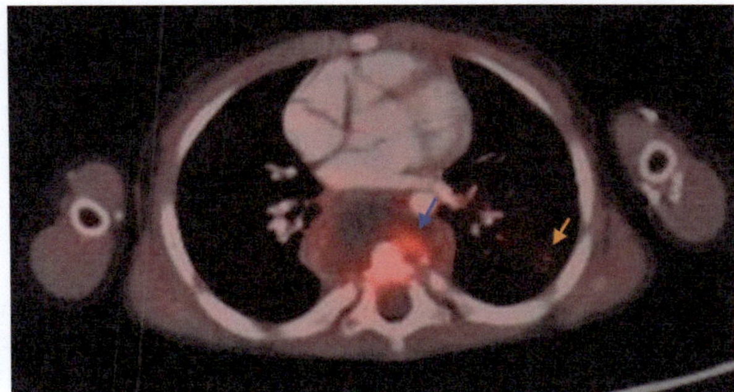

Red Flags in this Case
- Child has immigrated from an endemic area.
- Persistent back pain in young child.
- Chronic fever despite antibiotic treatment.
- Parents continued to bring him to health-care providers.
- Physicians became focused on one diagnosis.
- Kyphotic deformity developed as well as the persistent back pain.

Final Diagnosis

Tuberculosis involving the thoracic spine

Summary

The last 50 years have brought about remarkable advances in the understanding of the natural history, diagnosis, and treatment of spinal tuberculosis. The most impactful advance has been that of anti-tuberculous chemotherapy. In the modern era, the vast majority of spinal tuberculosis is treated medically without the need for surgical management. The availability of advanced imaging and real-time PCR has allowed more rapid diagnosis and initiation of treatment. The prevalence of drug resistance has limited the efficacy of medical management in certain endemic regions. The natural history of tubercular kyphosis has been well elucidated; however, the treatment of tubercular kyphotic deformity remains a challenge in low-income nations. Due to the degree of globalization in our world today, it remains critical for the contemporary physician to have a high index of suspicion in order to diagnose and treat spinal tuberculosis.

Editor Discussion

Tuberculosis is an immense health problem in low-income nations, and it remains a health-care challenge in high-income nations. Tuberculosis can affect virtually any organ system in the body. Diagnosis is often difficult. Tuberculosis is a "great mimicker" as its manifestations can simulate numerous other diseases across the body systems. However, recognition and understanding of the common and uncommon clinical and radiologic manifestations of tuberculosis including back pain and spinal involvement as illustrated in this comprehensive chapter should alert the physician to consider tuberculosis in high-risk patients in order to make a timely diagnosis and administer appropriate treatment.

W.L. Hennrikus

Although tuberculosis typically involves the lungs and rarely the bones or the spine, tuberculosis of the spine remains a significant worldwide problem. Tuberculosis is the leading cause of paralysis in the developing world. A child or adult may have years of no or inadequate medical treatment that eventually causes vertebral body and disc collapse. Combined with an abscess, the spinal cord can become compressed, with myelopathic symptoms developing. If significant enough anterior collapse, the posterior elements can dislocate, creating further instability. Even after successful medical treatment, if the deformity is great enough, further kyphotic (gibbus) deformity can continue with slowly worsening myelopathy. Given the current interest in international relief work, pediatric health-care workers traveling to endemic areas may see spinal tuberculosis. Immigrant children from endemic areas may also be seen in one's usual practice, so tuberculosis should always be considered possible.

R.M. Schwend

References

1. Taylor GM, Murphy E, Hopkins R, Rutland P, Chistov Y. First report of Mycobacterium bovis DNA in human remains from the Iron age. Microbiology 2007;153(Pt 4):1243–1249.
2. Herzog H. History of tuberculosis. Respiration. 1998;65(1):5–15.
3. Global tuberculosis report 2018. Geneva: World Health Organization; 2018.
4. Schirmer P, Renault CA, Holodniy M. Is spinal tuberculosis contagious? Int J Infect Dis. 2010;14(8):e659–66.
5. Esteves S, Catarino I, Lopes D, Sousa C. Spinal tuberculosis: rethinking an old disease. J Spine. 2017;6:358.
6. Zumla A, Raviglione M, Hafner R, Fordham von Reyn C. Tuberculosis. N Engl J Med. 2013;368(8):745–55.
7. Olson NA, Davidow AL, Winston CA, Chen MP, Gazmararian JA, Katz DJ. A national study of socioeconomic status and tuberculosis rates by country of birth, United States, 1996-2005. BMC Public Health. 2012;12:365.
8. Lawn SD, Zumla AI, Raviglione M, Hafner R, von Reyn CF. Tuberculosis Lancet. 2013;
9. McKenna MT, McCray E, Onorato I. The epidemiology of tuberculosis among foreign-born persons in the United States, 1986 to 1993. N Engl J Med. 1995;332(16):1071–6.
10. Cain KP, Benoit SR, Winston CA, Mac Kenzie WR. Tuberculosis among foreign-born persons in the United States. JAMA - J Am Med Assoc. 2008;300(4):405–12.
11. Garg RK, Somvanshi DS. Spinal tuberculosis: a review. J Spinal Cord Med. 2011;34(5):440–54.
12. Jain AK, Dhammi IK. Tuberculosis of the spine: a review. Clin Orthop Relat Res. 2007;460:39–49.
13. Shetty A, Kanna RM, Rajasekaran S. TB spine-current aspects on clinical presentation, diagnosis, and management options. Semin Spine Surg. 2016;28(3):150–62.
14. Rajasekaran S, Kanna RM, Shetty AP. Pathophysiology and treatment of spinal tuberculosis. JBJS Rev. 2014;2(9)
15. Teo ELHJ, Peh WCG. Imaging of tuberculosis of the spine. Singap Med J. 2004;45(9):439–44. quiz 445
16. Jain AK, Kumar J. Tuberculosis of spine: neurological deficit. Eur Spine J. 2013;22(Suppl 4):624–33.
17. Hodgson AR, Yau A. Pott's paraplegia: a classification based upon the living pathology. Paraplegia. 1967;5(1):1–16.
18. Jain AK. Tuberculosis of the spine: a fresh look at an old disease. J. Bone Jt. Surg. - Ser. B. 2010;92(7):905–13.
19. Rajasekaran S. Natural history of Pott's kyphosis. Eur Spine J. 2013;22(Suppl 4):634–40.
20. Rajasekaran S. The natural history of post-tubercular kyphosis in children. J Bone Jt Surg - Ser B. 2001;83(7):954–62.
21. Rajasekaran S. The problem of deformity in spinal tuberculosis. Clin Orthop Relat Res. 2002;398:85–92.
22. Rajasekaran S. Kyphotic deformity in spinal tuberculosis and its management. Int Orthop. 2012;36(2):359–65.
23. Rajasekaran S. The natural history of post-tubercular kyphosis in children. Radiological signs which predict late increase in deformity. J Bone Joint Surg Br. 2001;83(7):954–62.
24. Rajasekaran S, Shanmugasundaram TK. Prediction of the angle of gibbus deformity in tuberculosis of the spine. J. Bone Jt. Surg. - Ser. A. 1987;69(4):503–9.
25. Cormican L, Hammal R, Messenger J, Milburn HJ. Current difficulties in the diagnosis and management of spinal tuberculosis. Postgrad Med J. 2006;82(963):46–51.
26. Kotil K, Alan MS, Bilge T. Medical management of Pott disease in the thoracic and lumbar spine: a prospective clinical study. J Neurosurg Spine. 2007;6(3):222–8.
27. Jain AK, Sinha S. Evaluation of systems of grading of neurological deficit in tuberculosis of spine Spinal Cord. 2005;43(6):375–80.

28. Agarwal A, Bhat MS, Kumar A, Shaharyar A, Mishra M, Yadav R. Lymphocyte/monocyte ratio in osteoarticular tuberculosis in children: a haematological biomarker revisited. Trop Dr. 2016;46(2):73–7.
29. Mazurek M, Jereb J, Vernon A, LoBue P, et al. Updated guidelines for using interferon gamma release assays to detect Mycobacterium tuberculosis infection - United States, 2010. MMWR Recomm Rep. 2010;59(RR-5):1–25.
30. Hodgson AR, William W, Yau AC. X-ray appearances of tuberculosis of the spine: Thomas; 1969.
31. Gouliouris T, Aliyu SH, Brown NM. Spondylodiscitis: update on diagnosis and management. J Antimicrob Chemother. 2010;65(Suppl 3):iii11–24.
32. Barry CE, Boshoff HI, Dartois V, Dick T, Ehrt S, Flynn JA, et al. The spectrum of latent tuberculosis: rethinking the biology and intervention strategies. Nat Rev Microbiol. 2009;7(12):845–55.
33. Mondal A. Cytological diagnosis of vertebral tuberculosis with fine-needle aspiration biopsy. J Bone Jt Surg - Ser A. 1994;76(2):181–4.
34. Handa U, Garg S, Mohan H, Garg SK. Role of fine-needle aspiration cytology in tuberculosis of bone. Diagn Cytopathol. 2010;38(1):1–4.
35. Pandey V, Chawla K, Acharya K, Rao S, Rao S. The role of polymerase chain reaction in the management of osteoarticular tuberculosis. Int Orthop. 2009;33(3):801–5.
36. Colmenero JD, Morata P, Ruiz-Mesa JD, Bautista D, Bermudez P, Bravo MJ, et al. Multiplex real-time polymerase chain reaction: a practical approach for rapid diagnosis of tuberculous and brucellar vertebral osteomyelitis. Spine (Phila Pa 1976). 2010;35(24):E1392–6.
37. Berk RH, Yazici M, Atabey N, Ozdamar OS, Pabuccuoglu U, Alici E. Detection of Mycobacterium tuberculosis in formaldehyde solution-fixed, paraffin-embedded tissue by polymerase chain reaction in Pott's disease. Spine (Phila Pa 1976). 1996;21(17):1991–5.
38. Francis IM, Das DK, Luthra UK, Sheikh Z, Sheikh M, Bashir M. Value of radiologically guided fine needle aspiration cytology (FNAC) in the diagnosis of spinal tuberculosis: a study of 29 cases. Cytopathology. 1999;10(6):390–401.
39. Tuli SM. Historical aspects of Pott's disease (spinal tuberculosis) management. Eur Spine J. 2013;22(Suppl 4):529–38.
40. Varghese M. Drug therapy in spinal tuberculosis. In: Rajasekaran S, editor. Spinal infect. Trauma. Delhi: Jaypee Bros Med Publishers; 2011:133–141.
41. Konstam PG. Spinal tuberculosis in Nigeria. Ann R Coll Surg Engl. 1963;32:99–115.
42. Konstam PG, Blesovsky A. Ambulant treatment of spinal tuberculosis. Lancet. 1962;280(7268):1280.
43. Tuli SM, Kumar K, Sen PC. Penetration of antitubercular drugs in clinical osteoarticular tubercular lesions. Acta Orthop. 1977;48(4):362–8.
44. Kumar K. The penetration of drugs into the lesions of spinal tuberculosis. Int Orthop. 1992;16(1):67–8.
45. Hodgson AR, Stock FE, Fang HS, Ong GB. Anterior spinal fusion. The operative approach and pathological findings in 412 patients with Pott's disease of the spine. Br J Surg. 1960;48:172–8.
46. Hodgson AR, Yau A, Kwon JS, Kim D. A clinical study of 100 consecutive cases of Pott's paraplegia. Clin Orthop. 1964;36:128–50.
47. Hodgson AR, Stock FE. Anterior spinal fusion a preliminary communication on the radical treatment of Pott's disease and Pott's paraplegia. Br J Surg. 1956;44(185):266–75.
48. Tuli SM. Results of treatment of spinal tuberculosis by "middle-path" regime. J Bone Jt Surg Br. 1975;57(1):13–23.
49. Jain R, Sawhney S, Berry M. Computer tomography of vertebral tuberculosis: patterns of bone destruction. Clin Radiol. 1993;47(3):196–9.
50. Jain AK. Treatment of tuberculosis of the spine with neurologic complications. Clin Orthop Relat Res. 2002;(398):75–84.
51. Jutte PC, van Loenhout-Rooyackers JH. Routine surgery in addition to chemotherapy for treating spinal tuberculosis. Cochrane Database Syst Rev. 2006;(5):CD004532.

52. Nene A, Bhojraj S, Ortho D. Results of nonsurgical treatment of thoracic spinal tuberculosis in adults. Spine J. 2005;5(1):79–84.
53. Nussbaum ES, Rockswold GL, Bergman TA, Erickson DL, Seljeskog EL. Spinal tuberculosis: a diagnostic and management challenge. J Neurosurg. 1995;83(2):243–7.
54. Moon MS. Spine update tuberculosis of the spine: controversies and a new challenge. Spine (Phila Pa 1976). 1997;22(15):1791–7.
55. World Health Organization. Companion handbook to the WHO guidelines for the programmatic management of drug-resistance tuberculosis. World Health Organization. 2014.
56. Van Loenhout-Rooyackers JH, Verbeek ALM, Jutte PC. Chemotherapeutic treatment for spinal tuberculosis. Int J Tuberc Lung Dis. 2002;6(3):259–65.
57. Dickinson JM, Mitchison DA. In vitro studies on the choice of drugs for intermittent chemotherapy of tuberculosis. Tubercle. 1968;49:66–70.
58. Nguyen L. Antibiotic resistance mechanisms in M. tuberculosis: an update. Arch Toxicol. 2016;90(7):1585–604.
59. Mohan K, Rawall S, Pawar UM, Sadani M, Nagad P, Nene A, et al. Drug resistance patterns in 111 cases of drug-resistant tuberculosis spine. Eur Spine J. 2013;22(Suppl 4):647–52.
60. Turgut M. Spinal tuberculosis (Pott's disease): its clinical presentation, surgical management, and outcome. A survey study on 694 patients. Neurosurg Rev. 2001;24(1):8–13.
61. Dunn R, Zondagh I, Candy S. Spinal tuberculosis: magnetic resonance imaging and neurological impairment. Spine (Phila Pa 1976). 2011;36(6):469–73.
62. Park DW, Sohn JW, Kim E-H, Cho D-I, Lee J-H, Kim K-T, et al. Outcome and management of spinal tuberculosis according to the severity of disease: a retrospective study of 137 adult patients at Korean teaching hospitals. Spine (Phila Pa 1976). 2007;32(4):E130–5.

Chapter 31
Complementary and Alternative Medicine (CAM) to Back Pain

Eva Seligman and Teri M. McCambridge

Introduction

"Complementary and alternative medicine" (CAM) approaches to health care are popular in our society, and so there is no surprise that patients and their families may turn to alternative methods when treating back pain. In the United States, the overall rate of CAM use by children ages 4–17 years has been 12% for the past decade [1]. According to the CDC's National Health Interview Survey (NHIS), nearly half of these families reported using CAM for a specific health condition, with acupuncture being most common [1]. The most common health complaints for which parents decided to try a CAM for their child were back or neck pain, head or chest cold, musculoskeletal conditions, anxiety or stress, and ADHD [1]. Despite the popularity of CAM modalities, there is little evidence to justify their use. The studies that do exist often focus on adults. Therefore, determining the true efficacy of each CAM intervention in children is challenging. In this chapter, we review common types of CAM modalities that can be considered for managing back pain, including defining each intervention and the theory behind its potential efficacy, review evidence for use when available, and delineate possible risks associated with its use.

Back pain in children and adolescents can represent significant pathology and should be taken seriously. A thorough history and physical exam with determination of "red flag symptoms" (Table 31.1) and any indicated lab work and imaging (Table 31.2) are completed to rule out these diagnoses before turning to CAM therapies that focus on the treatment of nonspecific musculoskeletal back pain.

E. Seligman (✉)
Department of Pediatrics, Johns Hopkins University School of Medicine, Baltimore, MD, USA

T. M. McCambridge
Department of Pediatrics and Orthopedics, University of Maryland Medical System, Baltimore, MD, USA

© Springer Nature Switzerland AG 2021
R. M. Schwend, W. L. Hennrikus (eds.), *Back Pain in the Young Child and Adolescent*, https://doi.org/10.1007/978-3-030-50758-9_31

Table 31.1 Red flag symptoms for back pain

Patient characteristics/symptoms	Physical exam findings
Fevers or chills	Refusal/inability to ambulate
Malaise	Petechial or purpuric rash
Weight loss or anorexia	Hepatosplenomegaly
Pain at night or pain that wakes from sleep	Abnormal neurologic exam
Radicular pain	Midline spinal tenderness or step-offs
Dysuria	Progressive or severe spinal curvature
Loss of bowel or bladder control	
Easy bruising or bleeding	
Bone pain at other locations	
Age 4 years or younger	
Duration of symptoms longer than 6 weeks	

Table 31.2 Potential laboratory and radiographic studies for back pain

Laboratory studies	Radiographic studies
Complete blood count with differential	Spinal x-ray (minimum two views)
Erythrocyte sedimentation rate	Pelvis x-ray
C-reactive protein	Spine MRI
Comprehensive metabolic panel	

Case Presentation

Case No. 1

A 15-year-old healthy girl had low back pain for 3 months. She is an avid swimmer and a member of the high school swim team. She had no specific injury to her back; however, one day, she started having tightness and pain after swim practice. She never had any radiating pain, numbness or tingling, loss of bowel or bladder control, fevers, or weight loss. She was initially seen by her primary care doctor, who noted lumbar paraspinal muscle tenderness and no vertebral point tenderness. The physician recommended scheduled heat packs and NSAIDs. Despite using these interventions around the clock, she continued to have low back pain. Due to continued pain, she had radiographs of the lumbar spine, which were normal. A family friend recommended that she try yoga or Pilates. She decided to enroll in a local yoga studio and has been taking yoga class weekly for the past 10 weeks. Her pain gradually improved and almost entirely resolved.

Yoga

Definition and Theory of Efficacy

Yoga is a series of movements, postures, breathing, and meditation that originated in India over 5000 years ago as a part of Ayurvedic medicine. There are a variety of styles of yoga [2]. Many postures in yoga aim to improve core strength and spinal flexibility (Fig. 31.1), which may improve low back pain in pediatric patients as this condition is often associated with poor trunk muscle endurance, poor trunk muscle strength, and limited spinal flexibility [3].

Epidemiology

Yoga practice is gaining worldwide popularity, and 8.4% of US children report taking yoga classes or receiving formal training in yoga in the past 12 months according to the National Health Interview Survey 2017 [4]. Yoga is more commonly tried in older children (ages 12–17 years), girls, non-Hispanic whites, and children of parents that have higher than a high school level of education [1].

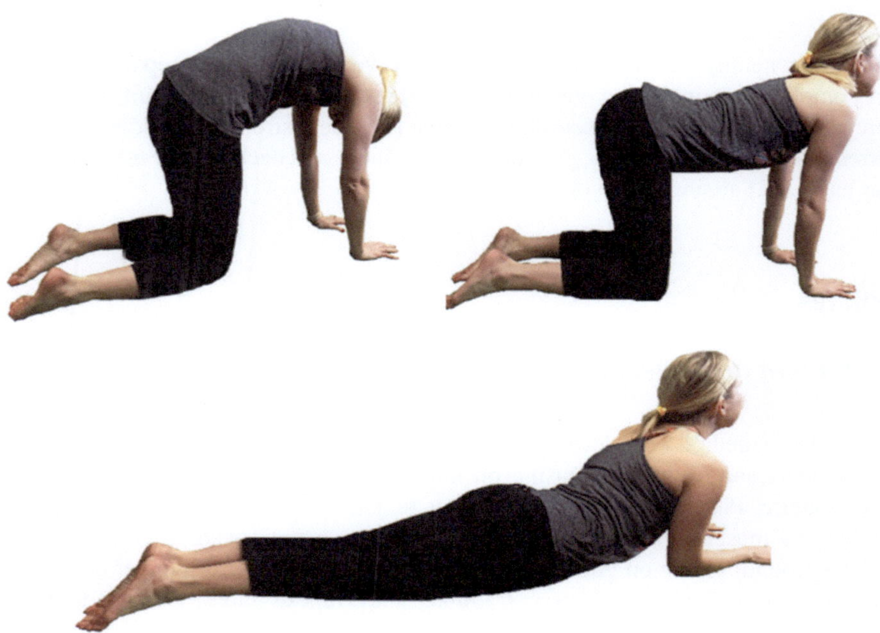

Fig. 31.1 Yoga poses that may improve paraspinal muscle strength and flexibility

Data on Efficacy

With the growing concerns of the opioid epidemic and realization that most low back pain improves regardless of treatment, in 2017, the American College of Physicians recommended "non-pharmacologic treatment" as the initial management for chronic low back pain, specifically naming yoga and exercise among the possible acceptable first interventions [5]. Studies are limited, resulting in a low-quality evidence to justify yoga for low back pain. All studies are based on adult patients. Common outcomes include a variety of pain scores, disability scores, and spinal flexibility scores. When practiced at least weekly for up to 2 years, yoga may relieve pain and improve functional disability. It is unclear if these benefits differ from other exercise programs including physical therapy [6]. However, studies have demonstrated non-inferiority of yoga to physical therapy [7]. Modest effects in pain reduction are seen in multiple studies with short term, daily, or weekly yoga use over months. In one study comparing multiple daily sessions of yoga to daily exercises, the spinal flexibility improved and pain decreased with both interventions. However, the effect was greatest with daily yoga [8].

Possible Harm

Yoga is generally safe and well tolerated. However, there are case reports in adults of complications including pneumothorax [9] and pneumomediastinum from deep breathing exercises with concurrent Valsalva [10], heat stroke, and sudden cardiac arrest [11]. More commonly, patients describe increased back pain or other muscular pains [12] arising from yoga.

Pilates

Definition and Theory of Efficacy

The Pilates method was developed by Joseph Pilates in the 1920s as a series of movements and exercises focusing on improving strength and flexibility of core musculature. Pilates uses small movements to activate the paraspinal, gluteal, and abdominal muscles using only body weight. Pilates exercises are often performed on the ground relying on gravity to create resistance; however, a number of Pilates machines (e.g., Reformer, Tower, Cadillac, and Trapeze Table) are also used to facilitate these exercises [13, 14]. Pilates differs from yoga as it focuses on muscle relaxation and the strengthening of small muscle groups without the emphasis on meditation or flexibility. Pilates exercises are designed to strengthen core muscles, which is hypothesized to reduce nonspecific low back pain by improving posture and balance [13] and lumbopelvic stabilization [15].

Epidemiology

Pilates exercise saw a particular rise in popularity in the early 2000s. At that time, an estimated 10.5 million Americans were participating in Pilates [16].

Data on Efficacy

The studies examining the efficacy of Pilates on low back pain focus on heterogenous groups of adult patients with different Pilates regiments and outcome measures. The majority of studies demonstrate some benefit in pain and disability scores, particularly in the short term [14, 17–19]. There may also be interval improvement in pain with more frequent Pilates sessions (up to 2–3 times per week) [20]. In general, Pilates appears to be as effective at improving low back pain when compared to other movement-based interventions such as yoga or physical therapy.

Possible Harm

There is insufficient evidence to describe specific harm associated with Pilates.

Case Presentation

Case No. 2

A 14-year-old boy presents to his pediatrician with back stiffness and low back pain for 1 month. He notes pain in his right lower back that is exacerbated when climbing stairs or when bending forward. He denies fevers, weight loss, or trauma. On exam, he has tenderness over the bilateral sacroiliac (SI) joints (right greater than left) that is worsened with forward bend and right leg flexion, abduction, and external rotation (FABER). His pediatrician also notes a mild leg length inequality. A workup including radiograph and MRI of the pelvis and lumbar spine, complete blood count, and inflammatory markers is normal, ruling out L5 spondylolysis and sacroiliitis. He seeks care with a local chiropractor, and his pain improves with six sessions of spinal manipulation.

Spinal Manipulation/Chiropractic

Definition and Theory of Efficacy

The foundation of chiropractic practice lies in the connection between the body's structure and function. A focus is given to spinal alignment through manual manipulation. Spinal manipulation involves application of direct, forceful pressure to various joints to improve alignment and mobility. These techniques are also performed by osteopathic doctors and physical therapists [21]. Chiropractors are licensed by state governing bodies and trained at institutions accredited by the Council on Chiropractic Education Commission of Accreditation.

Epidemiology

Care by chiropractors has become so common that some chiropractors have advocated that these forms of treatment no longer be classified as CAM. In the United States, self-reported rates of chiropractic care reach 10% of the overall adult population and nearly 3.5% in children [21]. The majority of patients seek chiropractic care for low back pain [22].

Data on Efficacy

There are many randomized trials comparing chiropractic adjustments to a variety of other forms of treatment ranging from muscle relaxants to acupuncture. The heterogeneity of these studies, including type of back pain, outcomes, and rating scales, makes it difficult to draw conclusions about the overall efficacy of chiropractic spinal manipulation. In adults, studies demonstrate trends toward improvement in low back pain, including greater efficacy than placebo, muscle relaxant, and sham manipulation [23]. Another study found that active manipulation reduced pain in adult patients with acute back pain and sciatica with disc protrusion [24].

Possible Harm

Despite the relative frequency of spinal manipulation, a formal reporting system for adverse events associated with chiropractic manipulation does not exist, and adverse events reported in children are limited to case series and reports. Though rarely reported, spinal manipulation has resulted in severe complications, including subarachnoid hemorrhage, paraplegia, and severe headache. More commonly, patients reported mid-back soreness after manipulation. In the only systematic review to examine adverse events associated with pediatric spinal manipulation, Vohra et al. identified 20 cases of delayed or missed diagnoses of severe pathology, including neuroblastoma, meningitis, and rhabdomyosarcoma [25]. As such, all patients should undergo a thorough medical evaluation to rule out serious structural or medical causes of back pain prior to chiropractic evaluation. Radiographs should also be obtained prior to manipulation to rule out structural abnormalities that may be harmed by chiropractic spinal manipulation (i.e., spondylolisthesis, avulsion fracture, etc.)

Case Presentation

Case No. 3

A 12-year-old girl with mild (12 degree) thoracic scoliosis has had low back pain for several months. All laboratory and radiologic testing has been normal. She has tried Pilates, a chiropractor, and physical therapy but continues to have pain. She and her mother are interested in CAM approaches to care and are wondering what other modalities might improve back pain.

Acupuncture

Definition and Theory Behind Efficacy

Acupuncture involves the insertion of needles into the soft tissue at points along meridian lines defined in traditional Chinese medicine that correspond to organs, emotions, and sensations (Fig. 31.2). There is a variety of techniques within acupuncture, and the depth and location of needle insertion, use of additional

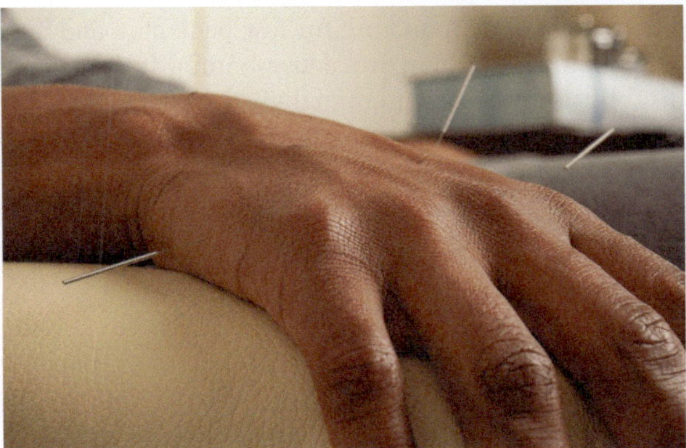

Fig. 31.2 Acupuncture points used for back pain (image courtesy of Sarah O'Leary, Acupuncturist)

movements of the needle, and the addition of laser or electricity will vary depending on the specific technique employed by the practitioner. Several theories exist to explain the potential efficacy of acupuncture. Stimulation of specific points along the meridian lines is thought to realign energy balance within the body. Since many of the acupuncture points are located near neural centers, another theory asserts that insertion of the needle may block the transmission of pain through neural gates. Functional MRI studies demonstrate increased blood oxygen flow to areas of needle insertion, which may also explain effect [26]. Cherkin et al. found no difference between acupuncture and sham procedure (insertion of needle at non-acupuncture points) and hypothesized that touch of the skin alone may stimulate mechanoreceptors and hormone release that decreases pain [27].

Epidemiology

The National Health Interview Survey 2017 does not contain data specifically regarding rates of acupuncture use in the pediatric population. An analysis of the 2012 survey found that, overall, acupuncture was the most commonly used CAM modality with particular health concerns such as back or neck pain, stress and anxiety, head or chest cold, and attention deficit hyperactivity disorder [1]. In the United States, it is estimated that over 6% of adults have tried acupuncture at some point in their lives [28].

Data on Efficacy

Acupuncture has been demonstrated to be effective in pediatric chemotherapy-related nausea and postoperative nausea. There are no studies investigating the role of acupuncture for pediatric back pain; however, many adult studies exist that include adolescents. Multiple randomized trials have attempted to delineate the efficacy of acupuncture for low back pain and have concluded that traditional acupuncture and sham procedures similarly result in a reduction in back pain and disability scores when compared to a "usual care" approach of medication and physical therapy [27, 29, 30]. The similarity in effect of acupuncture and sham (i.e., superficial needling in soft tissue at non-acupuncture points) calls into question the theory by which acupuncture provides back pain relief as discussed above [29]. The duration of therapy required for effect remains unclear, with positive effects ranging from a single session [31] to several months of therapy [32, 33].

Possible Harm

Side effects of acupuncture are generally very mild and include pain or bruising at the needle insertion site and worsening of overall symptoms. Severe complications are exceedingly rare and have been described as skin infection, pneumothorax, and a single case of cardiac rupture [34].

Cupping

Definition and Theory of Efficacy

The practice of cupping is central to traditional Chinese medicine and has been used in many eastern medicine practices for over 2000 years. Cupping is practiced in the United States in the Hmong communities in Wisconsin and California. There are two primary varieties of cupping: wet and dry. In dry cupping, a heated cup is placed on the skin creating a suction effect as the air cools. Wet cupping employs similarly heated cups; however, small incisions are made on the skin prior to placement of the cups. Blood is drawn out through these incisions as the suction phenomenon occurs. Suctioning is thought to stimulate blood flow to that area, promoting the elimination of tissue toxins. Another theory postulates that the transfer of pain from one area to a new area (i.e., the location of cup placement) can cure the individual of the original pathology [35]. The theories to explain the potential effect of cupping have not been scientifically substantiated.

Epidemiology

Cupping has gained popularity in western society in the past decade, particularly as it is used more frequently among high-profile athletes such as Michael Phelps. Estimates of use in the United States are not available.

Data on Efficacy

Randomized trials on cupping for back pain are limited. One study in Iran, including older teenagers, found sustained improvement in pain, reduced disability, and decreased medication use after three sessions of wet cupping compared to typical management of rest, NSAIDs, and avoidance of heavy lifting [36]. Another study in Korea demonstrated decrease in acetaminophen use and similar improvement in pain and disability scores compared to the standard of care [37]. A 2017 meta-analysis by Yun-Ring Wang et al. included six randomized controlled trials and concluded that cupping significantly reduced back pain and disability scores when compared to medication and "usual care." The studies included in this meta-analysis focused on adults and employed a variety of cupping techniques and durations of therapy [38].

Possible Harm

Minimal adverse effects are reported with cupping and primarily involve dermatologic complications. Pain at the cupping site, bleeding, changes in skin pigmentation, and local skin infections are the most commonly reported adverse events. Vasovagal syncope and anemia have also occurred [36, 38].

Kinesio Taping

Definition and Theory of Efficacy

Kinesio tape was developed by Dr. Kenzo Kase in the 1970s. It is an adhesive with a unique grain and elasticity that is purported to have an increased tensile force that can lift fascia and soft tissue [39]. The tape is thought to improve muscle function by gentle repositioning of the fascia and promoting blood circulation to the skin. Another theory postulates that application of the tape results in the stimulation of mechanoreceptors and proprioceptors that improve joint function and movement.

Epidemiology

Estimates of use in the United States are not available; however, over 150 thousand medical providers worldwide report using Kinesio tape [40].

Data on Efficacy

Studies on Kinesio taping are limited and none focus on pediatric patients. One study in adults added Kinesio tape as an adjunct to therapeutic ultrasound, hot packs, transcutaneous nerve stimulation, and therapeutic exercises and found that these patients had improvement in back pain, flexibility, and endurance directly after each intervention session [41]. A systematic review of Kinesio taping for back pain found that the taping alone or with another treatment was no more effective than physical therapy alone for improving pain or disability scores [42]. This study found limited evidence to suggest that Kinesio tape improved anticipatory postural control of transverse abdominal muscles [42].

Possible Harm

Adverse effects associated with Kinesio taping are not described in the literature. There are theoretical risks of skin irritation and resultant infection.

Meditation

Definition and Theory of Efficacy

Meditation is a practice that involves training the mind to change one's level of consciousness or awareness. There are a variety of techniques that include guided and independent breathing and thought techniques. Chronic back pain in children and adults has been associated with stress and anxiety, which meditation and mindfulness techniques attempt to reduce. Studies of mindfulness meditation, a particular form of meditation that focuses on building nonjudgmental awareness of sensory stimuli, have demonstrated an effect on endogenous opioid pathways though the practice does not itself seem to produce endogenous opiates [43].

Epidemiology

The overall use of meditation also increased significantly from 0.6% in 2012 to 5.4% in 2017 [4]. Self-reported rates of "relaxation therapy" in the US pediatric population are reported to be nearly 3%. In this patient population, the most common reasons for using relaxation therapy were reduction of stress and anxiety (31%) and back/neck pain (15%) [44].

Data on Efficacy

There are no studies that focus on meditation for back pain in the pediatric population. Studies are emerging in adults, which include older teens. In a randomized clinical trial, Cherkin et al. found that meditation and cognitive behavioral therapy were equally effective in reducing low back pain and disability scores and that both were more effective than "usual care" [45]. There are a number of pilot studies investigating the role of meditation, mindfulness exercises, and electronic-based relaxation techniques on low back pain with promising results [46–48].

Possible Harm

There are no described adverse events associated with meditation.

Brief Summary

While the literature to support or refute CAM interventions for back pain is growing, the majority of studies do not include pediatric patients. It is therefore impossible to draw conclusions about the effectiveness in children of each CAM interventions. In general, adverse events are uncommon.

Editor Discussion

The use of CAM in pediatrics is growing. For example, chiropractic is now a common choice for families seeking alternative medical care. Unfortunately, there is little information in the literature examining the safety and efficacy of CAM such as chiropractic for pediatric orthopedic disorders. The parents' perception of CAM is often very positive. However, delayed referral, misdiagnosis, adverse events from manipulative therapy, and ineffective treatments have been reported [49]. More research is needed to validate the safety and efficacy of CAM in children.

W.L. Hennrikus

Children often have poor core muscle strength when specifically tested. Ask a child to do 10 push-ups with a quality plank body posture, hands near the sides of the chest, thorax just barely touching the surface. It is surprising how often even an athletic child cannot do this well. This provides a direct indication and visual that there is weakness of the core shoulder, trunk, and hip muscles. The parents and child may be more accepting of this discussion after seeing for themselves that these muscles are indeed weak. If the child has a slouched forward posture, supine hyperextension stretching over a bolster or an exercise ball can lengthen the anterior thorax and decrease the stress on the posterior extensor muscles, which become fatigued with a kyphotic posture. Yoga and Pilates are CAM modalities that the child can actively perform. Active participation in posture and stretching is better than passive.

R.M. Schwend

References

1. Black LI, Clarke TC, Barnes PM, Stussman BJ, Nahin RL. Use of complementary health approaches among children aged 4-17 years in the United States: National Health Interview Survey, 2007-2012. Natl Health Stat Report. 2015;78:1–19. Available from: http://www.ncbi.nlm.nih.gov/pubmed/25671583.
2. Natural Medicines - Professional. 2018 [cited 2019 Jan 10]. Available from: https://natural-medicines-therapeuticresearch-com.proxy1.library.jhu.edu/databases/health-wellness/professional.aspx?productid=1241.
3. Potthoff T, de Bruin ED, Rosser S, Humphreys BK, Wirth B. A systematic review on quantifiable physical risk factors for non-specific adolescent low back pain. J Pediatr Rehabil Med. 2018;11(2):79–94. Available from: http://www.medra.org/servlet/aliasResolver?alias=iospress&doi=10.3233/PRM-170526.
4. Black LI, Barnes PM, Clarke TC, Stussman BJ, Nahin RL. Use of yoga, meditation, and chiropractors among U.S. children aged 4–17 years key findings. [cited 2019 Feb 7]. Available from: https://www.cdc.gov/nchs/data/databriefs/db324_table-508.pdf#3.
5. Qaseem A, Wilt TJ, McLean RM, Forciea MA. Clinical guidelines committee of the American college of physicians. Noninvasive treatments for acute, subacute, and chronic low back pain: a clinical practice guideline from the American college of physicians. Ann Intern Med. 2017;166(7):514. Available from: http://www.ncbi.nlm.nih.gov/pubmed/28192789.
6. Holtzman S, Beggs RT. Yoga for chronic low back pain: a meta-analysis of randomized controlled trials. Pain Res Manag. 2019;18(5):267–72. Available from: http://www.ncbi.nlm.nih.gov/pubmed/23894731.
7. Saper RB, Lemaster C, Delitto A, Sherman KJ, Herman PM, Sadikova E, et al. Yoga, physical therapy, or education for chronic low back pain. Ann Intern Med. 2017;167(2):85. Available from: http://www.ncbi.nlm.nih.gov/pubmed/28631003.
8. Tekur P, Singphow C, Nagendra HR, Raghuram N. Effect of short-term intensive yoga program on pain, functional disability and spinal flexibility in chronic low back pain: a randomized control study. J Altern Complement Med. 2008;14(6):637–44. Available from: http://www.liebertpub.com/doi/10.1089/acm.2007.0815.
9. Johnson DB, Tierney MJ, Sadighi PJ. Kapalabhati pranayama: breath of fire or cause of pneumothorax? A case report. Chest. 2004;125(5):1951–2. Available from: http://www.ncbi.nlm.nih.gov/pubmed/15136413.
10. Kashyap AS, Anand KP, Kashyap S. Complications of yoga. Emerg Med J. 2007;24(3):231. Available from: http://emj.bmj.com/cgi/doi/10.1136/emj.2006.036459.
11. Boddu P, Patel S, Shahrrava A. Sudden cardiac arrest from heat stroke: hidden dangers of hot yoga. Am J Med. 2016;129(8):e129–30. Available from: https://linkinghub.elsevier.com/retrieve/pii/S0002934316303588.
12. Wieland LS, Santesso N. A summary of a Cochrane review: yoga treatment for chronic non-specific low back pain. Eur J Integr Med. 2017;11:39–40. Available from: http://www.ncbi.nlm.nih.gov/pubmed/29057019.
13. Sorosky S, Stilp S, Akuthota V. Yoga and pilates in the management of low back pain. Curr Rev Musculoskelet Med. 2008;1(1):39–47. Available from: http://www.ncbi.nlm.nih.gov/pubmed/19468897.
14. Lin H-T, Hung W-C, Hung J-L, Wu P-S, Liaw L-J, Chang J-H. Effects of pilates on patients with chronic non-specific low back pain: a systematic review. J Phys Ther Sci. 2016;28(10):2961–9. Available from: http://www.ncbi.nlm.nih.gov/pubmed/27821970.
15. Mazloum V, Sahebozamani M, Barati A, Nakhaee N, Rabiei P. The effects of selective Pilates versus extension-based exercises on rehabilitation of low back pain. J Bodyw Mov Ther. 2018;22(4):999–1003. Available from: https://www.sciencedirect.com/science/article/pii/S136085921730236X.

16. Di Lorenzo CE. Pilates: what is it? Should it be used in rehabilitation? Sports Health. 2011;3(4):352–61. Available from: http://www.ncbi.nlm.nih.gov/pubmed/23016028.
17. Yamato TP, Maher CG, Saragiotto BT, Hancock MJ, Ostelo RW, Cabral CM, et al. Pilates for low back pain. Cochrane Database Syst Rev. 2015;7:CD010265. Available from: http://www.ncbi.nlm.nih.gov/pubmed/26133923.
18. Wells C, Kolt GS, Marshall P, Hill B, Bialocerkowski A. The effectiveness of Pilates exercise in people with chronic low back pain: a systematic review. PLoS One. 2014;9(7):e100402. Available from: http://www.ncbi.nlm.nih.gov/pubmed/24984069.
19. Hasanpour-Dehkordi A, Dehghani A, Solati K. A comparison of the effects of Pilates and McKenzie training on pain and general health in men with chronic low back pain: a randomized trial. Indian J Palliat Care. 2017;23(1):36–40. Available from: http://www.ncbi.nlm.nih.gov/pubmed/28216860.
20. Miyamoto GC, Franco KFM, van Dongen JM, Franco YR dos S, de Oliveira NTB, Amaral DDV, et al. Different doses of Pilates-based exercise therapy for chronic low back pain: a randomised controlled trial with economic evaluation. Br J Sports Med. 2018;52(13):859–68. Available from: http://www.ncbi.nlm.nih.gov/pubmed/29525763.
21. National Center for Complementary and Integrative Health. Chiropractic: In Depth|NCCIH. 2012. Available from: https://nccih.nih.gov/health/chiropractic/introduction.htm.
22. Rowe DE, Feise RJ, Crowther ER, Grod JP, Menke JM, Goldsmith CH, et al. Chiropractic manipulation in adolescent idiopathic scoliosis: a pilot study. Chiropr Osteopat. 2006;14:15. Available from: http://www.ncbi.nlm.nih.gov/pubmed/16923185.
23. Hoiriis KT, Pfleger B, McDuffie FC, Cotsonis G, Elsangak O, Hinson R, et al. A randomized clinical trial comparing chiropractic adjustments to muscle relaxants for subacute low back pain. J Manip Physiol Ther. 2004;27(6):388–98. Available from: http://linkinghub.elsevier.com/retrieve/pii/S0161475404000983.
24. Santilli V, Beghi E, Finucci S. Chiropractic manipulation in the treatment of acute back pain and sciatica with disc protrusion: a randomized double-blind clinical trial of active and simulated spinal manipulations. Spine J. 2006;6(2):131–7. Available from: http://www.ncbi.nlm.nih.gov/pubmed/16517383.
25. Vohra S, Johnston BC, Cramer K, Humphreys K. Adverse events associated with pediatric spinal manipulation: a systematic review. Pediatrics. 2007;119(1):e275–83. Available from: http://www.ncbi.nlm.nih.gov/pubmed/17178922.
26. MacPherson H, Green G, Nevado A, Lythgoe MF, Lewith G, Devlin R, et al. Brain imaging of acupuncture: comparing superficial with deep needling. Neurosci Lett. 2008;434(1):144–9. Available from: http://www.ncbi.nlm.nih.gov/pubmed/18294772.
27. Cherkin DC, Sherman KJ, Avins AL, Erro JH, Ichikawa L, Barlow WE, et al. A randomized trial comparing acupuncture, simulated acupuncture, and usual care for chronic low back pain. Arch Intern Med. 2009;169(9):858. Available from: http://www.ncbi.nlm.nih.gov/pubmed/19433697.
28. Austin S, Ramamonjiarivelo Z, Qu H, Ellis-Griffith G. Acupuncture use in the United States: who, where, why, and at what price? Health Mark Q. 2015;32(2):113–28. Available from: http://www.tandfonline.com/doi/full/10.1080/07359683.2015.1033929.
29. Haake M, Müller H-H, Schade-Brittinger C, Basler HD, Schäfer H, Maier C, et al. German Acupuncture Trials (GERAC) for chronic low back pain: randomized, multicenter, blinded, parallel-group trial with 3 groups. Arch Intern Med. 2007;167(17):1892–8. Available from: http://www.ncbi.nlm.nih.gov/pubmed/17893311.
30. Brinkhaus B, Witt CM, Jena S, Linde K, Streng A, Wagenpfeil S, et al. Acupuncture in patients with chronic low back pain. Arch Intern Med. 2006;166(4):450. Available from: http://www.ncbi.nlm.nih.gov/pubmed/16505266.

31. Inoue M, Kitakoji H, Ishizaki N, Tawa M, Yano T, Katsumi Y, et al. Relief of low back pain immediately after acupuncture treatment—a randomised, placebo controlled trial. Acupunct Med. 2006;24(3):103–8. Available from: http://www.ncbi.nlm.nih.gov/pubmed/17013356.

32. Manheimer E, White A, Berman B, Forys K, Ernst E. Meta-analysis: acupuncture for low back pain. Ann Intern Med. 2005;142(8):651–63. Available from: http://www.ncbi.nlm.nih.gov/pubmed/15838072.

33. Ceccherelli F, Gagliardi G, Barbagli P, Caravello M. Correlation between the number of sessions and therapeutical effect in patients suffering from low back pain treated with acupuncture: a randomized controlled blind study. Minerva Med. 2003;94(4 Suppl 1):39–44. Available from: http://www.ncbi.nlm.nih.gov/pubmed/15108610.

34. Golianu B, Yeh AM, Brooks M. Acupuncture for pediatric pain. Child (Basel, Switzerland). 2014;1(2):134–48. Available from: http://www.ncbi.nlm.nih.gov/pubmed/27417472.

35. Yoo SS, Tausk F. Cupping: east meets west. Int J Dermatol. 2004;43(9):664–5. Available from: http://doi.wiley.com/10.1111/j.1365-4632.2004.02224.x.

36. Farhadi K, Schwebel DC, Saeb M, Choubsaz M, Mohammadi R, Ahmadi A. The effectiveness of wet-cupping for nonspecific low back pain in Iran: a randomized controlled trial. Complement Ther Med. 2009;17(1):9–15. Available from: http://www.ncbi.nlm.nih.gov/pubmed/19114223.

37. Kim J-I, Kim T-H, Lee MS, Kang JW, Kim KH, Choi J-Y, et al. Evaluation of wet-cupping therapy for persistent non-specific low back pain: a randomised, waiting-list controlled, open-label, parallel-group pilot trial. Trials. 2011;12(1):146. Available from: http://www.ncbi.nlm.nih.gov/pubmed/21663617.

38. Wang YT, Qi Y, Tang FY, Li FM, Li QH, Xu CP, et al. The effect of cupping therapy for low back pain: a meta-analysis based on existing randomized controlled trials. J Back Musculoskelet Rehabil. 2017;30(6):1187–95.

39. Wilson V, Douris P, Fukuroku T, Kuzniewski M, Dias J, Figueiredo P. The immediate and long-term effects of Kinesiotape® on balance and functional performance. Int J Sports Phys Ther. 2016;11(2):247–53. Available from: http://www.ncbi.nlm.nih.gov/pubmed/27104058.

40. Drouin JL, McAlpine CT, Primak KA, Kissel J. The effects of kinesiotape on athletic-based performance outcomes in healthy, active individuals: a literature synthesis. J Can Chiropr Assoc. 2013;57(4):356–65. Available from: http://www.ncbi.nlm.nih.gov/pubmed/24302784.

41. Köroğlu F, Çolak TK, Polat MG. The effect of Kinesio® taping on pain, functionality, mobility and endurance in the treatment of chronic low back pain: a randomized controlled study. J Back Musculoskelet Rehabil. 2017;30(5):1087–93. Available from: http://www.medra.org/servlet/aliasResolver?alias=iospress&doi=10.3233/BMR-169705.

42. Nelson NL. Kinesio taping for chronic low back pain: a systematic review. J Bodyw Mov Ther. 2016;

43. Zeidan F, Adler-Neal AL, Wells RE, Stagnaro E, May LM, Eisenach JC, et al. Mindfulness-meditation-based pain relief is not mediated by endogenous opioids. J Neurosci. 2016;36(11):3391–7. Available from: http://www.ncbi.nlm.nih.gov/pubmed/26985045.

44. Ndetan H, Evans MW, Williams RD, Woolsey C, Swartz JH. Use of movement therapies and relaxation techniques and management of health conditions among children. Altern Ther Health Med. 2014;20(4):44–50. Available from: http://www.ncbi.nlm.nih.gov/pubmed/25141362.

45. Cherkin DC, Sherman KJ, Balderson BH, Cook AJ, Anderson ML, Hawkes RJ, et al. Effect of mindfulness-based stress reduction vs cognitive behavioral therapy or usual care on back pain and functional limitations in adults with chronic low back pain. JAMA. 2016;315(12):1240. Available from: http://www.ncbi.nlm.nih.gov/pubmed/27002445.

46. Zgierska AE, Burzinski CA, Cox J, Kloke J, Singles J, Mirgain S, et al. Mindfulness meditation-based intervention is feasible, acceptable, and safe for chronic low back pain requiring long-

term daily opioid therapy. J Altern Complement Med. 2016;22(8):610–20. Available from: http://www.ncbi.nlm.nih.gov/pubmed/27267151.
47. Carson JW, Keefe FJ, Lynch TR, Carson KM, Goli V, Fras AM, et al. Loving-kindness meditation for chronic low back pain. J Holist Nurs. 2005;23(3):287–304. Available from: http://www.ncbi.nlm.nih.gov/pubmed/16049118.
48. Blödt S, Pach D, Roll S, Witt CM. Effectiveness of app-based relaxation for patients with chronic low back pain (Relaxback) and chronic neck pain (Relaxneck): study protocol for two randomized pragmatic trials. Trials. 2014;15(1):490. Available from: http://www.ncbi.nlm.nih.gov/pubmed/25511185.
49. Awwad AB, et al. Pediatric orthopaedic consults from chiropractic care. J Surg Orthop Adv. 2018;27(1):58–63.

Chapter 32
A Girl with Lower Back Pain at Night and Scoliosis: Osteoblastoma as an Example of an Aggressive Benign Tumor

Richard M. Schwend

Brief Case Presentation

Chief Complaint

A 3-year history of worsening lower back and night pain.

History

This 12-year-old girl had been having back pain for about 3 years. Pain has slowly progressed and now often wakes her at night. She is having more daytime pain as well and has missed school several times because of the pain. It is getting very frustrating and is starting to cause depressive symptoms. Mom has been giving her oxycodone from her "secret" supply. This past month, she has had "leaky" urine, accidents, and stress incontinence. There have been no bowel complaints or lower extremity symptoms. Her past medical history included a breech presentation, C-section delivery, and normal physical development. There has been no menses. Family history is negative for scoliosis. On review of symptoms, family was not aware that she had scoliosis.

R. M. Schwend (✉)
Department of Orthopaedic Surgery, Children's Mercy Hospital, Kansas City, MO, USA
e-mail: rmschwend@cmh.edu

© Springer Nature Switzerland AG 2021
R. M. Schwend, W. L. Hennrikus (eds.), *Back Pain in the Young Child and Adolescent*, https://doi.org/10.1007/978-3-030-50758-9_32

Physical Examination

Weight 34.5 kg, height 131.3 cm, and BMI 20. She is healthy, developmentally normal, and Tanner 0 and has good nutrition. No unusual ligamentous laxity. She was noted to have a lumbar scoliosis with mid-lumbar tenderness. On forward bend, there was 7 degrees of thoracic rotation and 13 degrees of lumbar rotation on the scoliometer, with marked stiffness on forward flexion and extension. Screening neurological examination and gait were normal.

Imaging and Radiographic Studies (Figs. 32.1 and 32.2)

Questions About the Case the Reader Should Consider
1. Scoliosis is typically not painful or associated with mechanical pain with normal activity. What is the reason for the pain at night?

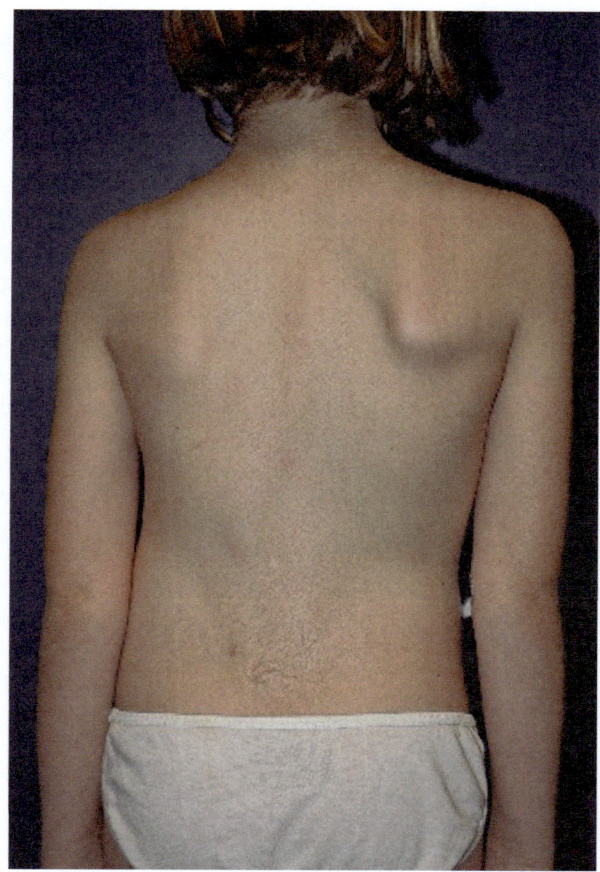

Fig. 32.1 Standing posterior spine. Notice high right shoulder, slight shift of her thorax to the right, prominent right scapula due to rotation of the thorax, and prominent left lumbar paraspinal muscles from rotation of the lumbar spine

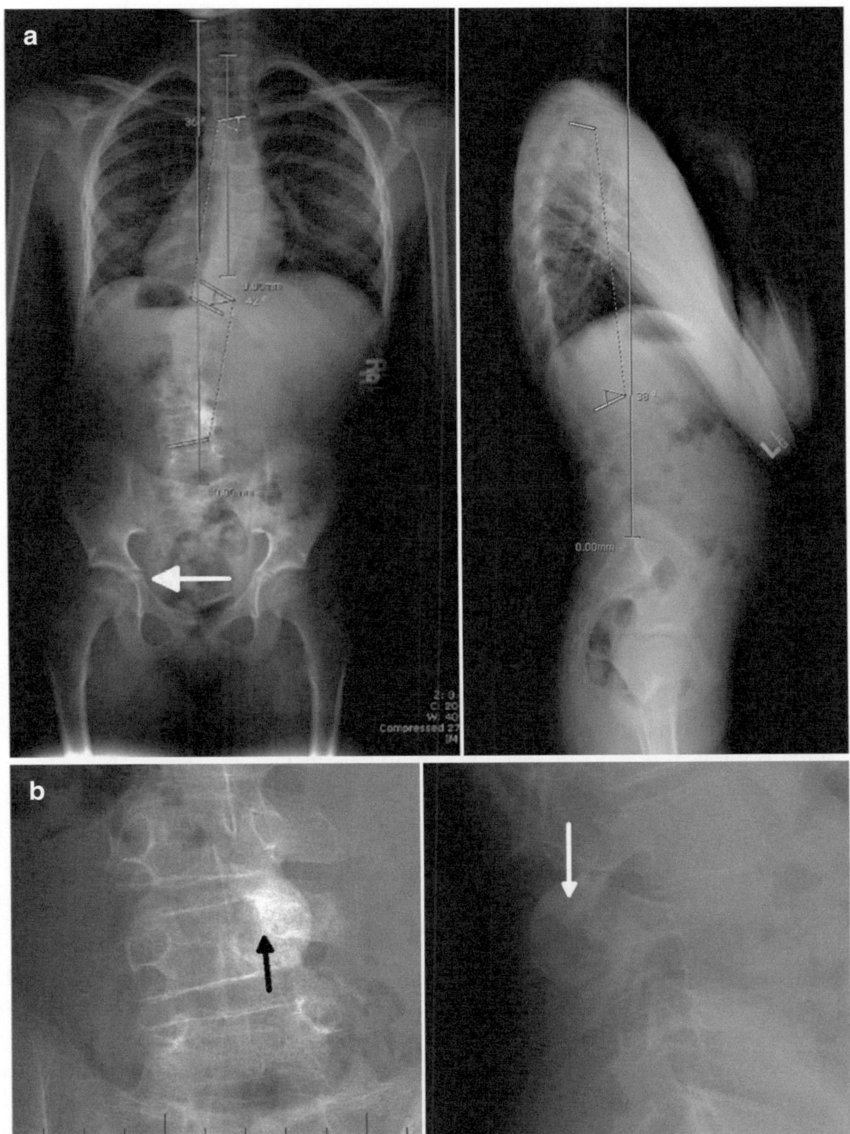

Fig. 32.2 (**a**) Posteroanterior (PA) and lateral standing radiographs. Note the thoracic (36 degrees) and the lumbar (42 degrees) scoliosis and imbalance of the thorax to the right. Initially, there was not felt to be any soft tissue or bone abnormalities, and the scoliosis was felt to be idiopathic. Note also the open triradiate cartilage (*white arrow*). (**b**) On closer inspection, there is sclerosis of the right L4 pedicle (*black arrow*), and the L4 pedicle appearance is obscured by the new bone formation. On closer view of the lateral image, there is expansion of the lamina and posterior elements (*white arrow*). (**c**) CT image of lumbar 4 vertebrae. Note that the lesion is in the posterior elements with greatly expanded right L4 pedicle and lamina. This caused impingement into the vertebral canal and may have affected bladder function

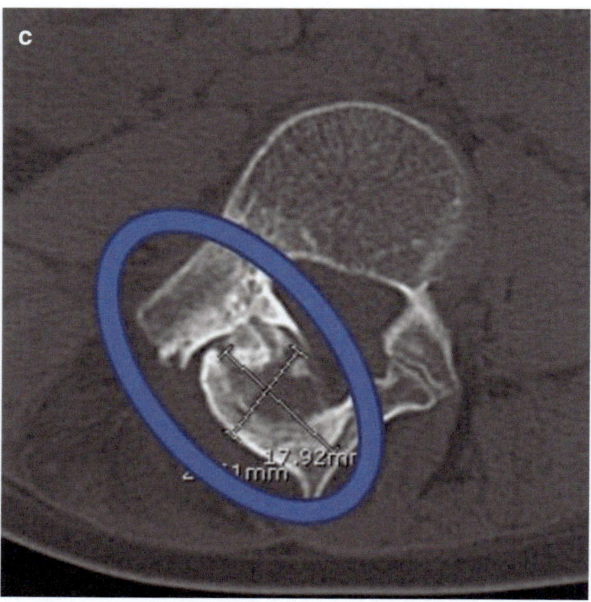

Fig. 32.2 (continued)

2. What is a possible explanation for her bladder symptoms?
3. Why was the bone lesion at L4 initially missed?
4. What is the next diagnostic test that should be considered?
5. What is appropriate referral and treatment in this case?

Discussion

Scoliosis is typically not painful or only mildly painful. It is rarely painful at night and does not usually wake a child out of her sleep. Severe back pain at night should make you consider an inflammatory condition, either an infection or a tumor [1]. Mechanical pain from the stresses of the day is usually relieved with sleep, whereas the pain of underlying inflammation becomes more severe at night [2].

The larger the lesion, the more likely there will be nerve compression. Osteoid osteoma is a benign tumor commonly found on the posterior elements of the spine, is less than 1 cm in size, and hurts at night [3, 4]. However, because the lesion is small and well contained in the bone, it rarely causes neural irritation symptoms or neurological findings. On the other hand, osteoblastoma, which is a bone-forming tumor greater than 2 cm, can greatly expand the bone of the posterior elements of the spine and create nerve compression or inflammation. Forty percent of osteoblastomas involve the spine, especially the cervical and lumbar regions, usually involving the posterior elements [5]. They are also seen in the axial skeleton, including the pelvis, sacrum, clivus, and ribs. This bone lesion, although benign, can be very aggressive and compress or irritate the spinal cord or nerve roots of the lumbar spine. Symptoms can include weakness, radicular pain, and sensory and bladder symptoms that includes incontinence [6]. However, this child has been taking opioid pain medication and may have chronic constipation, which can itself be a cause of bladder symptoms and dysfunction. When dealing with chronic pain, always ask about narcotic use—which can be a red flag (see below). Findings can be stiffness, spine imbalance, scoliosis, and lower extremity radicular findings or weakness [7, 8].

When looking at a radiograph, it is important to have a systematic method to examine all important aspects of the image. These include the areas outside the spine such as overall spine balance, evaluation of the soft tissues of the chest and abdomen, and other bones beyond the spine such as the pelvis, ribs, and long bones. It is very possible, even for an experienced radiologist reading many films during a typical day, to miss one seemingly small detail, such as the appearance of a pedicle. Pedicles on the AP film can be either missing or sclerotic. Unless one is actively looking at each pedicle, it is possible even for the most experienced of observers to miss such details. Once a radiology report describes "normal anatomy," further questioning by the clinician may not happen. We encourage the primary care doctor to review the image in person with the radiologist if any questions arise.

When a bone lesion is suspected based on biplanar radiographs, it is important to visualize the anatomy in the axial plane. CT imaging is ideal for visualizing bone lesions in the spine so is the next best test to obtain. Even though the radiation is greater than magnetic resonance imaging, modern pediatric imaging, as recommended by *Image Gently* (https://www.imagegently.org/), has decreased the effective dose. CT will show the bone structure and the lesion in great detail. MRI may show excessive soft tissue involvement, falsely suggesting a malignant tumor, when the tumor is in fact benign [9]. In this case, it would be very appropriate to refer the patient to the surgical specialists before advanced imaging studies are obtained. The surgeon may then order the appropriate study as well as specify technical detail (which test, which levels, contrast or no contrast).

In this case, the CT scan more accurately demonstrated that this was a 2.5 cm lesion of the right L4 lamina and pedicle consistent with an osteoblastoma. Posterior surgical excision of the lesion was performed. Pathology confirmed a benign but aggressive lesion. Her pain, stiffness, and urinary symptoms resolved, although the scoliosis continued to progress and eventually needed spinal fusion and instrumentation. Once a scoliosis is over 30 degrees before the onset of puberty, it has a tendency to continue to increase in severity with further growth [10]. For idiopathic scoliosis, a brace can be effective in 80% of children if used more than 15 hours/day; however, for scoliosis related to a syndrome or an underlying condition, bracing may not be as effective [11].

How to Approach the Case

Always be suspicious of night pain, which may indicate infection or tumor. Spinal stiffness is also an abnormal finding. When the pain is unusual in location, quality, or timing, such as night pain, consider the scoliosis to be atypical. Careful history, physical examination, and review of plain radiographs are the essential three aspects of making an accurate diagnosis. Advanced imaging studies such as MRI or CT scan should be used to more accurately define and *confirm* the underlying diagnosis, rather than to *search* for a diagnosis.

Red Flags for Back Pain with Scoliosis
- Younger child—under age 10 years
- Night pain
- Neural symptoms
- Neurological findings
- Large degree of scoliosis
- Atypical appearing scoliosis
- Chronic use of narcotics

Short Differential Diagnosis
- Infection: whenever tumor is suspected, also suspect infection, always.
- Osteoid osteoma: these lesions are also painful at night but are <1 cm in diameter and not typically associated with neurological signs.
- Osteoblastoma: Night pain, usually >2 cm in diameter, and as such can have associated neural symptoms and pain. Often seen in the spine, typically in the posterior elements.

Other lesions: aneurysmal bone cysts, malignant bone tumors, and tumors of the neural elements.

Final Diagnosis

Osteoblastoma L4 posterior elements (Fig. 32.3).

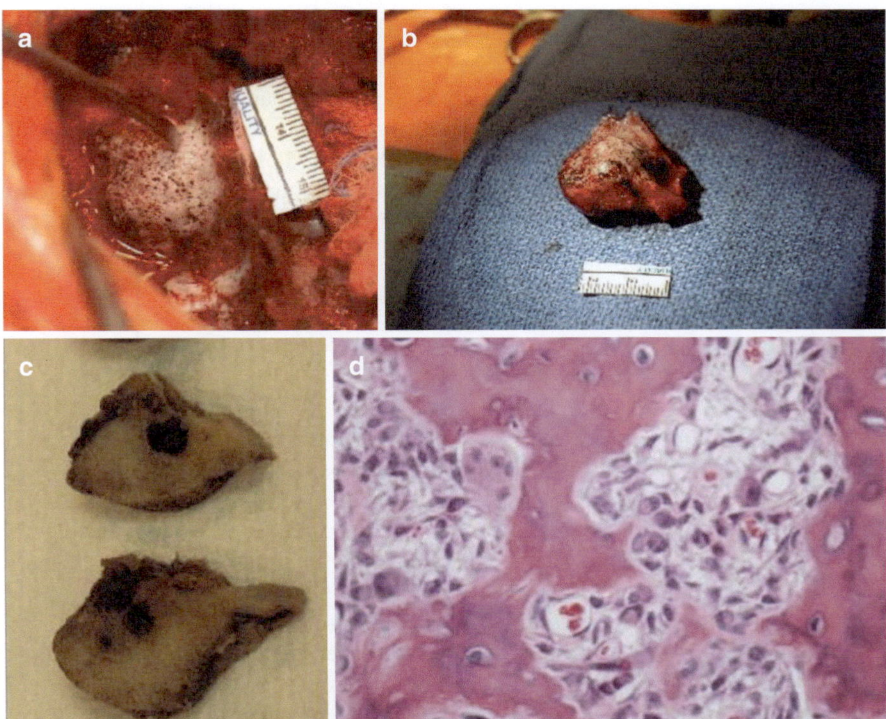

Fig. 32.3 (**a**) Appearance of right L4 lamina during surgery. Note the expanded but benign appearance of the bone. (**b**) Excised osteoblastoma of L4 posterior elements. Lesion is greater than 2 cm. (**c**) Cut section of the lesion showing the hollow "geode" appearance (from the Greek word meaning "earth like"—typically round rocks with a hollow center). (**d**) High-power micrograph showing osteoid (pink) being formed from large benign rimming osteoblasts

Natural History and Treatment Considerations

Osteoblastomas can recur if not fully removed. Since so much of the posterior elements are involved, surgical removal can lead to instability and further deformity, especially in the growing child. With time, scoliosis can worsen, as happened to this child, and spinal fusion and instrumentation were necessary. Scoliosis that is greater than 25 degrees in a growing child may benefit by brace treatment. However, if there is an underlying condition present, surgical treatment may be necessary. In this child before puberty with a 42-degree lumbar scoliosis, even with excision of the bone lesion, there was already enough deformity that the scoliosis continued to worsen and she later required surgical fusion and instrumentation.

Referral: When and to Whom?

Scoliosis that has atypical features such as significant pain, night pain, and neurological symptoms or that has progressed to more than 25 degrees in a growing child should be referred to an orthopedic surgeon who has training, expertise, and experience in treating spinal deformities. If a specific diagnosis of osteoblastoma of the spine has been made, referral to a surgeon with expertise in benign tumors of the spine is appropriate.

Brief Summary

Back pain in children can occasionally be chronic and relentless. When it occurs at night, has neurological symptoms or findings, is associated with a large degree of scoliosis or atypical scoliosis, or is seen in a young child, there is further cause for concern. Pain at night may be indicative of inflammation, from either infection or a tumor. Neurological findings suggest that there is a physical or structural explanation such as nerve compression, irritation, or stretch. Back pain in a *young* child under age 10 years is further reason for concern. History, physical examination, and careful review of plane radiographs are essential when evaluating a child with these types of symptoms and findings. Although rare, osteoblastoma is a classic lesion of the posterior elements of the spine that may have a constellation of these types of symptoms. Since osteoblastoma is a relatively large lesion, greater than 2 cm, and is associated with excess bone formation, it can be diagnosed on mindful review of plain radiographs. Refer to surgeon with pediatric spine experience.

Key Features and Pearls
- Bone formation in a child that is not in a typical location for that much bone is suspicious for tumor or sometimes infection. The tumor can be benign (osteoid osteoma), benign but aggressive (osteoblastoma), or malignant (osteosarcoma or Ewing sarcoma).
- A bone-forming lesion less than 1 cm in diameter is suspicious for osteoid osteoma. These lesions can be very painful, especially at night, but small enough to not be noticed on plain radiographs or even CT or MRI. You should be suspicious if there is persistent night pain, but the imaging studies are normal.
- A bone-forming lesion greater than 2 cm is suspicious for osteoblastoma. When seen in the spine, they are typically in the posterior elements. Due to its larger size and aggressive nature, there may be associated neurological findings with osteoblastoma.

Editor Discussion

Many years ago, Dr. Bob Hensinger taught us that back pain can be a symptom of infection or tumor, especially in a child under 5 years of age. Night pain is always a worry in a child of any age. Pain with other findings such as scoliosis, spine stiffness, neural symptoms, neurologic findings, or specific bone lesions seen on plane radiographs is also of concern.
  W.L. Hennrikus

It is very possible for a radiologist or a clinician to miss noticing a lesion on a plain radiograph. It is especially possible if the radiologist has given the image a "normal read" that the clinician will be influenced by the radiologist's report and either not directly examine the images or accept the normal report as accurate. When the clinical findings do not seem straightforward, or there are sufficient atypical findings, go back over the history, physical and plain imaging studies, preferably with a wise colleague, and re-examine the evidence. It is highly recommended to review unusual or atypical cases directly with the radiologist.
  R.M. Schwend

References

1. Hensinger RN. Acute back pain in children. Instructional Course Lect. 1995;44:111–26.
2. Payne WK, Ogilvie JW. Back pain in children and adolescents. Pediatr Clin N Am. 1996;43(4):899–917. Review
3. Raskas DS, Graziano GP, Herzenberg JE, Heidelberger KP, Hensinger RN. Osteoid osteoma and osteoblastoma of the spine. J Spinal Disord. 1992;5(2):204–11. Review
4. Pettine KA, Klassen RA. Osteoid-osteoma and osteoblastoma of the spine. J Bone Joint Surg Am. 1986;68(3):354–61.
5. Berry M, Mankin H, Gebhardt M, Rosenberg A, Hornicek F. Osteoblastoma: a 30-year study of 99 cases. J Surg Oncol. 2008;98(3):179–83.
6. Arkader A, Dormans JP. Osteoblastoma in the skeletally immature. J Pediatr Orthop. 2008;28(5):555–60.
7. Saifuddin A, White J, Sherazi Z, Shaikh MI, Natali C, Ransford AO. Osteoid osteoma and osteoblastoma of the spine. Factors associated with the presence of scoliosis. Spine. 1998;23(1):47–53.
8. Marsh BW, Bonfiglio M, Brady LP, Enneking WF. Benign osteoblastoma: range of manifestations. J Bone Joint Surg Am. 1975;57(1):1–9.
9. Chakrapani SD, Grim K, Kaimaktchiev V, Anderson JC. Osteoblastoma of the spine with discordant magnetic resonance imaging and computed tomography imaging features in a child. Spine. 2008;33(25):e968–70.
10. Canavese F, Dimeglio A. Normal and abnormal spine and thoracic cage development. World J Orthop. 2013;4(4):167–74.
11. Weinstein SL, Dolan LA, Wright JG, Dobbs MB. Effects of bracing in adolescents with idiopathic scoliosis. N Engl J Med. 2013;369(16):1512–21.

Annotated Bibliography

Akbar F, AlBesharah M, Al-Baghli J, Bulbul F, Mohammad D, Qadoura B, Al-Taiar A. Prevalence of low back pain among adolescents in relation to the weight of school bags. BMC Musculoskelet Disord. 2019;20(1):37.

Cross section study of high school students interviewed in Kuwait. Six-month prevalence of back pain was 70%. The perceived backpack weight rather than the actual backpack weight was associated with LBP (p < 0.001).

Alqarni AM, Schneiders AG, Cook CE, Hendrick PA. Clinical tests to diagnose lumbar spondylolysis and spondylolisthesis: a systematic review. Phys Ther Sport. 2015;16(3):268–75.

15 different clinical tests for these two conditions were evaluated. The one-legged hyperextension test had no value to diagnose patients with spondylolysis. Palpation of the lumbar spinous processes for tenderness had high specificity (87–100%) and moderate to high sensitivity (60–88%) to diagnose lumbar spondylolisthesis. However, there were not enough quality studies to do a meta-analysis.

Auerbach J, Ahn J, Zgonis M, Reddy SC, Ecker ML, Flynn JM. Streamlining the evaluation of low back pain in children. Clin Orthop Relat Res. 2008;466(6):1971–7.

In a review of 100 consecutive children with no worrisome night pain or constitutional symptoms, the following clinical and radiograph tests were factors highly predictive of distinguishing organic from mechanical back pain: Painless hyperextension combined with negative plain radiographs and MRI predicted mechanical back pain. For those with non-neurologic back pain of less than 6-month duration, bone scan was the most accurate, accessible and inexpensive, as well as practical over MRI because it did not require sedation in the younger child.

Batley S, Aartun E, Boyle E, Hartvigsen J, Stern PJ, Hestbæk L. The association between psychological and social factors and spinal pain in adolescents. Eur J Pediatr. 2019;178(3):275–86.

Cross sectional study of 1279 Danish adolescents. 86% reported any spine pain and 28% reported substantial pain. Spinal pain in adolescents is strongly associated

© Springer Nature Switzerland AG 2021
R. M. Schwend, W. L. Hennrikus (eds.), *Back Pain in the Young Child and Adolescent*, https://doi.org/10.1007/978-3-030-50758-9

with later spinal pain in adulthood. In this study, those adolescents with spinal pain reported higher frequency of psychological factors and loneliness, whereas those patients with increased frequency of psychological factors had increased odds of reporting substantial spinal pain.

Beck NA, Miller R, Baldwin K, Zhu X, Spiegel D, Drummond D, Sankar WN, Flynn JM. Do oblique views add value in the diagnosis of spondylolysis in adolescents? J Bone Joint Surg Am. 2013;95(10):e65.

Radiographs of 50 adolescents with L5 spondylolysis were reviewed. There was no difference in sensitivity or specificity between 4 view radiographs that included 2 oblique views versus 2 view AP and lateral lumbar spine films. Due to additional cost and radiation without obvious diagnostic benefit, routine oblique views of the lumbar spine are not needed.

Berger RG, Doyle SM. Spondylolysis 2019 update. Curr Opin Pediatr. 2019;31(1):61–8.

Comprehensive overview of spondylolysis, a common cause of low back pain in the young athlete. Recommended reading.

Biagiarelli FS, Piga S, Reale A, Parisi P, et al. Management of children presenting with low back pain to emergency department. Am J Emerg Med. 2019;37(4):672–9.

7-year cohort study of children presenting to their emergency department with LBP. They specifically described children with non-traumatic, primary musculoskeletal pain with severe prognosis conditions (red flags). These children were more likely to have an earlier onset with longer symptom duration and more likely to be hospitalized. An evaluation algorithm is described.

Bhatia NN, Chow G, Timon SJ, Watts HG. Diagnostic modalities for the evaluation of pediatric back pain. J Pediatr Orthop. 2008;28(2):230–3.

73 children with primary back pain with duration greater than 3 months were prospectively studied. 78% ended with no specific diagnosis. When a diagnosis was made, most commonly it was spondylolysis (9), followed by Scheuermann disease (2), osteoid osteoma (1) and herniated disc (1). Most of these diagnoses were made by clinical examinatin or initial plain radiographs. The authors conclude that exhaustive diagnostic protocols are not needed to diagnosis pediatrci routine back pain that does not have red flags.

Brooks TM, Friedman LM, Silvis RM. Back pain in a pediatric emergency department: etiology and evaluation. Pediatr Emerg Care. 2018;34(1)e1–e6.

One-year review of 177 children presenting to an emergency department with the chief complaint of back pain. Non-pathologic diagnosis was found in 77% of visits, with back or muscle strain the most common diagnosis, pathologic seen in only 2.3% of the visits. Plain radiographs were the only finding associated with a pathologic diagnosis. When CT or MRI was performed, no abnormalities were noted.

Burton AK, Clarke RD, McClune TD, Tillotson MK. The natural history of low back pain in adolescents. Spine (Phila Pa 1976). 1996;21(20):2323–8.

216 children were given a structured questinonaire about back pain at 11 years of age and annually for 4 additional years. Annual incidence increased from 12% at the initial interview to 22% at age 15+ years, with cumulative prevalalence increasing from 12% initially to 50% at age 15+ years. Recurrent pain was common, boys had more pain than girls and few required any treatment.

Calvo-Munoz I, Gomez-Conesa A, Sanchez-Meca J. Prevalence of low back pain in children and adolescents: a meta-analysis. BMC Pediatr. 2013;13:14.

In this meta-analysis, 59 articles met their selection criteria. The mean point prevalence of 10 studies was 12%, 12-month period prevalence in 13 studies was 34%, and the mean 1-week period prevalence from 30 studies was 40%. More recent studies and those with better methodology showed higher prevalence rates than earlier or poorer studies.

Calloni SF, Huisman TA, Poretti A, Soares BP. Back pain and scoliosis in children: when to image, what to consider? Neuroradiol J. 2017;30(5):393–404.

This free PMC article discusses the role of different imaging techniques in the diagnosis of back pain and scoliosis. It reviews imaging features of many of the common as well as more rare conditions related to back pain and spine deformity.

DiFiori JP, Benjamin HJ, Brenner JS, Gregory A, Jayanthi N, Landry GL, et al. Overuse injuries and burnout in youth sports: a position statement from the American Medical Society for Sports Medicine. Br J Sports Med. 2014;48(4):287–8.

Systematic, evidence-based review that assists clinicians recognize young athletes at risk for overuse injuries, identify risk factors for overuse injuries as well as for burnout, identifies high risk overuse injuries that may have long-term health consequences and provides recommenations on overuse injury prevention. Very comprehensive summary and practical recommendations are presented in this consensus statement avialable open access.

Feldman DE. Risk factors for the development of low back pain in adolescence. Am J Epidemiol. 2001;154(1):30–6.

Prospective cohort of 502 high school students in Montreal Canada was evaluted 3 times over 1.5 year period. Cumulative incidence of back pain was 17%. Risk factors for new onset back pain were rapid grwoth, smoking, thigh muscle tightness and working during the school year. The authors suggested stretching and lifestyle modifications could help prevent progression of pain into adulthood.

Feldman DS, Straight JJ, Badra MI, Mohaideen A, Madan SS. Evaluation of an algorithmic approach to pediatric back pain. J Pediatr Orthop. 2006;26(3):353–7.

87 children with non-traumatic thoracic and or lumbar backpain were treated utilizing this algorithm. 24% had an abnormal radiograph (such as spondylolysis) and received appropriate treatment. 29% of those with a negative radiograph had red flags which led to an MRI evaluation which was abnormal in ½ of these children. Thus 36% of the entire group received a specific diagnosis, more than other studies have reported. If a child had radicular pain, an abnormal neurologic examination or night pain, these clinical findings were highly predictive finding an underlying pathology. Lumbar pain had the highest negative predictive value for non-pathology.

Feng Q, Wang M, Zhang Y, Zhou Y. The effect of a corrective functional exercise program on postural thoracic kyphosis in teenagers: a randomized controlled trial. Clin Rehabil. 2018;32(1):48–56.

This single blinded randomized controlled trial in China demonstrated that a functional exercize program was able to improve exaggerated thoracic postural kyphosis in teenagers.

Garg S, Dormans JP. Tumors and tumor-like conditions of the spine in children. J Am Acad Orthop Surg. 2005;13(6):372–81.

Skeletal pathology is frequently a cause of back pain in children, more so than in adults. Most of these conditions in children are benign, but nevertheless may require surgical management. The authors emphasize that early diagnosis possible based on only clinical history, physical examination and plain radiographic imaging. The editors agree with their conclusion.

Jones GT, Macfarlane GJ. Epidemiology of low back pain in children and adolescents. Arch Dis Child. 2005;90(3):312–6.

At least 80% of the population will experience low back pain at some period in their lives. Over 7% of adults see clinician for back pain each year. The greatest known predictor of future back pain is a previous history of back pain.

Haus BM, Micheli LJ. Back pain in the pediatric and adolescent athlete. Clin Sports Med. 2012;31(3):423–40.

Most back pain in the young athlete can be diagnosed and treated with simple sport-specific history, careful physical examinaiton and appropriate image studies, typically plain radiographs. Most of the problems identified are benign and are treated non-surgically. The goal is to be able to get athletes back to their sports life, while preventing long-term disability.

Hestbaek L, Leboeuf-Yde C, Kyvik KO, Manniche C. The course of low back pain from adolescence to adulthood: eight-year follow-up of 9600 twins. Spine. 2006;31(4):468–72.

Classic Danish study of nearly 10,000 twins born between 1972 and 1982 surveyed for general health and symptoms. There was high association of low back pain as adolescent and into adulthood (Odds ratio 4) as well as association of more days of pain during adolescence associated with more days of back pain as an adult. This study indicates need to evaluate the pediatric population for prevention measures of adult back pain.

Kamada M, Abe T, Kitayuguchi J, Imamura F, Lee I-M, Kadowaki M, et al. Dose–response relationship between sports activity and musculoskeletal pain in adolescents. Pain. 2016;157(6):1339–45.

This study of Japanese adolescent athletes demonstrated a linear relationhip between hours of organized sports participation and the development of musculoskeletal pain, both traumatic and non-truamatic. All anatomic locations were represented. Athletes can expect to experience increased pain when they compete.

Kang HM, Choi EH, Lee HJ, et al. The etiology, clinical presentation and long-term outcome of spondylodiscitis in children. Pediatr Infect Dis J. 2016;35:e102–6.

This small study from South Korea demonstrated some unique features of this condition. Back pain was most common presenting symptom with fever in only 52%. However, for those less than 3 years old, irritability was more common than back pain. Staphylococcus aureus (40%) and Mycobacterium tuberculosis (32%) were the two most common organisms. Blood culture was not very effective for the diagnosis (19%); however, percutaneous biopsy (71%) and especially surgical biopsy (100%) were better able to make the diagnosis. Longer delay in making the diagnosis led more frequently to needing surgical management.

Klein G, Mehlman CT, McCarty M. Nonoperative treatment of spondylolysis and grade I spondylolisthesis in children and young adults: a meta-analysis of observational studies. J Pediatr Orthop. 2009;29(2):146–56.

In this study of pooled data of 665 patients, 84% of those treated non-operatively had a successful clinical outcome at 1 year. Those diagnosed and treated during the acute stages were much more likely to heal with conservative treatment than chronic defects. Unilateral defects were more likely to heal (71%) than bilateral (18%). Bracing did not make a difference in the eventual outcome. Although most patients improved, clinically very few demonstrated radiographic healing.

Miller R, Beck NA, Sampson NR, Zhu X, Flynn JM, Drummond D. Imaging modalities for low back pain in children: a review of spondyloysis and undiagnosed mechanical back pain. J Pediatr Orthop. 2013;33(3):282–8.

This classic study follows the principles of ALARA (As Low as Reasonably Achievable) and the Institutes of Medicine "Choosing Wisely". Undiagnosed mechanical low back pain (UMLBP) is the most common cause of low back pain in adolescents; it typically requires no imaging and two or less office visits. Of those with UMLBP, 7.8% eventually received the diagnosis of spondylolysis. For 86% of those with spondylolysis, the diagnosis was made by 2 view plain (AP and lateral) radiographs of the lumbar spine. This study showed that oblique radiographs were not useful in the diagnosis of spondylolysis and should be abandoned. Bone scans exposed children to more radiation than CT, so also should be reconsidered in the evaluation of spondylolysis. Because of cost and ionizing radiation, these two studies should be infrequently used in children.

Murray PM, Weinstein SL, Spratt KF. The natural history and long-term follow-up of Scheuermann kyphosis. J Bone Joint Surg Am. 1993;75(2):236–48.

Patients with Scheuermann kyphosis averaging 71 degrees were evaluated at a mean of 32 years later. Although they had more back pain and less phyically demanding jobs, there were no diffences from control patients in education, work abscense, self-esteem or social limitations. Nor was pulmonary function affected. Patients with mild to moderate untreated Scheuermann kyphosis can live very functional, although not pain-free, lives.

MacDonald J, Stuart E, Rodenberg R. Musculoskeletal low back pain in school-aged children: a review. JAMA Pediatr. 2017;171(3):280.

This concise and clear review provides the message that general knowledge of the pediatric spine and pelvis, a proper history and physical examination will provide the pediatrician with the essential tools to care for these children.

Moore MJ, White GL, Moore DL. Association of relative backpack weight with reported pain, pain sites, medical utilization, and lost school time in children and adolescents. J Sch Health. 2007;77(5):232–9.

5th through 12th grade students were interviewed to determine backpack weight and prevalence of back pain. Smaller children and girls more often experienced pain related to their backpack. 10% body weight was the cutoff weight recommended for maximum backpack weight for school age children.

Nielsen E, Andras LM, Skaggs DL. Diagnosis of spondylolysis and spondylolisthesis is delayed six months after seeing non-orthopedic providers. Spine Deform. 2018;6(3):263–6.

This retrospective study noted 24 weeks between onset of symptoms and initial presentation for spondylolysis and spondylolisthesis. However, there was then a 15-week average delay between initial presentation to a health care provider and diagnosis. This time was one week for an orthopaedic surgeon and 25 weeks for a non-orthopaedic provider. The authors recommend training for greater awareness and appropriate referral, since early diagnosis can lead to earlier resolution of symptoms and return to sports and other activities.

Premkumar A, Godfrey W, Gottschalk MB, Boden SD. Red flags for low back pain are not always really red: a prospective evaluation of the clinical utility of commonly used screening questions for low back pain. J Bone Joint Surg Am. 2018;100(5):368–74.

In this adult study, positive responses to red flag questions were helpful in making the diagnosis of a serious underlying condition. However, a negative response was not always reassuring. For example, 64% of patients with a spinal malignancy did not have associated red flags in the history. Clinicians need to be cautious when evaluating the responses to these questions. A similar study has not been performed in children.

Ramirez N, Johnston CE, Browne RH. The prevalence of back pain in hcildren who have idiopathic scoliosis. J Bone Joint Surg. 1997;79:364–8.

Retrospective study of scoliosis and back pain at major referal orthopaedic hospital. 23% of children initially presenting with scoliosis were noted to have back pain and additional 9% developed back pain during observtion. Although there was positive association of pain with increasing age, the degree of scoliosis was not associated. Only 9% of those with back pain had an underlying diagnosis, typically spondylolysis, spondylolisthesis, Scheurmann kyphosis, syrinx, herniated disc, hydromyelia, tehtered cord and intraspinal tumor. A painful left thoracic curve or neurologic findings curves were associated with underlying condition, but only in 24%. The authors stress that history, physical examination and plain radiographs should suffice for the majority of children with scoliosis and back pain. MRI should be reserved for those children with red flag fiindings of left thoracic curve or neurologic findings.

Ramirez N, Flynn JM, Hill BW, Serrano JA, Calvo CE, Bredy R, et al. Evaluation of a systematic approach to pediatric back pain: the utility of magnetic resonance imaging. J Pediatr Orthoped. 2015;35(1):28–32.

Prospective 2-year cohort study of all patients presenting to an academic pediatric orthopaedic clinic at a major children's hospital with a chief complaint of back pain. Back pain was the chief complaint in 8.6% of the total patients. MRI was done for "red flags" in the history or on physical examination, such as constant or night pain, neurological symptoms or findings and if the clinical exam and plain radiographs did not demonstrate a diagnosis. An eventual diagnosis was made in only 34% of the patients seen for back pain, by clinical findings and plain radiographs in 8.8% and MRI in another 25%. Lumbar pain and constant pain were the most sensitive red flags for finding underlying pathology.

Ring D, Johnston CE 2nd, Wenger DR. Pyogenic infectious spondylitis in children: the convergence of discitis and vertebral osteomyelitis. J Pediatr Orthop. 1995;15(5):652–60.

Classic study showed that "discitis" in children is basically pyogenic infectious spondylitis and makes recommendation for using antibiotics for all patients with these findings. The condition in children resembles adult spondylitis.

Schwend RM, Hennrikus W, Hall JE, Emans JB. Childhood scoliosis: clinical indications for magnetic resonance imaging. J Bone Joint Surg Am. 1995;77(1):46–533.

In scoliosis patient, if criteria for obtaining MRI was restricted to neck pain and headache with exertion and neurological findings such as weakness, ataxia, cavus foot, all serious abnormalities requiring neurosurgical evaluation would have been found.

Shah SA, Saller J. Evaluation and diagnosis of back pain in children and adolescents. J Am Acad Orthop Surg. 2016;24(1):37–45.

The most identifiable clinical entities in pediatric back pain are: spondylolysis, spondylolisthesis, Scheuermann kyphosis, overuse syndromes, disc herniation, apophyseal ring fracture, spondylodiscitis, vertebral osteomyelitis and neoplasm. The most common of these conditions can be evaluated with history, physical examination and plain radiographs. The more rare ones may have neurologic findings or suggestive clinical presentation to indicate MRI use.

Skaggs DL, Early SD, D'Ambra P, Tolo VT, Kay RM. Back pain and backpacks in school children. J Pediatr Ortho. 2006;26(3):358–63.

Population-based sample of middle school children in Los Angeles in which the majority used ab backpack. Heavier backpack, younger age and scoliosis was associated with back pain in multivariate analysis. Recommendation to have lighter backpack and lockers.

Sousa T, Skaggs DL, Chan P, Yamaguchi KT Jr, Borgella J, Lee C, Sawyer J, Moisan A, Flynn JM, Gunderson M, Hresko MT, D'Hemecourt P, Andras LM. Benign natural history of spondylolysis in adolescence with midterm follow-up. Spine Deform. 2017;5(2):134–8.

Retrospective study of 295 adolescent patients with spondylolysis who were treated conservatively. The Micheli Functional Scale Survey was administered at a minimum follow up of 2 years, average of 8 years. 90% were able to return to sports, although 42% had continued pain that interfered with activity in 67%. Radiographic healing did not determine pain or ability to return to sports. Although 58% had no pain, 22% reported pain of at least 4/10.

Stallknecht SE, Strandberg-Larsen K, Hestbæk L, Andersen A-MN. Spinal pain and co-occurrence with stress and general well-being among young adolescents: a study within the Danish National Birth Cohort. Eur J Pediatr. 2017;176(6):807–14.

Large Danish National Birth Cohort sudy of 45,371 adolescents between ages 10 and 14 years. Using newly developed and validated Young Spina Quaestionnaire, spine pain is a common finding at this age and co-occurs with stress and poor general well-being.

Szita J, Boja S, Szilagyi A, Somhegyi A, Varga PP, Lazary A. Risk factors of non-specific spinal pain in childhood. Eur Spine J. 2018;27(5):1119–26.

Prospective cohort study done in Hungary using a newly developed patient-reported questionnaire (PRQ). Using multivariate logistic regression models and predictive performance of the final model using the receiver operating characteristic (ROC) method, seven predictive risk factors were found: age > 12 years, watching TV more than 2 hour/day, uncomfortable school desk, problems with sleep, general overall discomfort and family medical history.

Taimela S, Kujala UM, Salminen JJ, Viljanen T. The prevalence of low back pain among children and adolescents. Spine (Phila Pa 1976). 1997;22(10):1132–6.

Population study in Finland schools of childen and adolescents completing a validated questionnaire. Low back pain is common complaint by adolescence, often becoming recurrent or chronic by age 14 years.

Tyagi R. Spinal infections in children: a review. J Orthop. 2016;13:254–8.

Good review of this topic. PDF of the article is free through Pubmed. Be aware of antimicrobial resistant bacterial strains and the increasing incidence of Kingella kingae infections.

Tofte JN, CarlLee TL, Holte AJ, Sitton SE, Weinstein SL. Imaging pediatric spondylolysis: a systematic review. Spine. 2017;42(10):777–82.

Bone scans had up to 9 times the effective radiation dose of 2 view plain films, whereas CT was double. 2 view plain films were the most cost effective and safest initial imaging study recommended. MRI is recommended early to detect spondylolysis and stress reactions and CT in more established and chronic cases. However, the poor quality of the studies makes it difficult to establish clinical practice guidelines.

Wang TY, Harward SC, Tsvankin V, et al. Neurological outcomes after surgical or conservative management of spontaneous spinal epidural abscesses: a systematic review and meta-analysis of data from 1980 through 2016. Clin Spine Surg. 2019;32:18–29.

Large systematic review of 808 patients from 20 studies. Surgical treatment is not always indicated or performed. However, when surgery was needed and was delayed, the outcomes were worse. The decision to operate should be individualized; however, when surgery is needed, do it sooner than later. Also beware of post-laminectomy kyphosis when surgery is required in young children, especially at the cervical thoracic junction.

Wieland LS, Santesso N. A summary of a cochrane review: yoga treatment for chronic non-specific low back pain. Eur J Integr Med [Internet]. 2017 [cited 2019 Jan 10];11:39–40. Available from: http://www.ncbi.nlm.nih.gov/pubmed/29057019.

12 clinical trials of 1080 participants. Yoga was not associated with serious adverse events compared to other back focused exercises, so was considered safe. There is need for higher quality research to more confidently show efficacy in chronic non-specific low back pain.

Yamato TP, Maher CG, Traeger AC, Wiliams CM, Kamper SJ. Do schoolbags cause back pain in children and adolescents? A systematic review. Br J Sports Med. 2018;52(19):1241–5.
Systematic review of 69 higher level evidence studies, 5 prospective longitudinal and 64 cross-sectional or retrospective of 72,627 school-aged children. By evaluating combined data from the highest quality studies, there was no convincing evidence that backpack use increased the risk of back pain. This study is good reminder of the importance of larger series and higher level of evidence.

Yang S, Werner BC, Singla A, Abel MF. Low back pain in adolescents: a 1-year analysis of eventual diagnoses. J Pediatr Orthop. 2017;37(5):344–7.
This is an important study in that it came from a very large national insurance database (PearlDiver Patient Records Database) of 10–19 year-olds with back pain. At up to 1 year after initial presentation, over 80% had no identifiable diagnosis. The most common diagnoses were lumbar strain/spasm (8.9%), scoliosis (4.7%), lumbar degenerative disk disease (1.7%), lumbar disk herniation (1.3%). All of the other conditions seen in pediatric orthopaedics (spondylolysis, spondylolisthesis, infection, fracture) were only seen in <1%. This is a good reminder that in the primary care population, the rates of specific diagnosis are much lower than from highly referred specialty orthopaedic academic practices.

Helpful Websites

www.aap.org/.../Pages/AAP-Policy-Statements.asp

This website provides access to >50 subject collections including >200 American Academy of Pediatric Policy Statements, Clinical Reports and Technical Reports. Each statement or report is updated every 5 years.

Policy Statements

Organizational principles to guide and define the child health care system and/or improve the health of all children.

Clinical Reports

Provide guidance for the clinician in rendering pediatric care

Technical Reports

Background information to support Academy policy.

orthoinfo.aaos.org/.../back-pain-in-children

This website provides tips and pearls for the evaluation of back pain in children provided by the American Academy of Orthopaedic Surgeons.

www.healthychildren.org

HealthyChildren.org is a parenting website backed by the American Academy of Pediatrics and committed to the attainment of optimal physical, mental, and social health and well-being for all infants, children, adolescents, and young adults. This site provides general information related to child health and specific guidance on parenting issues on all aspects of a child's health including back complain.

posna.org/Patient-Education/OrthoInfo

This website from the Pediatric Orthopaedic Association of North America provides patient education and handouts on multiple musculoskeletal problems including back pain in children.

www.scoliosis.org

This website provides valuable information about scoliosis and other back problems.

The National Scoliosis Foundation (NSF) is a patient-led nonprofit organization dedicated since 1976 to helping children, parents, adults and health-care providers

© Springer Nature Switzerland AG 2021

R. M. Schwend, W. L. Hennrikus (eds.), *Back Pain in the Young Child and Adolescent*, https://doi.org/10.1007/978-3-030-50758-9

to understand the complexities of spinal problems such as scoliosis including providing patient support and resources.

orthokids.org/Condition/Back-Pain-in-Children

This website from the Pediatric Orthopaedic Society of North America provides overviews of pediatric orthopaedic treatments for common musculoskeletal problems such as back pain.

thrive.kaiserpermanente.org/care-near-you/...

Example of back pain exercises for the teenager or young adult with mechanical back pain

(schwend revised 5/24/20)

Index